Technological Basis of Radiation Therapy: Practical Clinical Applications

Technological Basis of Radiation Therapy:
Practical Clinical Applications

Seymour H. Levitt, M.D.

Professor and Head
Department of Therapeutic Radiology
University of Minnesota Hospitals
Minneapolis, Minnesota

Norah duV. Tapley, M.D.

Professor of Radiotherapy
Department of Radiotherapy
The University of Texas System Cancer Center
M.D. Anderson Hospital and Tumor Institute
Houston, Texas

Lea & Febiger   1984   Philadelphia

Lea & Febiger
600 South Washington Square
Philadelphia, Pa. 19106
U.S.A.

Library of Congress Cataloging in Publication Data

Main entry under title:

Technological basis of radiation therapy.
  Bibliography: p.
  Includes index.
  1. Cancer—Radiotherapy. I. Levitt, Seymour H.
II. Tapley, Norah duV. III. Title. [DNLM: 1. Radio-
therapy—Methods. 2. Neoplasms—Radiotherapy. QZ 269 T255]
RC271.R3T43 1984   616.99′406424   83-9889
ISBN 0-8121-0898-1

Printed in the United States of America

Print Number: 3 2 1

This book is dedicated to my children—
Mary Jeanne, Jennifer Gaye, and Scott
Haden—who are my inspiration. Their
sacrifice of my time has made it possible
for me to pursue my career and this book.

This book is also dedicated in memo-
riam to Norah duVernet Tapley, M.D.,
physician, colleague, and friend.

Foreword

As I began preparation of the third edition of the *Textbook of Radiotherapy*, it became obvious that the number of pages would have to be increased due to the expanded radiobiology and clinical background. At that time, I decided to add only a minimal amount to the previous edition on clinical physics and special techniques. I soon realized, however, that each "organ" chapter could have included more details on tumor localization, treatment planning, and some of the more recent advances in CT scanning. Not only would such expansion have made the book bulky but it would have diluted the book's specific goals, which were to integrate the treatment of the various diseases into the background of radiobiology and clinical experience. In order for all of this additional material to be presented properly and given the treatment and space it called for, I encouraged Dr. Levitt and Dr. Tapley to write *The Technological Basis of Radiation Therapy: Practical Clinical Applications* as a companion text to the *Textbook of Radiotherapy*. In these times of increasing complexity, a volume such as theirs should prove to be an invaluable source of information to all those involved in the field of practical clinical radiation therapy.

Gilbert H. Fletcher, M.D.

Preface

The concept of this book originated here at the University of Minnesota during the development of the annual postgraduate conferences entitled, "Current Concepts in Radiation Therapy." With the guidance and inspiration of Dr. Gilbert H. Fletcher, Dr. Norah duV. Tapley and I undertook to develop this text which we saw as a complement to Dr. Fletcher's *Textbook of Radiotherapy*. We felt that there was a need for a companion volume to provide more detailed information concerning the actual rationale for and techniques of treatment. With the cooperation of the colleagues who have contributed chapters, we have finally brought this text to publication.

The untimely death of Dr. Norah Tapley was a great loss to society in general, to the radiation therapy community, and to me personally. Dr. Tapley was a great human being, a superb physician, and a compassionate and understanding friend and colleague. Her contributions to this text are immense and it could not have come into being without her.

The chapters herein contain the experiences and advice of individual authors at various institutions whom we felt had a great deal of experience in the practical aspects of the treatment of the cancer patient. The recent growth of and improvement with computerized tomography has had great impact on radiation therapy treatment planning. Although work on this book was initiated a number of years ago, we have tried to update it insofar as possible to include information relative to the utilization of computerized tomography for treatment planning.

I would caution the reader to carefully evaluate the techniques described herein and compare them to their own for evaluation of the validity of the technique in relationship to their own experience and equipment. It is possible that the techniques described are not appropriate for the equipment that the individual institution has. The guidelines are essentially general, and it should be possible for the radiation therapist to modify the techniques to suit the equipment available in the individual department.

Our hope in developing this book was that it would contribute to better treatment for the cancer patient and subsequently improve survival. The accurate localization, adequate treatment, and the ability to duplicate fields used in daily treatment are essential to quality radiation therapy. It is our hope that this volume will provide the radiation therapist with the tools to provide this type of quality radiation therapy to his or her patients.

Minneapolis, Minnesota   Seymour H. Levitt, M.D.
Houston, Texas   Norah duV. Tapley, M.D.

Contributors

Malcolm A. Bagshaw, M.D.
Professor and Chairman
Department of Radiology
Director
Division of Radiation Therapy
Stanford University School of Medicine
Stanford, California

Chu Huai Chang, M.D.
Professor of Radiology
College of Physicians and Surgeons, Columbia University
Director
Division of Radiation Oncology
Columbia-Presbyterian Medical Center
New York, New York

Luis Delclos, M.D., D.M., D.M.R.T.,
  F.A.C.R.
Professor of Radiotherapy
The University of Texas System Cancer Center
Radiotherapist
M.D. Anderson Hospital and Tumor Institute
Houston, Texas

Miriam M. Gitterman, M.S.
Associate in Radiation Therapy
Harvard Medical School
Assistant Radiation Biophysicist
Massachusetts General Hospital
Boston, Massachusetts

Eli Glatstein, M.D.
Professor of Radiology
Uniformed Services University for Health Sciences
Chief
Radiation Oncology Branch, National Cancer Institute
Bethesda, Maryland

Sadek K. Hilal, M.D., Ph.D.
Professor of Radiology
College of Physicians and Surgeons, Columbia University
Director
Division of Neuroradiology
Neurological Institute, Columbia-Presbyterian Medical Center
New York, New York

Henry S. Kaplan, M.D.
Maureen Lyles D'Ambrogio Professor of Radiology and Oncology
Stanford University School of Medicine
Director
Cancer Biology Research Laboratory
Stanford, California

Faiz M. Khan, Ph.D.
Professor of Therapeutic Radiology
University of Minnesota Medical School
Director
Radiation Physics Section, University Hospitals
Minneapolis, Minnesota

Tae H. Kim, M.D.
Associate Professor
Department of Therapeutic Radiation
Department of Pediatrics
University of Minnesota Medical School
Director of Clinical Service
Department of Therapeutic Radiation, University Hospitals
Minneapolis, Minnesota

Francisca Lee, M.D.
Department of Radiation Oncology
St. John's Mercy Hospital
St. Louis, Missouri

John G. Maier, Ph.D., M.D.†
Former Professor of Radiation Oncology
George Washington University
Washington, D.C.
Former Director
Department of Radiation Oncology
Fairfax Hospital
Falls Church, Virginia

James E. Marks, M.D.
Professor of Radiology
Mallinckrodt Institute of Radiology, Washington University School
of Medicine
St. Louis, Missouri

Eleanor D. Montague, M.D.
Professor of Radiotherapy
The University of Texas System Cancer Center
Radiotherapist
M.D. Anderson Hospital and Tumor Institute
Houston, Texas

Mark E. Nesbit, M.D.
Professor
Department of Pediatrics
University of Minnesota Medical School
Department of Pediatrics, University Hospitals
Minneapolis, Minnesota

Carlos A. Perez, M.D.
Professor of Radiology, Residency Training Program Director
Mallinckrodt Institute of Radiology, Washington University School
of Medicine
Radiotherapist-in-Chief
Barnes Hospital, Washington University Medical Center
Radiotherapist
Missouri Baptist Hospitals
St. Louis, Missouri

Roger Alan Potish, M.D.
Assistant Professor
Department of Therapeutic Radiology, University of Minnesota
Medical School
Staff Radiotherapist
Department of Therapeutic Radiology, University Hospitals
Minneapolis, Minnesota

James A. Purdy, Ph.D.
Associate Professor and Chief
Physics Section
Mallinckrodt Institute of Radiology, Washington University School
of Medicine
St. Louis, Missouri

Don P. Ragan, Ph.D.
Associate Professor
Radiation Oncology Department and Department of Radiology
Wayne State University
Radiology Department, Harper-Grace Hospitals, Hutzel Hospital,
and Detroit Receiving Hospital
Detroit, Michigan

†Deceased

Aly Razek, M.D.
Assistant Professor of Radiology
Mallinckrodt Institute of Radiology, Washington University School
  of Medicine
St. Louis, Missouri

Vincent Sampiere
Assistant Physicist and Instructor
M.D. Anderson Hospital and Tumor Institute
Houston, Texas

William U. Shipley, M.D.
Associate Professor of Radiation Therapy
Harvard Medical School
Associate Radiation Therapist
Department of Radiation Medicine, Massachusetts General Hospital
Boston, Massachusetts

William J. Spanos, Jr., M.D.
Associate Professor of Radiation Oncology, Associate Director of
  Radiation Oncology
Radiotherapist
Loma Linda University Medical Center
Loma Linda, California

Charles Votava, Jr., M.D.
Associate Clinical Professor
Texas Tech University School of Medicine
Chief
Department of Radiation Therapy, Methodist Hospital
Lubbock, Texas

Robert L. White, M.D.
Assistant Professor
Department of Radiation Oncology, George Washington University
Washington, D.C.
Chairman
Department of Radiation Oncology, Fairfax Hospital
Falls Church, Virginia

Jeffrey Ford Williamson, Ph.D.
Assistant Professor of Therapeutic Radiology
University of Minnesota Medical School
Staff Physicist
Department of Therapeutic Radiology, University Hospitals
Minneapolis, Minnesota

Contents

Chapter 1

RATIONALE FOR TREATMENT PLANNING IN RADIATION THERAPY

Carlos A. Perez
James A. Purdy
Don Ragan

Irradiation is an effective antitumor agent that can completely eradicate a malignant process in the irradiated volume in patients treated with curative intent. It can also yield palliative relief to many patients with incurable cancer. The success of radiation therapy depends upon the delivery of an adequate dose to the tumor volume. This chapter reviews the principles of radiotherapeutic strategy and illustrates the significance and methodology of treatment planning.

Although the gross effects of radiation on most normal tissues have been documented, the intricate interrelationship of total dose, fraction size and number, mechanisms of injury repair, and correlation between acute and late effects have not been elucidated. The increasing use of chemotherapeutic agents in the treatment of cancer patients makes this problem more complex because the combination of irradiation with these agents usually results in greater effect on normal tissues. Furthermore, as indicated by Fletcher,[6] the tolerance of the normal tissues is related to the volume irradiated, the nature and function of organs within that volume, and stage of the cancer treated. Recent reports by Herring,[8] Perez et al.,[20] and Shukovsky et al.[22] indicate that there is a close correlation between the dose of radiation given and the probability of tumor control at the primary site or in metastatic lymph nodes. Fletcher has emphasized that such dose-response curves are valid only for homogeneous tumor populations.[6] The doses of radiation depend on the stage and the histologic nature of the tumor. Fletcher has stressed the concept that large masses of tumor require higher doses than small tumors or subclinical microscopic metastases, which are controlled with lower doses.[5] Herring[8] has discussed the theoretic consequences of dose-response curves for tumor control and normal tissue injury. The predicted consequences are based on the precision with which the dose and the volume irradiated are defined. An imprecise treatment system could lead to a high incidence of necrosis with a low probability of tumor control. Reducing radiation doses in an effort to avoid complications will further reduce the probability of achieving tumor control if such action is based on the wrong assumption that complications are only related to radiation dose levels.

Project Sponsored By USPHS Cancer Center Grant No. 5. Pol CA13053, National Cancer Institute, National Institutes of Health, USPHS

1

In addition to accurate treatment planning, adequate reposition and immobilization techniques are needed to translate the dose optimization formulated in a plan to actual delivery in the patient. Marks et al.[15,16] demonstrated, by systematic use of verification films, a high frequency of localization errors on patients irradiated for head and neck cancer or malignant lymphomas. These errors were corrected with improved immobilization of the patients.

The practice initiated by Baclesse of delivering higher doses of radiation through reducing fields is based on the principle that the center of a tumor contains more cells and a higher hypoxic cell population than the periphery.[6] Extreme care must be taken in defining the volume to be irradiated with this technique because small inaccuracies result in appreciable variations of dose in the critical volume.

Although treatment planning is extremely helpful in determining the best form of therapy, the responsibility for critical judgment and execution rests with the radiation therapist. To treat patients effectively, the therapist must:

1. Have sufficient training to interpret treatment-planning information and to guide the physicist or dosimetrist in achieving the best dose distribution;
2. Be competent to judge the quality of the dose distribution and the technical feasibility and accuracy of a proposed plan;
3. Have the understanding needed to suggest changes and available alternatives;
4. Have sufficient knowledge to select the best possible combination of dose and fractionation for a given site and volume;
5. Understand the capabilities and limitations of the computer in treatment planning.

It is important to emphasize that no computer calculation can correct the therapist's errors of clinical judgment, mis-understanding of physical concepts, or unsatisfactory execution of treatment.

LIMITATIONS OF RADIATION THERAPY

The goal of radiation therapy is to produce the highest possible uncomplicated local and regional control of the tumor. The failure to eradicate a tumor can result not only from suboptimal dosimetry and treatment-planning computations but from a variety of factors:

1. Clinical Factors
   a. Inadequate appraisal of the full extent of the tumor in the surrounding tissues, or inapparent regional lymph node metastases that are not irradiated.
   b. Clinically unrecognized distant metastases at the time of initial treatment are a major cause of failure in some tumors, such as breast or lung primary tumors, and their management requires a systemic therapeutic modality.
2. Physical and Technical Factors
   a. Inaccurate definition of tumor volume to be treated, including a safe margin (particularly in large infiltrating tumors), is a frequent cause of recurrence.
   b. Inadequate treatment planning with inhomogeneous dose distributions in critical target volumes.
   c. Unreliable patient repositioning and immobilization techniques, with faulty reproducibility in daily treatments resulting in inadequate doses or volumes treated.
   d. Lack of adequate in vivo verification-dosimetry techniques, except in cases in which small dosimeters can be introduced into the upper digestive tract, the bladder, and the rectum.
3. Biologic Factors
   a. Initial cell burden because small tumors are more easily eradicated than large tumors.

b. Hypoxic cell subpopulations, which require greater doses of irradiation. This problem is partially resolved by the reoxygenation that occurs between fractionated doses of irradiation.

c. Repair of sublethal or potentially lethal damage between fractions.

d. Limited tolerance of normal tissues to irradiation.

e. Type of supporting tissue involved by the malignant process; a tumor that has not extended into the adjacent soft tissues or the bone is more easily controlled by radiation.

f. Lack of knowledge of human-cell kinetics and biologic equivalents for various dose rate-fractionation regimens.[2,9]

4. Less well-defined factors include the general condition, nutritional status, metabolism, and immune response of the individual patient. This subject has been thoroughly summarized by Bush and Hill.[3]

CONDITIONS FOR OPTIMIZATION OF EXTERNAL-BEAM IRRADIATION

Kitebatake et al.[14] outlined definite requirements for optimal dose distribution with external irradiation in both tumor and normal tissues. The following is a slightly modified list of factors published by these authors:

1. Small entrance and exit dose (except with superficial tumors): Ideally, when the maximum dose is not required at the skin or the subcutaneous tissues, the optimal dose distribution should be at the target volume in the depth of the patient, with lower dose to the skin at the entrance and exit sites.

2. Small side-scattering dose: High-energy-photon beams produce minimal amounts of side-scattered irradiation.

3. Small differential tissue absorption:

It is known that with 250 KV x-rays there is significantly greater absorption of irradiation in bone than in soft tissues.[12] This phenomenon disappears with high-energy x-rays due to the decreasing importance of the photo-electric effect and the increasing Compton effect between 1 and 10 MV. At energies of 20 MeV, however, there is an increase of 5% to 10% in the dose in the soft tissues near a bone (high Z) interface.

4. Optimal tumor (target) dose: The aim of good treatment planning is to exploit the maximum therapeutic ratio of a beam arrangement. The target volume should receive a homogeneous dose while delivering as little

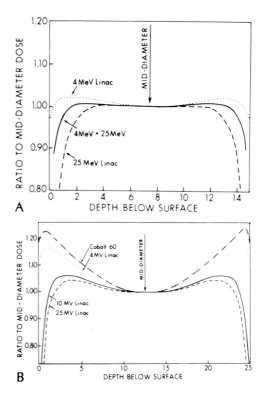

Fig. 1–1. Dose profiles for various energies with parallel opposing beams directed at anatomic areas of different thickness: *(A)* the head and neck, *(B)* the thorax or pelvis. Note the difference in maximum dose necessary to deliver the desired tumor dose (100%) at the midplane.

dose as possible to the surrounding normal tissue.

5. Small integral dose: The ideal situation should be represented by an optimal dose to the target volume with a minimum dose contribution to the rest of the patient.

Either superficial x-rays or low-energy electron beams are used for superficial skin or subcutaneous tumors. Whereas deeply seated tumors require high-energy photons, small cancers of the oral cavity or the genital tract can be treated by brachytherapy. Optimal dose distribution in many tumors requires more than one-beam energy or multiple-beam arrangements. A combination of external beam and intracavitary or interstitial therapy may also be required, depending on the location of the tumor and the beam type and energies used (Fig. 1–1). Optimal dose distribution may be achieved in such cases by a combination of multiple stationary beams or by moving-beam therapy, such as in arc or full-rotational techniques.

STEPS INVOLVED IN TREATMENT PLANNING (FIGURE 1–2)

The procedures involved in effective administration of radiation therapy comprise a complex, closely integrated operation that should include the following:

1. Thorough knowledge of the natural history and pathologic characteristics of the tumor.
2. Adequate evaluation of the patient and staging procedures to determine the full extent of the tumor.
3. Definition of treatment strategy, to select the best modality or combinations to be applied. This may depend on the stage, type of tumor to be treated, and the routes of spread.
4. Treatment simulation, with accurate definition of the tumor volume to be treated and the portals to be used.
5. Treatment planning, to determine the distribution of irradiation within the volume of interest.
6. Accurate and reproducible repositioning and immobilization techniques for daily treatment delivery.
7. Applicable dosimetry, portal localization, and verification procedures, to insure quality control throughout the therapy.
8. Periodic evaluation of the patient during and after therapy, to assess the effects of treatment on the tumor and the tolerance of the patient.

The treatment strategy must include, in addition to clinical, physical, and radiobiological concepts that may provide rational basis for the therapy, thoughtful consideration of the treatment's psychological repercussions, side-effects, and sequelae, all of which may affect the quality of life of the patient. Supportive care during treatment is important.

Even though general policies of treatment may be established and atlases com-

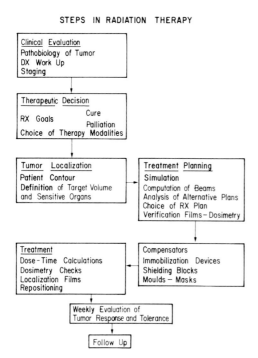

STEPS IN RADIATION THERAPY

Fig. 1–2. Steps involved in the treatment planning and delivery of radiation therapy.

piled, it is mandatory to remember that the treatment plan must be individualized to suit each patient's needs.

PROBLEMS WITH PRESENT TREATMENT-PLANNING TECHNIQUES

Several problem areas still exist in regard to treatment-planning computation. The most pertinent include: 1) surface and buildup doses; 2) the effect of tissue inhomogeneities;[17] 3) irregular field effects due to secondary blocking; 4) beam modifiers such as wedges and compensators;[1] 5) combination of interstitial and intracavitary isodoses with external-beam dose distributions; 6) tridimensional dose computations and display; and 7) dose optimization.

The effect of the patient's shape and of consequent oblique-beam incidence must be taken into account in treatment planning, as must the patient's internal anatomy and the differences among intervening tissues. Methods developed to handle the problem of oblique incidence include the effective source-to-skin-distance (SSD) method, the effective attenuation coefficient method, and the isodose curve shift method. All these methods are approximations and result in an inaccurate description of the surface dose and the dose in the build-up region. The surface dose

and the dose in the build-up region are largely determined by collimator design and diaphragm–surface distance and are therefore machine-specific. In the case of high-energy x-rays (25 MV) generated by a linear accelerator, the maximum dose depth changes from 4.0 cm for a 4 cm × 4 cm field size to 2.5 cm for a 25 cm × 25 cm field (Figure 1–3). Although this phenomenon is not well understood, we suspect that it is caused by electrons from the flattening filter and collimator jaws.

Correction for inhomogeneities in the medium is primarily done by the "isodose shift method." The isodose value is shifted to a distance proportional to the path length through the inconsistent medium (i.e., a downward shift if the inhomogeneity has a density of less than one or an upward shift if the inhomogeneity has greater than unit density). A method has been described using an absorption equivalent density and an inverse square law correction (effective density).[18] Interface effects, although important for high-energy photons (over 20 MV), are neglected in most cases.

The effect of a wedge or shielding block

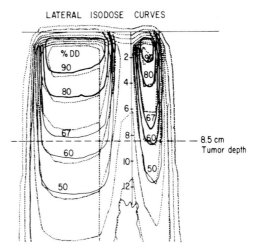

Fig. 1–4. Discrepancies between computer-generated isodose curves and measured isodose curves for a blocked field that includes a full-thickness spinal shield. Dashed lines represent computer-generated curves. The solid lines represent ionization measurements.

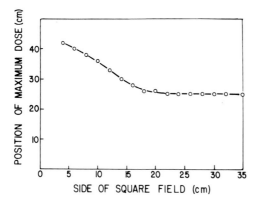

Fig. 1–3. Position of the maximum dose as a function of field size for 25 MeV linear-accelerator x-ray beam. Note the displacement toward the surface as the field size increases.

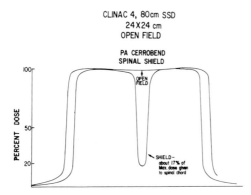

Fig. 1–5. The dose profile in a field treated by 4 MeV x-rays in which a 5 half-value layer (HVL) block is interposed in the middle (e.g., in the thorax PA portal to shield the spinal cord). Note that a 17% dose is delivered under the block at 10 cm depth. This is mostly contributed by scattered irradiation, although a small percentage is due to transmission through the shielding block. Neglecting to consider this 17% dosage contribution may result in significant inaccuracies in treatment planning.

on dose distribution is due to changes produced in the beam profile. In order for a beam-generation program to be related as closely as possible to the physical situation, the actual location, dimensions, and physical characteristics of the wedge or beam block must be entered into the program. Depending on the thickness and the attenuation coefficient of the wedge, attenuation factors can be calculated along various phantom lines applied to the primary dose and the scatter dose.

At present, irregular-field calculations are accomplished by dividing the dose at a given point into a primary component and a scatter component and determining each separately. This method, which is typified by the Toronto programs,[4] results in a dose calculation at a specific point. It is extremely time-consuming and impractical to use this method to construct a full isodose distribution. In addition, significant inaccuracies exist for points of interest within a centimeter of the field edges. When an isodose distribution is required, the method most commonly used is the "effective-square-field method" in which the irregular field is approximated by an effective rectangular field, isodose curves

are obtained using a rectangular field. Serious errors may result especially in the penumbra region or when special shielding blocks (e.g., full- or half-value-thickness spinal-cord shield) are used (Figs. 1–4 and 1–5).

Although the methods mentioned above are much faster than hand calculations, they still require considerable time in computation and final display. This problem is compounded by the need for interaction among the physicist, the physician, and the computer technologist. Plans are usually done by a treatment-planning technologist using a prescription given to him by the physician. The plans are given to the physician for review. Corrections are made, if needed, and the process is repeated. To circumvent these problems, small computers have been developed to allow the physician to participate directly in the treatment-planning process. In practice, though, most institutions still employ treatment-planning technologists to compute the treatment plans. An additional problem is that there is no wide agreement as to how to specify treatment-planning doses. The doses to the center of the tumor volume are normally used; other specifications include maximum, minimum, or modal dose. There are numerous arguments for and against the use of all of the above but none are totally satisfactory. Standardization in the specification of treatment-planning doses is a necessity if treatment planning optimization is to become a reality.

Most computerized treatment-planning systems have inherent errors of 5% to 15%, and lack of resolution of several millimeters. Lack of exact information on localization of tumor and normal tissue, and lack of clear patient-contour definition have greatly diminished the potential accuracy of the treatment-planning process for a large number of anatomic sites. Additional vagaries, inevitable in the delivery of successive treatments of radiation therapy, have resulted in the need for

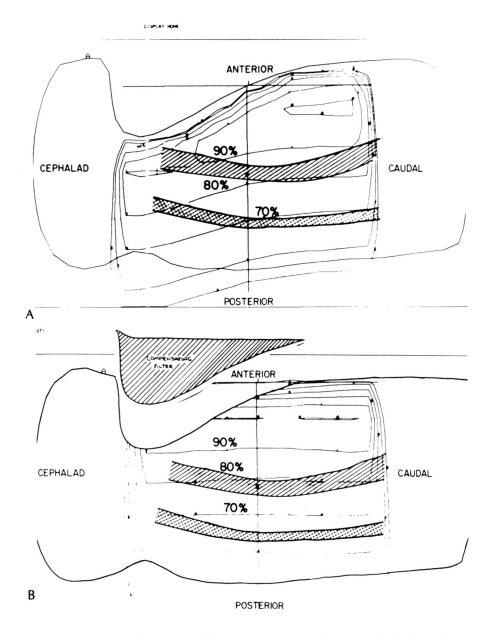

Fig. 1–6. *(A)* Inaccuracies that may result from present treatment planning methods. One isodose is usually obtained through the central axis (plane through line A). Such an isodose distribution does not illustrate that the spinal cord (crossed-hatched) receives the same dose as the tumor (plane through line B). *(B)* The effect of a compensating figure on dose distribution; the amount of radiation delivered to the spinal cord is significantly reduced.

wider, safer portal margins and have thereby diminished the effectiveness of precise treatment planning. Problems inherent in the specification of radiation-therapy beams have also contributed to the inaccuracies of the past, including the computations of beam characteristics for wedged or compensated fields, irregularly shaped fields, high-energy x-rays, electrons, and high linear energy transfer (LET) particles. Because of the difficulties of multiplanar patient definition and beam specifications, which require large computers, almost all computations have been limited to two-dimensional isodose representations that often fail to alert the clinician to problems in other areas of the beam (Fig. 1–6). With the increased use of shaped fields, the need for truly three-dimensional computations and graphic representation has become critical.

NEW APPROACHES TO TREATMENT PLANNING

Computer applications in treatment planning have improved dramatically.

Computer availability has increased also. There are over three hundred computer systems specifically engineered for treatment-planning in the United States;[10] there are as many multipurpose computer systems capable of treatment planning on a time-shared basis. This increased computer capability has not generally resulted in a greater amount of data process throughput (about 8 to 10 treatment plans per day on a job-specific computer) but rather, has increased our capability to solve complex problems. Recent advances, such as computerized tomography (CT), offer the possibility of overcoming many of the problems of treatment planning outlined in the previous sections. Even without direct interphasing of the CT-density-matrix information, CT scans can be combined with traditional patient contouring to improve the quality of present computer assisted treatment planning (Figs. 1–7 and 1–8).

The direct use of integrated multiple planes for three-dimensional reconstruc-

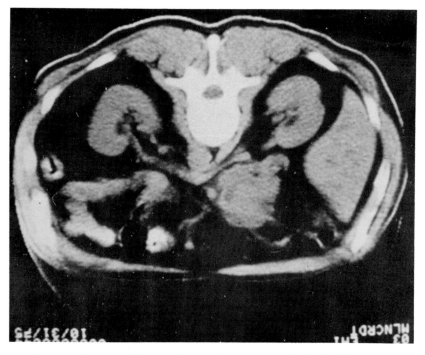

Fig. 1–7. CT scan of the upper abdomen showing a large tumor in the head of the pancreas.

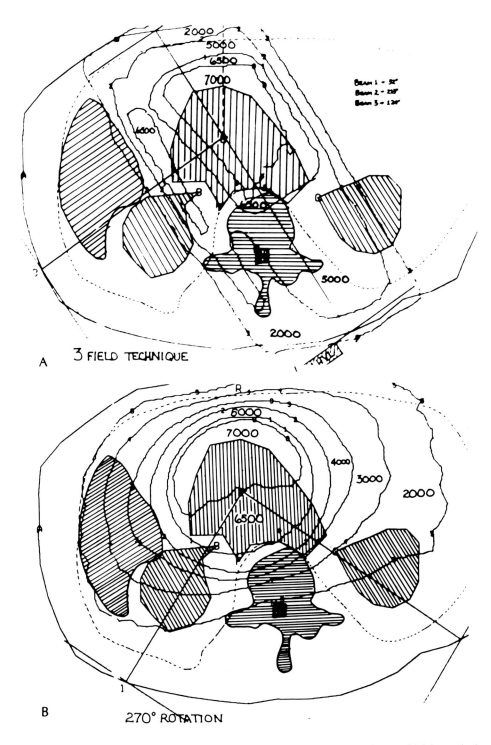

Fig. 1–8. Treatment plans with (A) stationary fields and (B) 270° arc rotation that would deliver a high dose of radiation to the pancreas without excessive dose to the kidneys. CT scanning is particularly useful in providing accurate delineation of tumor volume in certain anatomic locations.

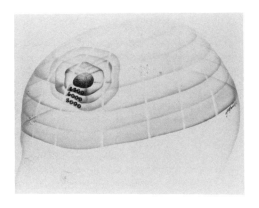

Fig. 1–9. Hypothetical tridimensional display of irradiation dose distribution.

tion of the patient's structure must be one of the goals of future treatment planning. Sterling et al.[23] created an interesting system for three-dimensional treatment-planning display that used computer-gener-

ated films projected in a rapid sequence to depict the dose distribution in a given volume. More practical systems must be developed to allow the radiation therapist to manipulate the information that can provide an integrated multiplanar, multidirectional representation of the patient and the dose distribution. Off-axis-beam information and multiple-plan isodoses throughout the irradiated volume can be made practical by the added information provided by CT scan. This information could be displayed in multiplanar isodose distributions or three-dimensional representation on video screens, and could be manipulated in different planes by the dosimetrist or physician (Fig. 1–9).

Technologic developments will eventually allow practical and inexpensive generation of tridimensional display of anatomic structures and isodose distri-

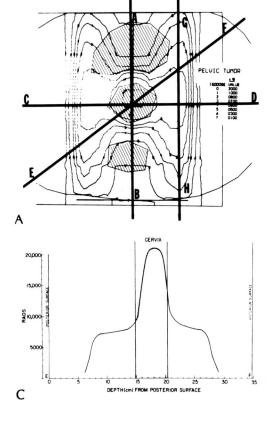

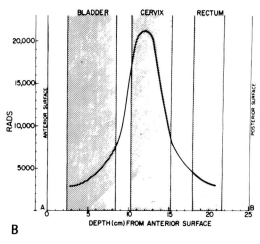

Fig. 1–10. *(A)* Isodose distribution in the midplane of the pelvis for a carcinoma of the uterine cervix treated with a combination of external beam 22 MeV photons (whole pelvis and parametrial portals with step wedge midline blocks) and two intracavitary insertions (7500–8000 mg hrs.); *(B)* Representation of dose-distribution profile through plane AB; *(C)* Dose profile through plane CD showing the dose delivered to the cervix, paracervical tissues, and the parametria.

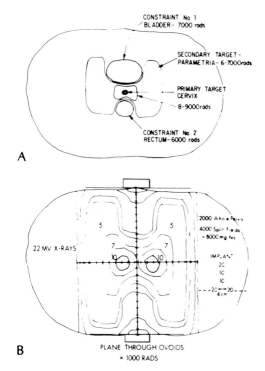

CONSTRAINT No 1
BLADDER - 7000 rods

SECONDARY TARGET -
PARAMETRIA - 6-7000 rods

PRIMARY TARGET
CERVIX
8-9000 rods

CONSTRAINT No 2
RECTUM - 6000 rods

A

2000 Whole Pelvis
4000 Split Fields
+ 8000 mg hrs

22 MV X-RAYS

IMPLANT
2C
1C
1C
--2C -- 20--
4 cm

B

PLANE THROUGH OVOIDS
× 1000 RADS

Fig. 1–11. *(A)* A treatment plan definition, for which tumor doses to be delivered to specific targets are required by the radiation therapist. Constraints to sensitive anatomical structures (the bladder anteriorly and the rectum posteriorly) are indicated. With this type of information, dose optimization may be achieved by a proper combination of external beams or by a combination of interstitial, intracavitary, and external-beam therapy. *(B)* The dose distribution accomplished with a combination of 2000 rads whole pelvis, additional 4000 rads parametrial dose delivered with midline step-wedge block combined with two intracavitary insertions that deliver about 7500 rads to the paracervical tissues (isodose curve number 1).

many factors that influence the dose prescription (Fig. 1–11). The formulation of applicable score functions must be developed to objectively evaluate alternative treatment plans.[11,13,19]

Other developing technologic advances in treatment planning include computerized methods of treatment-parameter verification, and automation of teletherapy,[24] or intracavitary-source equipment.

The use of computerized treatment planning and CT scans is not confined to patient treatment. The combination of these two techniques can provide an invaluable tool to further the investigation of clinical phenomena. Through accurate documentation of the sites irradiated and the doses delivered, additional conclusions may be drawn about the sensitivity of tumors and normal tissues to a spectrum of radiation doses.

Treatment planning is particularly valuable in the training of radiation therapists because it allows for a rapid and objective evaluation of proposed treatments. This has been enhanced by the small on-site computers with which the radiotherapist can quickly and easily interact.

As the degree of sophistication in computer design and application grows, there will be an increased need for trained personnel in computerized treatment planning at all levels of operation from physicist to dosimetrist to physician.

butions.[25] In the meantime, it is possible to obtain a significant amount of pertinent information by computing dose profiles in multiple planes[21] and combining them with information about the appropriate anatomic sites within the irradiated volume (Fig. 1–10).

Further work needs to be done toward dose optimization. Initial attempts at computer assistance in this area by such investigators as Hope and Orr,[11] and Gallagher,[7] were frustrated by the large amount of data needed to define the variables of the patient, the tumor, and the

REFERENCES

1. Boge, R.J., Edland, R.W., and Mattes, D.C.: Tissue compensators for megavoltage radiotherapy fabricated from hollowed styrofoam filled with wax. Radiology *111*:193, 1974.
2. Brown, B.W., et al.: Theoretical considerations of dose rate factors influencing radiation strategy. Radiology *110*:197, 1974.
3. Bush, R.S. and Hill, R.P.: Biologic discussions augmenting radiation effects and model systems. Laryngoscope *85*:1119, 1975.
4. Cunningham, J.R., Shrivastave, P.N., and Wilkinson, J.M.: Program IRREG—calculation of dose from irregularly shaped radiation beams. Comp. Programs Biomed. *2*:192, 1972.
5. Fletcher, G.H.: Clinical dose-response curves of human malignant epithelial tumours. Br. J. Radiol. *46*:1, 1973.

6. Fletcher, G.H. and Shukovsky, L.J.: The interplay of radiocurability of tolerance in the irradiation of human cancer. J. Radiol. Electrol. 5:383, 1975.

7. Gallagher, T.L.: Optimization of external radiation beams for therapy planning, Ph.D. Thesis. St. Louis, Washington University, 1967.

8. Herring, D.F.: The consequences of dose response curves for tumor control and normal tissue injury on the precision necessary in patient management. Laryngoscope 85:1112, 1975.

9. Hethcote, H.W. and Waltman, P.: Theoretical determination of optimal treatment schedules for radiation therapy. Radiat. Res. 57:150, 1973.

10. Holmes, W.F.: External beam treatment planning with the programmed console. Radiology 94:391, 1970.

11. Hope, C.S. and Orr, J.S.: Computer optimization of 4 MeV treatment planning. Phys. Med. Biol. 10:365, 1965.

12. Johns, H.E. and Cunningham, J.R.: *The Physics of Radiology*, 3rd ed. Springfield, Ill., Charles C Thomas, 1969.

13. Jones, D. and Washington, J.: The quantitative description of a radiation therapy plan. Radiology 115:451, 1975.

14. Kitabatake, T., Hattori, H., and Okumura, Y.: Optimum energy in supervoltage x-ray therapy. Strahlentherapie 137:158, 1969.

15. Marks, J.E. and Haus, A.G.: The effect of immobilization on localization error in the radiotherapy of head and neck cancer. Clin. Radiol. 27:175, 1976.

16. Marks, J.E., Haus, A.G., Sutton, H.G., and Griem, M.L.: Localization error in the radiotherapy of Hodgkin's disease and malignant lymphoma with extended mantle fields. Cancer 34:83, 1974.

17. Nelson, R.F.: Computerized treatment planning and inhomogeneities. Act Radiol. 11:161, 1972.

18. Nordberg, U.B.: Correction of isodose-diagrams for ^{60}Co and 35 MeV electron at penetration of lung tissue. Acta Radiol. 11:113, 1972.

19. Orr, S.: Radiation dose distributions and their optimization. Laryngoscope 85:1024, 1975.

20. Perez, C.A. et al.: Carcinoma of the tonsillar fossa. Significance of doses of irradiation in volume treated in the control of the primary tumor in metastatic neck nodes in carcinoma of tonsil. Int. J. Rad. Oncol. Biol. Phy. 1:817, 1976.

21. Powers. W.E. et al.: Dose Profile in Treatment Planning. To be published.

22. Shukovsky, L.J. and Fletcher, G.H.: Time–dose and tumor volume relationships in irradiation of squamous cell carcinoma of tonsillar fossa. Radiology 107:621, 1973.

23. Sterling, T.D., Perry, H., and Katz, L.: Automation of radiation treatment planning. IV. Derivation of a mathematical expression for the per cent depth dose surface of cobalt-60 beams and visualization of multiple field dose distributions. Br. J. Radiol. 37:544, 1964.

24. Takashashi, S.: Conformation radiotherapy. Acta Radiol. Suppl. 242:1, 1965.

25. Van de Geijn, J.: The computation of two and three dimensional dose distributions in cobalt-60 teletherapy. Br. J. Radiol. 38:369, 1965.

Chapter 2

TREATMENT AIDS FOR EXTERNAL-BEAM RADIOTHERAPY

Vincent A. Sampiere
Faiz M. Khan
Luis Delclos

Over the years, radiotherapists have sought supportive apparatus to help in the accurate delivery of radiation treatments. It has been demonstrated by several workers, and summarized in Section 7 of the International Commission of Radiological Units and Measurement (ICRU) Report 24, that the probability of tumor control is a very steep function of dose and that the minimum accuracy of the delivered dose should be ± 5% of the prescribed dose when the goal is eradication of the primary tumor. Because consistent accuracy of the daily patient setup is vital to maintaining good radiotherapy, we believe that a catalog of devices that have been designed to solve specific problems in the patient-setup routine is useful. These devices have been arranged into four general categories:

1. Patient restraints and positioning devices.
2. Field-blocking accessories and devices.
3. Tumor localization and treatment devices.
4. External-beam treatment setup devices.

PATIENT RESTRAINTS AND POSITIONING DEVICES (Figs. 2–1 through 2–12)

The devices discussed in this section aim to achieve the following:

1. Aid in daily-treatment setup and provide reproducibility
2. Assure immobilization of the patient or area under treatment with a minimum of discomfort for the patient
3. Achieve the conditions prescribed in the treatment plan
4. Enhance the precision of treatment with a minimum of additional setup time
5. Adapt, with minimum modification, to most patients

FIELD-BLOCKING ACCESSORIES AND DEVICES (Figs. 2–13 through 2–25)

Shaping of fields involves various steps and accessory devices. The discussion below involves block construction, block support, and prefabricated blocks.

There are two general methods of constructing individual lead blocks, divergent and nondivergent. If the source size is large (e.g., ^{60}Co), the divergence of the blocks does not appreciably improve the sharpness of the field edge because of inherent geometric penumbra. On the other hand, if the source size is small (e.g., linear accelerator x-ray beam), it is desirable to use divergent blocks, especially in situations where the tumor and the normal area to be spared are in close proximity.

When a blocking tray is used to suspend blocks in a radiation beam, there should be a 15- to 20-cm distance between the patient surface and the tray to maintain the skin-sparing effect of megavoltage beams.

In addition, the nondivergent blocks should be positioned closer to the patient to achieve sharp beam edges; this, however, results in a heavier block. A compromise is usually made for extended treatment distances, taking into consideration the weight of the blocks, surface buildup, and sharpness of beam edges. Pictured in this section are different designs of blocking trays that fulfill various treatment requirements. The thickness of the transparent plastic should be sufficient to support the maximum expected weight of blocks and should be large enough in size to accommodate peripheral blocks. Each tray should have a measured transmission factor available.

Some treatment setups require standard-shaped blocks (e.g., kidney shields, eye shields) that can be prefabricated to save time. A sufficient selection should be on hand to take into account variations among patients.

TUMOR LOCALIZATION AND TREATMENT SIMULATION DEVICES
(Figs. 2–26 through 2–33)

The devices discussed in this section relate to apparatus that are helpful in visualizing, demarking, or determining the location of the tumor in relation to treatment geometry. Devices for taking physical measurements of body contour and thickness are also included.

EXTERNAL-BEAM TREATMENT SETUP DEVICES (Figs. 2–34 through 2–48)

Auxiliary devices may be used to modify the beam in order to achieve a desired effect. Compensators and boluses are examples. Other apparatus discussed here are used to achieve accurate beam positioning for a specific treatment setup.

REFERENCES

1. Sampiere, V.A.: Radiation measurement and dosimetric practices. *In* Textbook of Radiotherapy, 3rd ed. Edited by G.H. Fletcher. Philadelphia, Lea & Febiger, 1980.
2. Tapley, N.duV.: Breast. *In* Clinical Applications of the Electron Beam. Edited by N.duV. Tapley. New York, John Wiley, 1976.
3. Edland, R.W. and Hansen, H.: Irregular field shaping for ⁶⁰Co teletherapy. Radiology 92:1567, 1969.
4. Powers, W.E. et al.: A new system of field shaping for external beam radiation therapy. Radiology 108:407, 1973.
5. Tapley, N.duV.: Skin and Lips. *In* Clinical Applications of the Electron Beam. Edited by N.duV. Tapley. New York, John Wiley, 1976.
6. Hussey, D.: Testis. *In* Textbook of Radiotherapy, 3rd ed. Edited by G.H. Fletcher. Philadelphia, Lea & Febiger, 1980.
7. Fletcher, G.H.: Squamous cell carcinoma of the uterine cervix. *In* Textbook of Radiotherapy 3rd ed. Edited by G.H. Fletcher. Philadelphia, Lea & Febiger, 1980.
8. Hall, E.J., and Oliver, R.: The use of standard isodose distributions with high energy radiation beams: The accuracy of a compensator technique in correcting for body contours. Br. J. Radiol. 34:43, 1961.
9. Santiago, A.: An intraoral stent for the direction of radiation beam therapy. J. Pros. Dent. 15:938, 1965.

PATIENT RESTRAINTS AND POSITIONING DEVICES

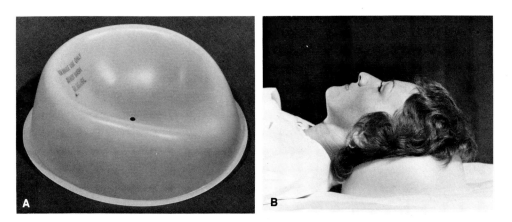

Fig. 2–1. Head holder. This disposable formed-plastic head holder *(A)* provides stability for the head when the patient is in the supine position. It allows the head to be close to the table top (B). Two sizes, pediatric and adult, are adaptable to most patients.

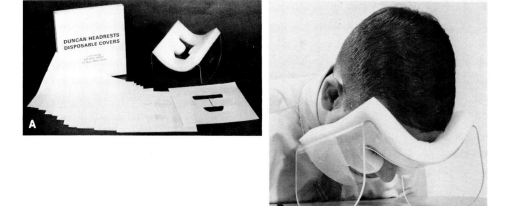

Fig. 2–2. Face-down stabilizer. This formed-plastic head holder *(A)* has a foam-rubber lining and disposable paper liners with an opening provided for the eyes, nose, and mouth of the patient. It allows comfort and stability as well as air access to the patient in prone position *(B)*. (Courtesy of M-G Equipment Co., St. Paul, Minnesota.)

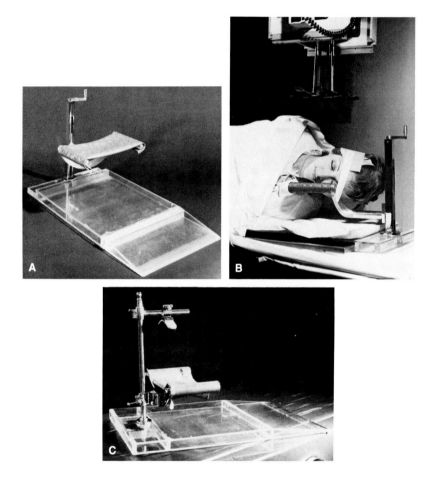

Fig. 2–3.   Head holder with tunnel for film cassette. This apparatus consists of a vinyl sheet suspended between two bars. It provides a secure holder for lateral positioning of the head *(A)*. Vertical adjustment is provided by a gear crank. A tunnel in the base of the holder accepts a film cassette for portal localization films. Placement and retrieval of the cassette is accomplished without disturbing the patient setup *(B)*. A second model (C) that has an adjustable head clamp to immobilize the head is shown. (A. From Sampiere: *In* Textbook of Radiology, 3rd ed. Edited by G.H. Fletcher. Philadelphia, Lea & Febiger, 1980. C. Courtesy of Delclos, L.)

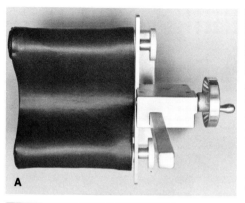

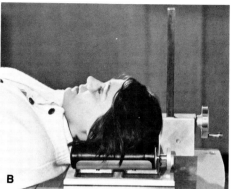

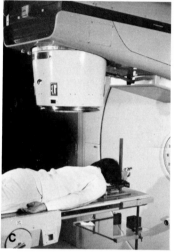

Fig. 2–4. Adjustable head and face holder. This apparatus is designed for proper positioning of the head or face. When the patient is in the supine position, the head rests on a vinyl sheet suspended between two bars *(A)*. Vertical height is adjustable to provide proper tilt or leveling of the head. For a patient in the prone position, the same device is used as a face rest *(B)*. The bars are covered with styrofoam and vinyl, and can be moved laterally to provide a comfortable and secure face rest without hindering breathing *(C)*. The adjustments are made easily by a gear crank arrangement.

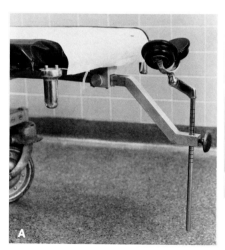

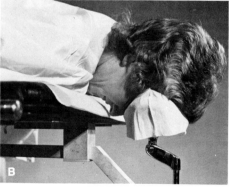

Fig. 2–5. Off-treatment-table head holder. A standard dental head rest is mounted at the end of a treatment table *(A)* to allow positioning of the head at a lower level than possible on the table top *(B)*. This provides adjustment in the vertical and superior-inferior axis.

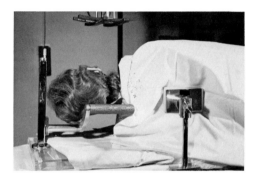

Fig. 2–6. Body brace. This brace for patients in a lateral position. It is mounted on a base that rests on the table top beneath the patient (see Fig. 2–14). Foam-rubber pads mounted on arms that can be moved vertically or horizontally are placed against the patient, adding stability to the positioning. Two braces are normally used, one anteriorly and one posteriorly.

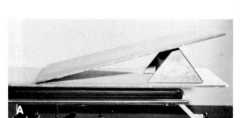
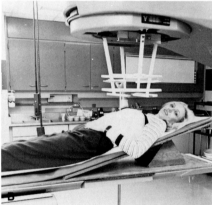

Fig. 2–7. Back support to tilt chest wall. An axillary table top is fabricated with a hinged section that can be positioned at various angles to the horizontal table top by means of a wedged brace (A). This arrangement allows positioning the sloping chest wall to be more appositional to a vertical beam (B).

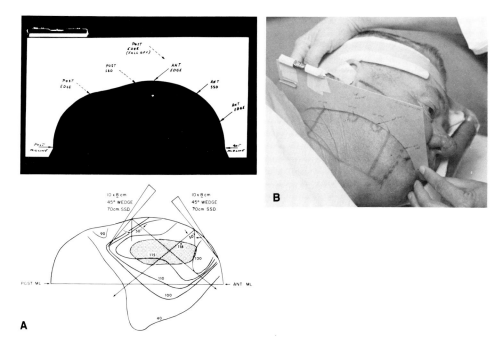

Fig. 2–8. Cardboard cutout. A cardboard cutout is made by transferring the patient's contour outline and the beam parameters on the treatment plan to a sheet of cardboard, using secretary's carbon paper *(A,B)*. This cutout, or template, can then be used to transfer the field edges, source-skin distance (SSD) positions, and anatomic landmarks from the treatment plan to the patient *(C)*. A pocket level attached to the upper surface of the cardboard, which is parallel to the base line in the treatment plan, provides a daily check of the patient's positioning relative to the prescribed treatment-field angulations. (From Sampiere: *In* Textbook of Radiology, 3rd ed. Edited by G.H. Fletcher. Philadelphia, Lea & Febiger, 1980.)

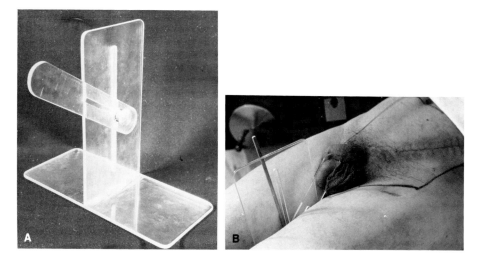

Fig. 2–9. Testicular retractor. This device excludes the (non-treated) testicle and scrotum from the direct beam while a portion of the scrotum is irradiated. The T-shaped device has a groove along the vertical support that allows a narrower blade, also with a groove *(A)*, to be positioned in any vertical or angled orientation to the patient. It is fixed in position by means of a locking screw *(B)*. (From Delclos. Radiologia *13*:283, 1971.)

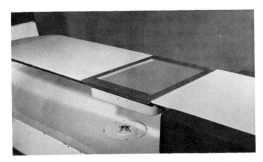

Fig. 2–10. Mylar-window table insert. A sheet of thin Mylar is stretched and mounted in a frame that fits into a treatment table that has a removable section. For opposing-beam portals, excellent patient support is provided with a minimum surface buildup effect, minimum reduction of beam intensity, and good visual access to the treatment surface.

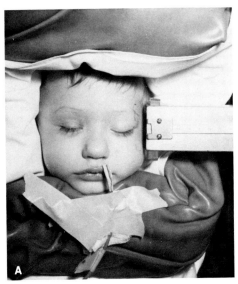

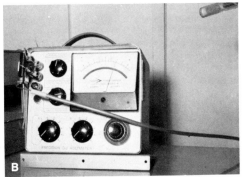

Fig. 2–11. Pediatric respiration indicator. The system consists of a sensitive differential voltmeter with a center scale reading, a fast-reacting thermistor, and a 22-volt battery, in series. The respiration rate of pediatric patients who are sedated during treatment can be constantly monitored by positioning a thermistor close to the patient's nose *(A)*. The thermistor senses the temperature change as breath is inhaled and exhaled, and indicates this by oscillation of the meter needle *(B)*. (From Tapley: *In* Textbook of Radiotherapy, 3rd ed. Edited by G.H. Fletcher. Philadelphia, Lea & Febiger, 1980.)

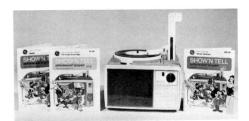

Fig. 2–12. Pediatric entertainers. Illustrated is a combination record player and slide projector. This entertainment device, positioned on a moveable cart, has been useful in distracting and calming children during the setup procedure and treatment interval.

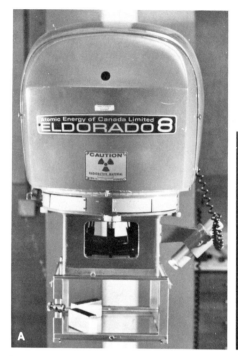
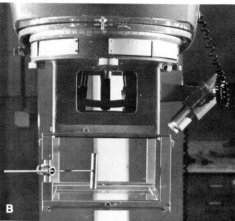

Fig. 2–13. *(A)* Machine-mounted tray for accessories (e.g., shielding blocks, wedge filters, compensators). The plexiglass plate may be interchanged with one with holes for lateral or angulated beam shielding. A universal clamp arrangement is mounted in the corner post of the tray to hold an eye shield at the end of a steel rod *(B)*. The eye block can be positioned anywhere in the beam.

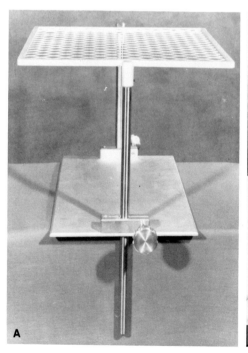
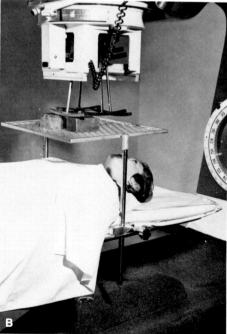

Fig. 2–14. Table-mounted blocking tray. This blocking tray is constructed to cover a larger area and support more weight than the machine-mounted tray. It can also be used at several treatment distances, still maintaining optimum blocking geometry. The base that locks the supporting columns *(A)* at the proper height lies beneath the patient on top of the treatment table *(B)*.

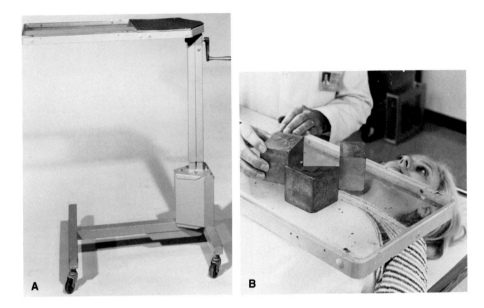

Fig. 2–15. Floor-mounted blocking tray. A patient over-bed tray *(A)* has been converted to a blocking tray. This is particularly useful when a patient is being treated on a stretcher. Tray height is adjusted with a crank gear. Lead blocks are placed on a plastic sheet attached to the blocking-tray frame *(B)*. Attenuation correction is made for the thickness of plastic used.

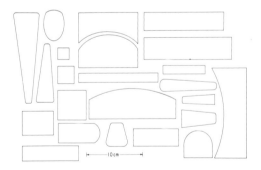

Fig. 2–16. Standard set of blocks. Each machine has an assortment of secondary blocks to accomplish the blocking needed for various irregularly shaped fields. The undersurface of the blocks can be covered with a thin layer of cork to minimize sliding and scratching of the plastic base when used with an angled blocking tray. The thickness of these blocks is specified by the radiotherapist.

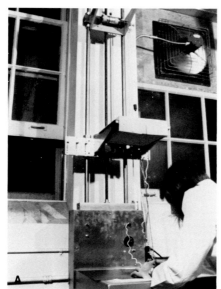

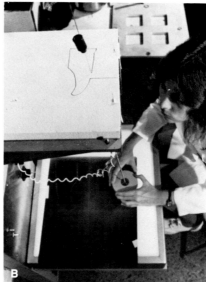

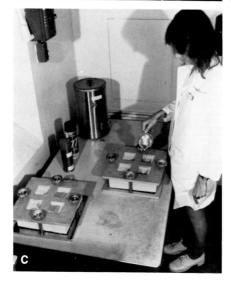

Fig. 2–17. Hot-wire apparatus for constructing blocks. The apparatus shown in the figure is based on the technique described by Edland and Hansen[3] for divergently cutting styrofoam with an electrically heated wire *(A,B)*. Several modifications were made in the device shown (e.g., motorization of distance adjustments, variable lateral placement of the styrofoam frame, and a reduction of the additional pull that is required to keep the wire under adequate tension). The low-melting alloy Cerrobend is used to cast lead block in the cut styrofoam cavity *(C)*.[4] The system has proved useful particularly in blocking the mantle field.

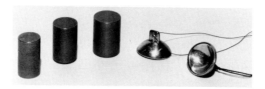

Fig. 2–18. Eye shields. Two types of eye shields[5] are shown. The eye shields on the right are inserted beneath the eye lids. They provide protection from superficial and orthovoltage x-ray and low-energy electrons (7 MeV or less). The eye shields on the left are lead cylinders in three different diameters (1.0, 1.5, 2.0 cm) that can be suspended above the patient on a Mylar tray. The appropriate thickness is specified by the radiotherapist.

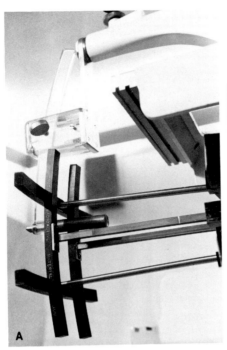

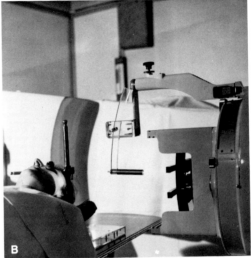

Fig. 2–19. Ocular protection satellite. Protection of selected eye structures, the whole eye ball, or the orbit is accomplished by the insert holder illustrated for any angled beam. The desired shield is attached to the end of a sliding arc *(A)*, whose vertex is at the center of the cobalt source. This is fixed to the mounting ring *(B)*, which is standard equipment on the Atomic Energy of Canada Limited (AECL) Theratron 60 or 80 units and Eldorado 6 or 8 units. (Courtesy of Delclos, L.)

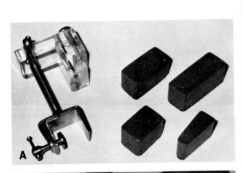

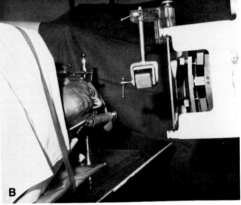

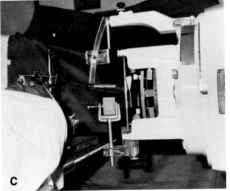

Fig. 2–20. Suspended secondary block holder. A lead block holder *(A)* that attaches to the collimator of the unit can provide blocking of any shape with vertical *(B)*, angled or horizontal beam. It can be used in combination with the ocular protection satellite and wedges *(C)*. (Courtesy of Delclos, L.)

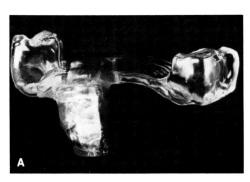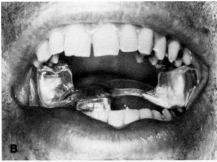

Fig. 2–21. Intraoral stents. The dentist can make a stent to the radiotherapist's specification that provides heavy-metal protection for the tongue and gingiva when the cheek and lip are treated with electrons. Stents are made of a dental acrylic that encompasses the heavy metal *(A)*. These stents can also be made to displace the tongue to a desired position *(B)*. (From Tapley: *In* Clinical Applications of the Electron Beam. Edited by N.DuV. Tapley. New York, John Wiley, 1976.)

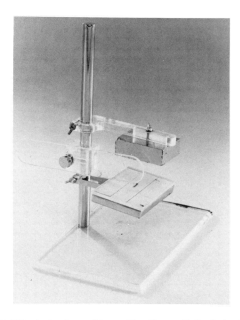

Fig. 2–22. Gonad shield. This device is used to position the genitalia during irradiation of the scrotum and the inguinal and pelvic lymph nodes in patients with malignant tumor of the testicle.[6] It retracts the penis and the remaining testicle out of the treatment field, while maintaining a fixed treatment volume of hemiscrotum at a fixed source–surface distance (SSD). It allows a more reliable estimate of dose to the remaining (untreated) testicle than was possible with previous systems. It attenuates the exit dose to the underlying perineum and proximal medial thighs. A shield of several half-value layers can be positioned directly over the testicle that is being held out of the treatment field.

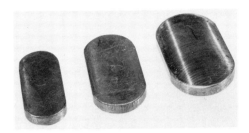

Fig. 2–23. Kidney shields. Shaped lead blocks made according to the specifications of the radiotherapist, are available in three sizes; these are used to shield kidney(s) during whole or strip abdominal irradiation. (From Delclos and Dembo: *In* Textbook of Radiotherapy, 3rd ed. Edited by G.H. Fletcher. Philadelphia, Lea & Febiger, 1980.)

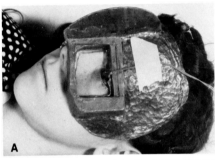

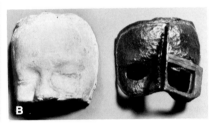

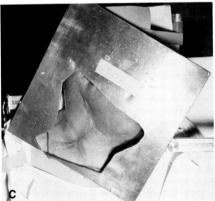

Fig. 2–24. Custom shielding. Lead shields can be custom fitted to individual patients *(A)* who present unusual blocking problems. Shown are examples of lead masks used with low-energy x-ray or electron beams *(B)*. These masks are molded to a dental-stone positive of the patient. Also shown is a lead cutout suspended above the patient *(C)* that collimates an irregular field that would otherwise be difficult to block. (C. From Almond: *In* Clinical Applications of the Electron Beam. Edited by N.duV. Tapley. New York, John Wiley, 1976.)

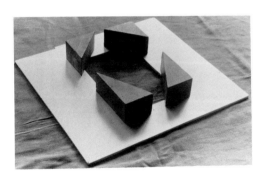

Fig. 2–25. Preshaped fields. Some irregularly shaped standard treatment fields (e.g., the pelvic field with blocked corners and the extended pelvic field covering the common iliac node areas) require secondary blocking. These standard-shaped fields[7] can be defined quickly by using preset blocks mounted on a base that can be inserted into the beam.

TUMOR LOCALIZATION AND TREATMENT SIMULATION DEVICES

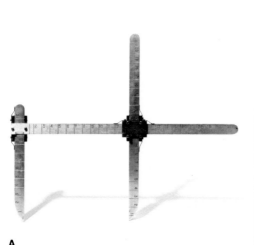

A

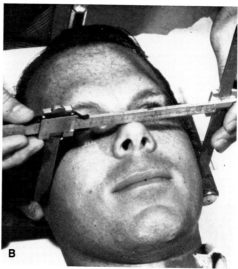

B

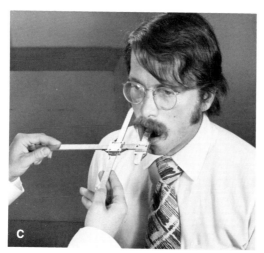

C

Fig. 2–26. Head and neck caliper (Pied-Cullis). Because of its size, the caliper is useful in head and neck measurements of either patient diameters *(A)* or surface-to-tumor depths *(B)*. The parallel arms move in both horizontal and vertical directions *(C)*, which allows the measurement of tumor or intraoral depths relative to lateral and anterior-posterior surfaces. (From Sampiere: *In* Textbook of Radiotherapy, 3rd ed. Edited by G.H. Fletcher. Philadelphia, Lea & Febiger, 1980.)

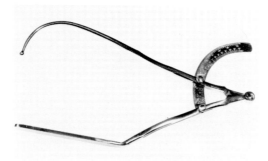

Fig. 2–27. Body caliper. A pelvimeter has been modified by attaching a straight base to one half of the caliper. This arrangement is most convenient for measuring trunk and abdomen diameters. A scale is included so that a given diameter can be read with the caliper in position.

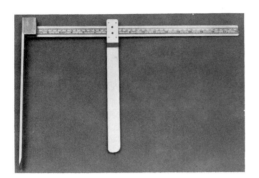

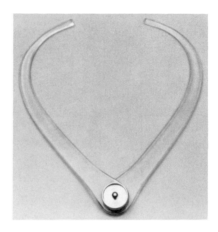

Fig. 2–28. Caliper. This caliper is designed to measure body thickness. The movable arm is parallel to the base arm and moves smoothly along the vertical bar by means of a nylon sleeve. The instrument has a millimeter scale.

Fig. 2–29. Caliper. This outside caliper is convenient for measuring diameters around head and neck areas. The arms can be locked in a separated position with the thumb screw shown.

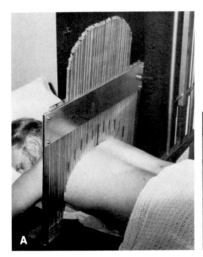

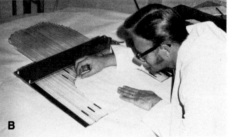

Fig. 2–30. Contour maker. The device is convenient for making external body contours required in treatment planning. The apparatus consists of low-friction nylon rods that move freely to conform to the contour included in the 180° cross section. The rods can be locked all at once *(A)*. Another feature is the central rod, graduated in centimeters, that is used to determine the anterior-posterior diameter of the patient. The ends of the outside supports provide the horizontal baseline for the resultant contour represented by the end of each nylon rod *(B)*. (From Kuisk: Radiology *101*:203, 1971.)

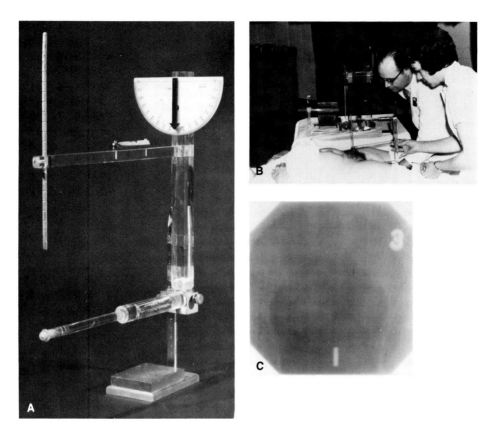

Fig. 2–31. Cervical localizer. This localization device consists of a lead-tipped rod that is inserted into the vagina against the lower edge of the tumor (cervical or vaginal). A rod is attached *(A)* that suspends above the anterior surface of the patient along a line directly above the lead tip, thus locating the lower edge of the tumor relative to the patient's surface *(B).* Levels are incorporated in the probe and the handle to keep both arms horizontal during the procedure. The lead insert on the tip shows clearly *(C)* on portal films and allows evaluation of treatment field margins. *(B,C.* From Fletcher: *In* Textbook of Radiotherapy, 3rd ed. Edited by G.H. Fletcher. Philadelphia, Lea & Febiger, 1980.)

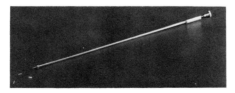

Fig. 2–32. Silver seed inserter. Inactive gold seeds or small silver wires can be positioned to identify selected areas of tumor with this modified 10-inch rigid radon seed implanter. A small flange has been soldered to the end so that seeds or wires can be implanted at the same depth. (From Delclos: Radiology 93:695, 1969.)

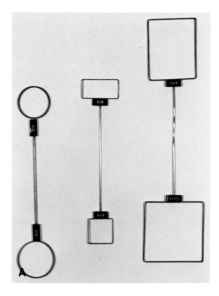
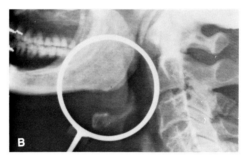

Fig. 2–33. Field demarcation wire frames for beam selection and localization on the photon- and electron-beam units. Wire frames *(A)* are available in an assortment of nominal field sizes and shapes corresponding to available cones. These are convenient to use either with the fluoroscopic beam to locate and mark the proper field boundaries on a patient's surface on the simulator, or for permanent localization films *(B)*.

EXTERNAL-BEAM TREATMENT SETUP DEVICES

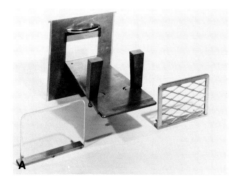
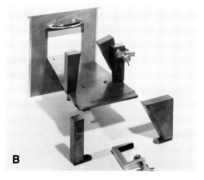

Fig. 2–34. Tangential breast beam collimator. To gain better beam characteristics for tangential breast treatments (i.e., minimal divergence and little penumbra through the lung transversed) a beam collimator that shields the bottom portion of the original beam is fabricated. With cobalt units it is important to place the shield below the center of the collimator one-half the diameter of the cobalt source to prevent any unwanted penumbra in the primary field. A brass plate attaches to the shield and projects to the treatment distance to provide penumbra blocking. The end of this plate is either a perpendicular plastic plate, used for the bolus treatment, or a straight extension to the SSD for the no-bolus treatments *(A)*. Side shielding of different angles is provided to block the sides of the tangential fields so that no overlap with the supraclavicular field occurs. Clamps *(B)* can be used to hold two side blocks together to achieve a more complex blocking arrangement. The clamps have rubber surfaces to better hold the blocks in position. (From Fletcher et al.: AJR *84*:761, 1960.)

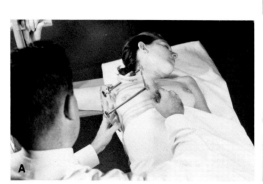
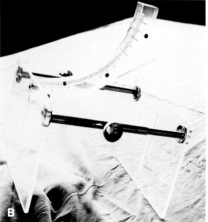

Fig. 2–35. Breast bridge with rolling-ball angle inclinometer. This breast bridge, used with tangential breast treatments, consists of a pair of plastic plates that can be locked at the appropriate separation as determined for an individual patient *(A)*. The attached rolling ball inclinometer *(B)* indicates the angle above or below the horizontal of the bridge baseline, so that correct machine angulation can be achieved. (From Fletcher et al.: AJR *84*:761, 1960.)

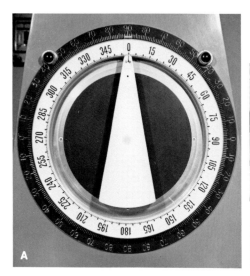
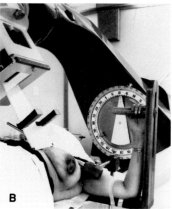

Fig. 2–36. The cobalt four-quadrant compass. Determining field angles for the tangential chest wall and breast portals using the 360° angle indicator that is standard equipment in many rotational units can be confusing and can result in errors. This supplementary angle indicator is divided into four quadrants. Zero degree is located on the horizontal and 90° is on the vertical *(A)*. Angles read off the breast bridge then apply directly to this scale *(B)*. (From Delclos: Radiologia *15*:327, 1973.)

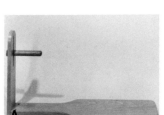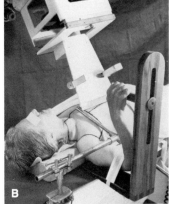

Fig. 2–37. Arm board for breast irradiation. The arm board *(A)* illustrated is positioned beneath the patient. The perpendicular support provides a hand grasp *(B)* that can be moved and then set to the proper height by a twist lock. (From Fletcher et al.: AJR *84*:761, 1960.)

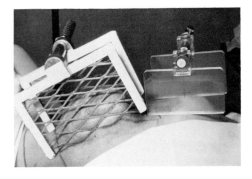

Fig. 2–38. Sqeeze bridge bolus and no-bolus. For those treatments where a squeeze boost to the tangential breast fields is needed, two bridges are available. One is a wire mesh frame used where no additional surface dose is wanted and the other is a plastic frame to provide buildup where more surface dose is desired. (From Fletcher and Montague: AJR *93*:573, 1965.)

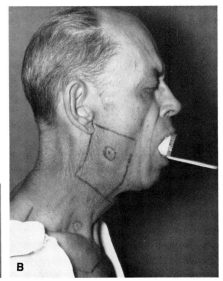

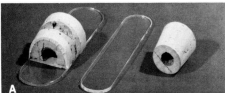

Fig. 2–39. Cork with tongue blade. A cork is mounted on a wooden or plastic tongue blade *(A)* to move the tongue out of a radiation field or insure inclusion of the tongue in the radiation field. A gum or tooth groove is cut in the top of the cork to better stabilize the cork in the mouth *(B)*. An air hole is drilled through the center of the cork. (From Fletcher: *In* Textbook of Radiotherapy, 3rd ed. Edited by G.H. Fletcher. Philadelphia, Lea & Febiger, 1980.)

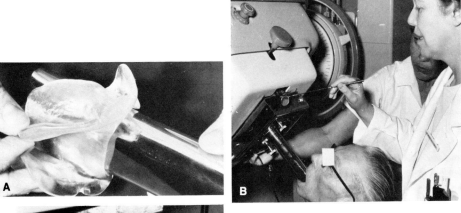

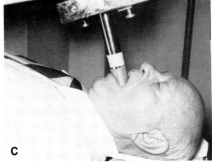

Fig. 2–40. Cone holder—intraoral. Positive placement of an intraoral cone[9] can be accomplished by the custom-fitting of a dental impression around the cone *(A,B,C)*. (From Santiago: J. Prosthet. Dent. *15*:938, 1965.)

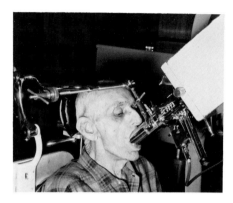

Fig. 2–41. Cone holder—external. This cone holder is attached to a chair that also has a dental head rest for patient stability. It holds the intraoral cone in the desired position before the cone is attached to the machine (orthovoltage or electron beam). (From Fletcher: *In* Textbook of Radiotherapy, 2nd ed. Edited by G.H. Fletcher. Philadelphia, Lea & Febiger, 1973.)

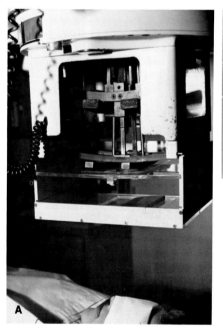

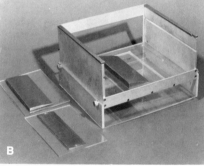

Fig. 2–42. Wedge holder. This wedge holder attaches to the collimator by sliding into available grooves. It provides a constant wedge placement in the radiation beam and prevents a 90° rotation of the wedge by its elongated rectangular shape. A groove in the upper position of the wedge holder allows placement of a tissue compensating filter in addition to the wedge *(B)*. A secondary blocking tray can be attached to the bottom of the wedge box *(A)* to allow convenient shaping of the treatment field.

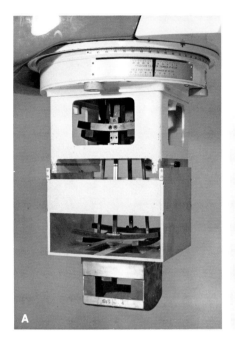
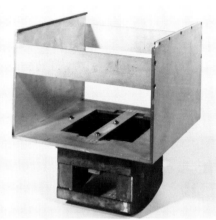

Fig. 2–43. Parametrial cone. This treatment cone was designed specifically for external-beam parametrial irradiation in combination with brachytherapy. It provides both compression and proper shielding *(A)*. At a depth of 10 cm, the central shields project a shadow 3-, 4-, and 5-cm wide and 10-cm long from the inferior edge of the field. The central shield is suspended in the cone base *(B)*, and can be moved off the center of the field to follow the displacement of a radium system off the midline of the patient. Each corner is blocked to reduce the irradiated volume. (From Fletcher: *In* Textbook of Radiotherapy, 3rd ed. Edited by G.H. Fletcher. Philadelphia, Lea & Febiger, 1980.)

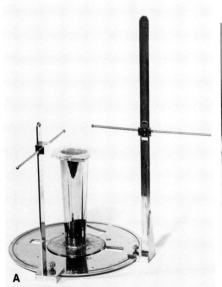
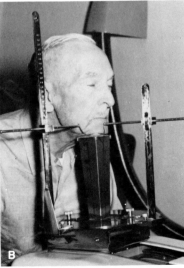

Fig. 2–44. Positioning device for submental treatments. This device attaches to the base of the cone holder *(A)*. Rods indicating the direction of the central ray can be rotated about the base of the device and conveniently positioned to indicate the relationship between the central ray and the patient's surface *(B)*. (From Tapley: *In* Textbook of Radiotherapy, 2nd ed. Edited by G.H. Fletcher. Philadelphia, Lea & Febiger, 1973.)

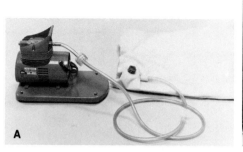

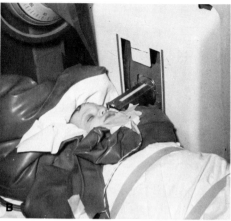

Fig. 2–45. Body immobilizer. This immobilizer device (developed by Picker X-Ray Corporation, White Plains, NY) is used mostly for pediatric patients who cannot be relied on to hold a critical position such as that necessary for treatment of retinoblastoma. The system consists of a vacuum pump and an outer rubber bag filled with plastic mini-spheres *(A)*. A vacuum line with a fine mesh filter evacuates the inner atmosphere, causing the plastic minispheres to "lock" together. The rubber bag with spheres is positioned around the child *(B)* and supported in this position. A vacuum is then applied and maintained during treatment.

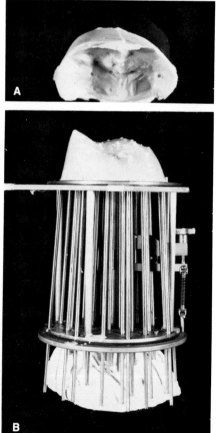

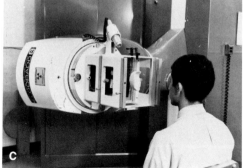

Fig. 2–46. Apparatus for constructing irregular surface compensators. The instrument generates the surface contour in three dimensions at a given distance from the surface and corrects for beam divergence *(A,B,C)*. The compensator is built on this surface with a suitable material of proper density. The details of the apparatus and its use have been discussed in the literature.[1,2] (From Khan, Moore, and Burns, *Radiology* 90:593, 1968.)

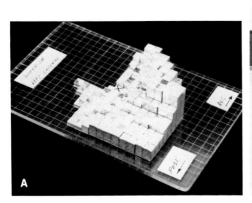
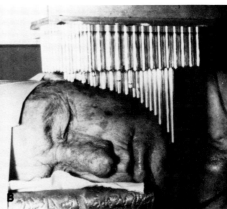

Fig. 2–47. Compensating filters. A system of tissue compensation similar to that described by Hall and Oliver[27] is shown. A matrix column of rods *(A)* attached to the collimator over the patient in treatment position is brought into contact with the patient's surface. The rod at the center of the beam is marked, as is the rod at the position on the patient's surface that indicates 0.0 cm tissue compensation and SSD position (usually the widest diameter). By substracting this 0-cm rod length from all other rod lengths, the thickness of tissue compensation at each rod position can be calculated. Aluminum rods with a 0.65 cm square cross section are used for the tissue compensator filter *(B)*. Each compensating rod is positioned on a square, which has a bolus thickness requirement determined by the previously mentioned method. The 0.65 cm square positioned in a constant geometry above the patient projects to a 1-cm square at the SSD distance. The compensating tissue ratio for ^{60}Co irradiation is 0.325 cm. AL: 1 cm tissue. (From Sampiere: *In* Textbook of Radiology, 3rd ed. Edited by G.H. Fletcher. Philadelphia, Lea & Febiger, 1980.)

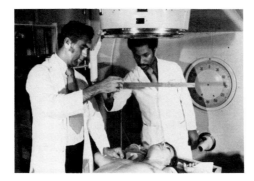

Fig. 2–48. Patient surface distance measuring device. A rod attachable to the head of the unit supports a horizontal arm that rotates freely around the axis of the rod and carries a roll of metallic tape that slides along the arm. A spirit level laid over the arm gauges the beam's perpendicularity. The vertical distance from the tape-case edge to the selected point on the patient's surface is measured by bringing the tape directly over the point. This distance is related to the vertical SSD. The device is specifically useful in measuring vertical SSDs at selected points in a large field (e.g., the mantle). The information is subsequently used to calculate the dose.

Chapter 3

COMPLEX FIELD ARRANGEMENTS: FIELD SHAPING AND SEPARATION OF ADJOINING FIELDS

Faiz M. Khan

FIELD SHAPING

Considerable time and effort are required in shaping irregular fields in radiation therapy. Complex shapes are achieved by intricate blocking of radiation to the normal and critical areas within the field. The frequency and complexity of field shaping varies from institution to institution. In using complex techniques involving elaborate blocking, it is necessary to establish an organized system of field shaping. This is particularly true for the mantle and some head and neck fields.

Standardized Lead Blocks

The construction of shielding blocks is a time consuming process. For relatively simple cases of shielding, however, it is desirable to have a stock of precut lead blocks of various geometrical shapes available. Some of the blocks may be contoured to block specific organs (e.g., kidneys, eyes, head of humerus, and skin edges).

Block Thickness

Shielding blocks are most commonly made of lead. The thickness of blocks depends on the beam energy and the allowed transmission through the block. A 5% transmission through the block is acceptable—that means a thickness corresponding to a little more than 4 half-value layers (HVL). In the case of ^{60}Co, 5-cm-thick lead is considered adequate. The radiation quantity of interest is the dose received in the shielded volume, which may be 10% to 15% of peak dose (D_{max}) because of the added contribution of radiation scattered from the adjoining open areas of the field.

Dose at a given point in the shielded volume also depends on the proximity of that point to the surrounding exposed volume. For example, when lungs are shielded in a mantle field, the shielded apex areas may receive 2 to 3 times the dose received under the middle of the shield. There is also a gradient of dose across the block edges where the dose changes from a full value in the open area to a low value within the shielded area. Sharpness of this gradient depends on many factors such as block divergence, position in the field, source size, block-to-surface distance (BSD), and beam energy.

It is not advantageous to increase the thickness of the blocks beyond what is needed for 5% transmission. The blocks get heavier without much further diminution of the dose in the shielded volume.

Block Divergence

Because the treatment beam is divergent, the blocks may be tapered with the sides conforming to the direction of rays. Straight (untapered) blocks, in general, produce a less sharp dose gradient at the edge than divergent blocks. The advantage is not very significant in the case of beams emanating from a large source such as ^{60}Co. The geometric penumbra in that case dominates the effect on dose gradient.

Divergent blocks are suitable for beams with small focal spots and especially when large BSDs are used. Another advantage is that, by employing divergent shields, the shields can be placed closer to the source, thus reducing the size of otherwise bulky and heavy blocks. This should be the consideration when the area to be shielded is large (e.g., lungs in a mantle field treatment).

Straight-cut blocks are easier to construct and are mostly prefabricated to various shapes and sizes. Because the sides of the blocks are not parallel to the rays (nondivergent), a partial transmission of beam results at the block edges. To minimize this effect, the blocks should be placed close to the patient surface. This calls for bigger blocks and introduces the problem of increased skin dose. A distance of 15 cm to 20 cm between the plastic block-supporting tray and the skin surface is a good compromise for most megavoltage beams.

The BSD is important from the point of view of set-up accuracy. If the BSD is too large, a small displacement in the position of the shield in the beam is magnified at the position of the shielded area. It is desirable to use a minimum BSD, provided the surface dose is kept within acceptable limits. Unless reduction in block size is a prime consideration, blocks (both divergent and straight) should be placed at a distance of about 15 cm from the patient.

Shadow Tray and Skin Sparing

The skin-sparing effect is one of the most desirable features of megavoltage beams. This effect may be reduced or lost if the photon beam is excessively contaminated with secondary electrons. In the case of ^{60}Co beams, it has been shown[9,20] that an air gap of 15 cm to 20 cm between the scatterer and the skin surface is required to maintain the skin-sparing effect (i.e., surface dose of less than 50%).

The surface dose also increases with field size and may become prohibitively excessive for extremely large fields; in one cobalt unit, the surface doses of 30% to 60% were measured respectively for field sizes of 5 cm × 5 cm and 30 cm × 30 cm, with no absorber in the beam.[22] The range of surface-dose values and build-up characteristics of a beam may vary from machine to machine. The effect of field size on surface dose has been discussed in the literature.[1,13,22]

The amount of electron contamination produced in the beam depends on the atomic number of the absorber or the electron scattering material. Low-atomic-number absorbers, such as a lucite shadow tray,

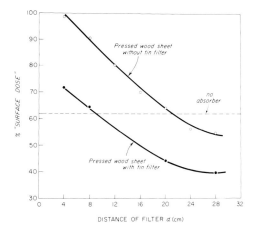

Fig. 3–1.   Percent surface dose vs. absorber to surface distance *(d)* for a pressed wood tray and tray plus tin filter. ^{60}Co beam; field size, 20 × 20 cm, SSD, 80 cm; source to diaphragm distance, 45 cm. (From Khan: AJR *111*:180, 1971.)

produce more forward scatter of electrons than the high-atomic-number materials and, therefore, give rise to a greater surface dose. It has been shown both theoretically and experimentally that the absorbers of an intermediate atomic number such as tin ($Z = 50$) produce minimum electron contamination.[7,8,12,13,22] A sheet of this material, known as electron filter, may be placed under the shadow tray to minimize skin dose. The thickness of electron filter should approximately equal the range of the secondary electrons produced in that material. For ^{60}Co gamma rays, a tin sheet of about 1-mm thickness is adequate. Figure 3–1 shows the effect of tin in reducing surface dose. Beam attenuation produced by the shadow tray and the electron filter must be taken into account in treatment calculations.

In practice, it is necessary to have a transparent shadow tray for treatment set-ups. In one of the arrangements used at the University of Minnesota, an accessory was designed with the shadow tray frame having tracks so that a tin sheet mounted on a pressed wood sheet could be slipped under the shadow tray. In this case, the tin filter must face the patient surface. Saylor and Quilin[22] have suggested that leaded glass, which is transparent and has a medium effective atomic number, be used as electron filter. However, the fragility of lead glass effectively negates its usefulness as electron filter.

Construction of Individualized Blocks

An elaborate and organized system of constructing blocks is required for individual patients and individual treatment fields. Although it is tedious and time-consuming to construct individualized blocks, the system is advantageous for various reasons. Complex fields require considerable block-stacking, which carries the risk of radiation leakage through gaps and toppling of blocks into the field or onto the patient. Treatment setups are tedious and less reproducible if field shaping is performed at every treatment session with an array of numerous blocks. An individually constructed block, on the other hand, is in one piece, is simple to use and eliminates or minimizes the aforementioned problems. Most individual blocks are divergently shaped and thus enhance sharpness of dose cutoff at the edge. In mantle fields, individually shaped lung blocks are essential to provide a precise shaping of the complex field.

Various methods have been proposed for the construction of individualized blocks. The reader is referred to several sources.[2,3,10,11,15,18,19] The method described here is currently used at the University of Minnesota and is more or less similar to the one described by Powers et al.[19]

A device for cutting styrofoam cavities divergently with an electrically heated wire is in common use today. Such a device is commercially available, as are styrofoam and Cerrobend lead. Outline of the treatment field is made on a simulator radiograph or a port film. The film, the styrofoam block, and the wire apparatus are adjusted so that the treatment geometry is obtained. The lower end of the wire traces the outline on the film. For lung blocks, cavities are cut in the styrofoam with the heated segment of the wire and subsequently filled with melted Cerrobend (an alloy of lead, bismuth and cadmium; melting point 70°C, density at 20°C = 9.4 g/cm^3). The required thickness of Cerrobend block (for 5% narrow-beam transmission) is about 3 inches, depending on energy, from ^{60}Co energy to 22 MV x-rays.[19] The material is poured slowly into the styrofoam cavities to prevent formation of air bubbles. The styrofoam block may be tightly pressed against a rubber pad at the bottom to avoid leakage of the liquid material. The inside of the cavities may be sprayed with silicone for easy release of the styrofoam from the block.

Making a "negative" block, with central area open and blocking around the periphery, is a bit more cumbersome. First the inner cut is made in the styrofoam block to outline the given field. An outer rectangular cut is made corresponding to the overall field (defined by the collimator) with 1 cm to 2 cm margin. The two cuts thus made give rise to three styrofoam pieces. The intermediate piece, corresponding to the areas to be shielded, is removed, retaining only the outermost and the innermost pieces. Alignment of pieces is carefully maintained relative to central axis. Cerrobend is then poured into the cavity between the inner and the outer pieces.

The blocks are mounted on a ¼″ plexiglass plate with cross-hairs drawn on the plate. One way of mounting blocks is to have fixed pegs on the plate. The plate is placed under the styrofoam blocks when the Cerrobend is poured, thus creating corresponding holes for the pegs in the lead block. These plates are individualized for each patient. Figure 3–2 shows blocks that were constructed for a mantle and a head and neck field.

It is not necessary to construct individualized divergent blocks for all cases. It has been my experience that custom blocking is beneficial for lung blocks in

mantle field and shielding for a few complex head and neck fields; satisfactory blocking can be achieved by standard, prefabricated lead blocks in most other cases.

Electron-Beam Shielding

Considerable beam shaping is required in treating superficial tumors with electron beams (6–15 MeV). Lead cutouts are often used to shape fields. The cutouts are usually molded and placed directly on the skin surface.

Electron beams require thicker lead sheets for 5% transmission than the superficial x-rays and the orthovoltage. Figure 3–3 gives the thickness of lead for transmitted surface doses for electrons. It can be seen that, if the lead is too thin, the surface dose may be enhanced rather than reduced (because of more scattering than attenuation).

X-ray contamination is slightly increased when lead shields are used due to the bremsstrahlung interactions. In treating small volumes, however, the x-ray contamination associated with lead shielding is not of much concern.

In some situations, such as the treatment of lip and buccal mucosa lesions, internal

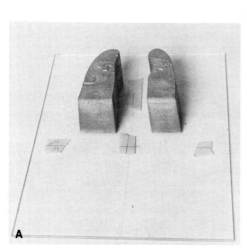
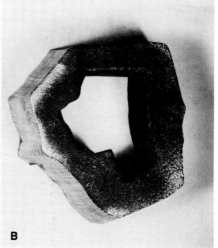

Fig. 3–2. Photographs of Cerrobend blocks: *(A)* lung blocks for a mantle field; *(B)* a block for shaping a head-and-neck field.

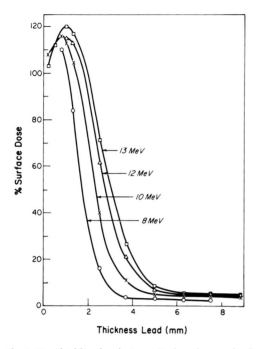

Fig. 3–3. Shielding for electrons. Surface dose vs. lead thickness as a percentage of the maximum dose in phantom without lead. Shielding thickness may be determined for 5% transmission. (From Khan, Moore, and Levitt: Br. J. Radiol. 49:883, 1976.)

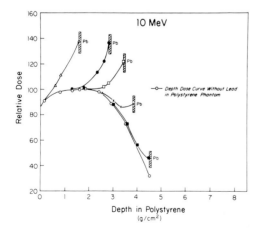

Fig. 3–4. Modification of depth dose by electron backscattering from lead placed at various depths in the phantom. Lead thickness = 1.7 mm. (From Khan, Moore, and Levitt: Br. J. Radiol. 49:883, 1976.)

shielding is useful to protect the internal structures. The problem with internal shielding is the electron backscatter (EBS) resulting in increase in dose at the lead–tissue interface of approximately 40% to 50% (Fig. 3–4). This effect has been discussed by Okumura et al.,[17] Saunders and Peters,[21] Nüsslin,[16] Weatherburn et al.[23] and Khan et al.[14] It has been suggested that 5 mm to 10 mm of tissue-equivalent bolus be interposed between the internal shield and the preceding tissue. The lead shield may alternatively be sheathed with 2 mm to 3 mm of aluminum to absorb the backscattered electrons of electron beams up to 15 MeV.

SEPARATION OF ADJACENT FIELDS

Adjacent fields are commonly used in external-beam radiotherapy. Many treatment techniques involve the junction of fields with the adjointing margins abutted or separated depending upon various circumstances. The radiation distribution in the junction volume is profoundly changed as a result. These changes can be easily observed by placing isodose charts side by side and summating the doses in the junction area. Because of a rapid falloff of the dose near the boundary of the field, a small change in the relative spacing of the field margins produces a large change in dose distribution in the junction volume. It is therefore important to know the distribution of dose at the junction so that the fields are arranged to avoid a junctional dose that either exceeds normal tissue tolerance or is inadequate to sterilize the tumor.

If the adjacent fields are abutted on the surface, the fields would overlap to an increasing degree with depth because of divergence. This causes a substantial increase in dose over a large area. In clinical practice, head and neck fields are most often abutted (provided the spinal-cord dose does not exceed its tolerance dose) because of relative superficiality of tumor. The fields of the thorax, pelvis, or such a critical structure as the spinal cord, are usually separated.

In some cases of adjacent fields, the doses at the junction are delivered over about twice the time period as the central axis dose for the individual fields. An example of this is the mantle and the inverted-Y fields. From the time-dose-effect perspective, it has been suggested that a somewhat higher dose at the junction may be desirable,[4] provided that the tolerance of the normal tissue or a critical organ is not exceeded.

Methods of Field Separation

Geometric. It is possible to achieve dose uniformity at the junction of two fields from geometric considerations, provided that the geometric boundary of the field is defined by the 50% decrement line (i.e., the line joining the points at the depth where the dose is 50% of the central-axis dose at the same depth). The separation of the fields at the surface can then be calculated so that the adjacent field boundaries join at the chosen depth.

If two adjacent fields are incident from one side only, and if the fields are separated to junction at a given depth, then the dose lateral to the junction is made uniform. The dose to the entrance side will be lower and the dose to the exit side will be higher than the junction dose.

In the four-field technique where two adjacent fields are incident from one side and two from the parallel opposed direction, the corresponding opposing fields are usually made to junction at the midline depth. This gives a uniform dose lateral to the junction and lower doses above and below the junction. Figure 3–5 compares abutting and geometrically separated fields. This example qualitatively applies to the mantle and inverted Y fields.

Figure 3–6 illustrates the calculation of field separation. Let L_1 and L_2 be the field lengths, d be the depth of the junction point at which dose uniformity is desired, *SSD* be the source–surface distance; the field separation S on the surface is then given by[4]:

$$S = \frac{L_1}{2}\left(\frac{d}{SSD}\right) + \frac{L_2}{2}\left(\frac{d}{SSD}\right)$$

Dosimetric. With the availability of computers for radiotherapy treatment planning, separation of fields to achieve uniform dose at a desired depth can be easily planned by optimizing the placement of fields on the contour and obtaining isodose curves in the plane containing the central axes of all the beams (see Chapter 9). This method is more informative in the sense that uniformity as well as "hot" and "cold" spots can be visualized in an individual patient. The accuracy of this method depends on the accuracy of the individual field isodose curves.

Compensating Wedges. It is possible to design compensating wedges so that an artificial dose falloff is created at the adjacent field borders which, when summated at a given depth, would give a uniform dose distribution. A similar technique has been used by Griffin et al.[6] for cranial-spinal irradiation.

Junction Shift. In this method, the fields are abutting on the surface but the junction is moved to different positions on different days of treatment, so that the hot spot is spread over a distance. This method may also be applied to field separation in order to avoid hot and cold spots occurring at one place.

Guidelines for Adjacent-Field Irradiation

The decision whether the fields should be abutted or separated should be based on dosimetric data and clinical considerations (e.g., the presence of a critical organ and under- or over-dosage of the tissues around the junction volume).

The site of field matching should be carefully chosen so that, as far as possible, it does not contain a tumor-involved area or a sensitive critical organ.

It is advisable not to use secondary

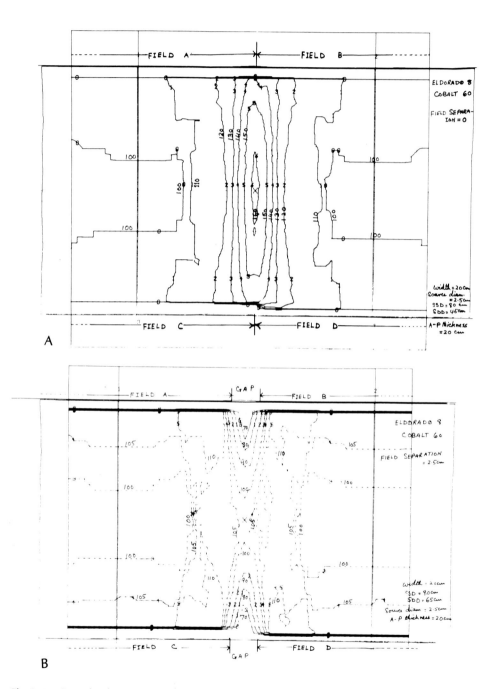

Fig. 3–5.   Dose distribution in the junction volume of two anterior and two posterior fields. *(A)* abutting fields, *(B)* fields geometrically separated to junction at the midline depth.

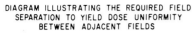

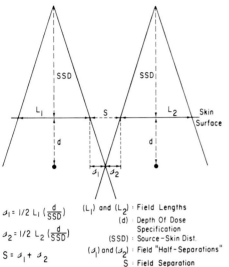

DIAGRAM ILLUSTRATING THE REQUIRED FIELD
SEPARATION TO YIELD DOSE UNIFORMITY
BETWEEN ADJACENT FIELDS

$$\jmath_1 = 1/2 \ L_1 \left(\frac{d}{SSD}\right)$$

$$\jmath_2 = 1/2 \ L_2 \left(\frac{d}{SSD}\right)$$

$$S = \jmath_1 + \jmath_2$$

(L_1) and (L_2) : Field Lengths
(d) : Depth Of Dose Specification
(SSD) : Source–Skin Dist.
$(\jmath_1)$ and $(\jmath_2)$: Field "Half–Separations"
S : Field Separation

Fig. 3–6. Geometric method for the calculation of separation between adjoining fields. (From Cundiff et al.: Dosimetry Workshop. Hodgkin's Disease. Chicago, American Association of Physicists in Medicine, 1970.)

blocking or penumbra trimmers at the adjacent edges.

In field separations calculated by geometric method, it must be known that the margin of the field coincides with the 50% decrement line. It is also essential that the radiation beam be accurately aligned with the beam-defining light.

REFERENCES

1. Dutreix, J., Dutreix, A., and Tubiana, M.: Electronic equilibrium and transition stages. Phys. Med. Biol. 10:177, 1965.
2. Earl, J.D. and Bagshaw, M.A.: A rapid optical method for preparation of complex field shapes. Radiology 88:1162, 1967.
3. Edland, R.W. and Hansen, H.: Irregular Field-Shaping for 60Co Teletherapy. Radiology 92:1567, 1969.
4. Faw, F.L. and Glenn, D.W.: Further investigations of physical aspects of multiple field radiation therapy. Am. J. Roentgenol. 108:184, 1970.
5. Glenn, D.W., Faw, F.L., Kagan, R., and Johnson, R.E.: Field separation in multiple portal radiation therapy. Am. J. Roentgenol. 102:199, 1968.
6. Griffin, T.W., Schumacher, D., and Berry, H.C.: A technique for cranial-spinal irradiation. Brit. J. Radiol. 49:887, 1976.
7. Hine, G.J.: Scattering of secondary electrons produced by gamma rays in materials of various atomic numbers. Phys. Rev. 82:755, 1951.
8. Hine, G.J.: Secondary electron emission and effective atomic numbers. Nucleonics 10:9, 1952.
9. Johns, J.E., Epp, E.R., Cormack, D.V., and Fedoruk, S.O.: Depth dose data and diaphragm design for Saskatchewan 1000 Curie cobalt unit. Brit. J. Radiol. 25:302, 1952.
10. Jones, D.: A method for the accurate manufacture of lead shields. Brit. J. Radiol. 44:398, 1971.
11. Karzmark, C.J. and Huisman, P.A.: Melting, casting and shaping lead shielding blocks: Method and toxicity aspects. Am. J. Roentgenol. 114:636, 1972.
12. Khan, F.M.: Use of electron filter to reduce skin dose in cobalt teletherapy. Am. J. Roentgenol. 111:180, 1971.
13. Khan, F.M., Moore, V.C., and Levitt, S.H.: Effect of various atomic number absorbers on skin dose for 10 MeV x-rays. Radiology 109:209, 1973.
14. Khan, F.M., Moore, V.C., and Levitt, S.H.: Field shaping in electron beam therapy. Brit. J. Radiol. 49:883, 1976.
15. Maruyama, Y., Moore, V.C., Burns, D. et al.: Individualized lung shields constructed from lead shot embedded in plastic. Radiology 92:634, 1969.
16. Nusslin, F.: Electron back-scattering from lead in a perspex phantom. Brit. J. Radiol. 48:1041, 1975.
17. Okumura, U., Mori, T., and Kitagawa, T.: Modifications of dose distributions in high-energy electron beam treatment. Radiology 99:683, 1971.
18. Parfitt, R.: Manufacture of lead shields. Brit. J. Radiol. 44:895, 1971.
19. Powers, W.E., Kinzie, J.J., Demidecki, A.J. et al.: A new system of field shaping for external-beam radiation therapy. Radiology 108:407, 1973.
20. Richardson, J.E., Kerman, H.D., and Brucer, M.: Skin dose from cobalt 60 teletherapy unit. Radiology 63:25, 1954.
21. Saunders, J.E. and Peters, V.G.: Backscattering from metals in superficial therapy with high energy electrons. Brit. J. Radiol. 47:467, 1974.
22. Saylor, W.L. and Quillin, R.M.: Methods for the enhancement of skin sparing in cobalt 60 teletherapy. Am. J. Roentgenol. 111:174, 1971.
23. Weatherburn, H., McMillan, K.T.P., Stedeford, B., and Durrant, K.R.: Physical measurements and clinical observations on back-scattering of 10 MeV electrons from lead shielding. Brit. J. Radiol. 48:229, 1975.

Chapter 4

DOSIMETRY OF IRREGULARLY SHAPED FIELDS

Faiz M. Khan

Irregular fields are encountered in radiotherapy when radiation-sensitive structures are shielded from the main beam or when the field extends beyond the irregularly shaped contour of the patient's body. Split fields, L-shaped or hockey-stick fields, inverted-Y, and mantle fields are examples of such fields. Because basic calculation data such as radiation output, backscatter factors (BSF) and percent depth doses (%DD) are usually available only for rectangular or square fields without blocking, special considerations apply to the dosimetry of irregular fields.

DEPTH-DOSE CALCULATIONS

Blocking changes dose distribution in the open portions of the field by reducing the radiation scatter from the shielded volume going into the open volume. The magnitude of the reduction for a given beam transmitted through the block depends on the size, shape, and proximity of the shielded area to the point considered. The effective field size for an irregular field is generally smaller than the overall field defined by the source-collimator projection.

The calculation of depth dose for irregular fields may be accomplished by approximation methods. These methods fall into two main categories: those based on phantom measurements with correction factors to accommodate variations in the actual treatment conditions from the phantom irradiation,[2,3,21,22] and those involving geometric approximations in which the given irregular field is approximated by a rectangular field.[10,17,23] Whereas approximation methods are often helpful in routine dosage calculations, their validity must be checked by measurements or by a standard method of calculations.[17]

More accurate methods have been developed for irregular field dosimetry.[6,13,15] These methods are suited for computers and will be discussed later in the chapter.

Geometric Approximation Method

It is difficult to formulate approximation rules that are valid in all cases of irregular fields. A procedure has been developed[17] that is helpful in making reasonable approximations.

(1) A rectangular portion of the field containing a given point is selected so that it includes most of the irradiated area surrounding the point and excludes only those areas that are remote from the point. In doing so, a shielded area may be included in the rectangle provided that this area is small and is remote from the point. Figure 4–1 illustrates this concept in a variety of irregularly shaped fields.

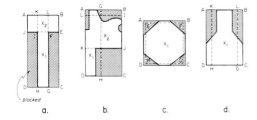

Fig. 4–1. Examples of various irregularly shaped fields. Approximate equivalent rectangles for points of interest are shown by dashed lines. Points vs. equivalent rectangles are:

a)	b)	c)	d)
1→GHKL	1→AGHD	1→EFGH	1→KLGH
2→ABEJ	2→LIJK		

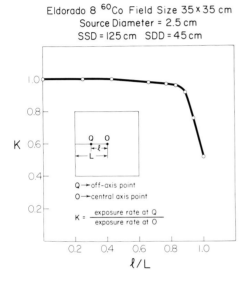

Eldorado 8 ^{60}Co Field Size 35 x 35 cm
Source Diameter = 2.5 cm
SSD = 125 cm   SDD = 45 cm

K

Q → off-axis point
O → central axis point

$$K = \frac{\text{exposure rate at } Q}{\text{exposure rate at } O}$$

ℓ/L

Fig. 4–2. A plot of K vs. l/L, representing off-axis diminution of exposure rate in the beam. (From Khan et al.: Radiology *106*:187, 1970.)

(2) The %DD and the BSF for the approximated rectangular field are determined from the regular depth dose tables.

(3) Suppose that in the above step, %DD was obtained at the given point for the nominal source to surface distance (SSD). The corrected %DD is given by

$$\%DD = (\text{uncorrected } \%DD) \times K$$

$$\times \left(\frac{SSD + d}{SSD + g + d} \right)^2 \times \frac{BSF_i}{BSF_o} \quad (1)$$

where K is the off-axis ratio in air of exposure rate at the point of calculation Q to that on central axis point in the same plane (Fig. 4–2); d is the depth below surface; g is the vertical distance between skin surface over Q and the nominal SSD plane*; BSF_i and BSF_o are the BSFs for the equivalent fields determined at point Q and the central axis point, respectively. The factor BSF_i/BSF_o approximates unity for most cases for high-energy photons. The corrected %DD represents depth dose as a percentage of the D_{max}, the maximum dose at central axis.

The sources of error in the above method are that an extremely irregular field may not be closely approximated by a rectangular field, and that, in step 2, it is assumed that the point is located at the center of the equivalent rectangle and that the dose at this point varies with depth as it does along the central axis of the rectangular field. The factor K in equation 1 compensates only for the change in exposure rate relative to the real central axis of the beam but does not include corrections for change in scattered dose if the assumed rectangle and the point considered are off-axis.

Examples of Calculations

Consider Figure 4–1a. This is one of the fields (posterior central nervous system) used in the treatment of acute lymphoblastic leukemia in children.[16] Suppose radiations are ^{60}Co gamma rays. Point 1 is the central axis of the beam irradiating the spine at a depth of 4 cm; point 2 is the midbrain at a depth of 8 cm. The overall field is ABCD. The effective field is slightly larger than HGKL for point 1 and approximately ABEJ for point 2.

Suppose the field dimensions are: AB = 13 cm; BC = 50 cm; HG = 5 cm; and BE = 16 cm; SSD at point 1 = 125 cm. From the output calibration chart, *Dose*

---

*g is positive or negative depending on whether SSD at the given point is respectively larger or smaller than the nominal SSD.

rate in free space for the overall field at SSD + 0.5 cm is 54.8 rad/min.; SSD at point 2 is 122 cm; off-axis ratios K from Figure 4–3 are 1.0 and 0.98 for points 1 and 2, respectively.

Suppose 150 rads are to be delivered at point 1. Find the treatment time, assuming a shadow-tray-transmission factor of 0.95. Find the dose received by point 2.

point 1:
effective field $\simeq$ 5 × 50 (eq. sq. = 9 × 9 cm)
uncorrected %DD = 85.4 at 4 cm depth
corrected %DD (from equation 1) = 85.4
BSF_o = 1.032

$$\text{treatment time} = \frac{150}{0.854} \times \frac{1}{54.8 \times 0.95 \times 1.032}$$

= 3.27 min.

point 2:
effective field $\simeq$ 13 × 16 (equivalent square = 14.3 × 14.3)
uncorrected %DD = 70.3 at 8 cm depth
K = 0.98; g = −3 cm; BSF_i = 1.049
corrected %DD (from equation 1)

$$= 70.3 \times 0.98 \times \left(\frac{133}{130}\right)^2 \times \frac{1.049}{1.032} = 73.3$$

This is relative to D_{max} at central axis.

$$D_{max} \text{ at point 1} = \frac{150}{0.854} = 175.6$$

Depth Dose received at point 2 = 175.6 × 0.733 = 128.8 rads

PRACTICAL FIELD EXAMPLES

The accuracy of the geometric approximation method depends on the degree of irregularity of the field. With relatively less complicated fields (e.g., L-shaped, split, and inverted Y fields) the approximation method is reasonably accurate (i.e., within 3% of the local dose for points well within the fields). For more complex fields, such as a mantle field, accuracy in general is not as good and depends on the location of the point of calculation. It is important to point out that the approximation method works better for higher-energy radiation (higher than ^{60}Co or 4 MV) where the variation of scatter or %DD with field size is small.

Although many different kinds of irregularly shaped fields are used in radiotherapy, the mantle and the inverted Y

fields are more complex and are discussed here as examples.

Mantle Field

Figure 4–3 is an example of a mantle field. The seven points shown in the diagram represent the sites of dosimetric interest. Approximate rectangular fields at each of these points are illustrated in the diagram. These rectangles can be converted to equivalent squares from the tables in reference 14 or area/perimeter (A/P) calculations.[19,24]

Specifically in mantle fields, the %DD at central axis is closely approximated (within 2%) by the rectangular field ABCD in Figure 4–3. The same effective field pertains to the BSF_o.

An important consideration in mantle-field dosimetry is the dose variation within the field. The dose at central axis, lower mediastinum, neck, supraclavicular regions, and axilla may be substantially different. The variation in dose is mainly due to the differences in thickness, SSD, location (off-axis distance) of different

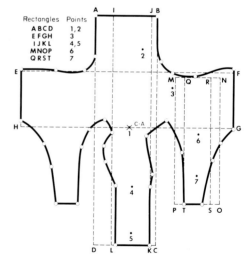

Fig. 4–3. Example of a mantle field. Solid line represents patient contour. Points denoted by the symbol 0 were selected to represent the contour to the computer. Calculations were made at points 1 through 7. Rectangles shown by dashed lines represent approximate equivalent fields. (From Khan et al.: Radiology *106*:187, 1970.)

points, and change in scattered dose due to the adjoining blocked areas. Although the use of a body-thickness compensator [4,5,9,18] and a flattening filter[26] reduces dose inhomogeneity, the dose distribution in various regions of the mantle field may be different because of significant differences in scatter. This later problem is less important in higher-energy radiation (above 4 MV x-rays).

Unless the dose distribution is made uniform, adjustment in dose must be made in various regions of the field. One way of doing this is to shield the areas that receive adequate dose during the course of treatment as seen in Figure 4–4. Although the blocking is changed for the last few treatments, the change in total dose distribution is not significant enough to necessitate recomputation.

Inverted Y

This field, which has the shape of an inverted Y, is used to irradiate the para-

aortic and pelvic lymph nodes in the treatment of Hodgkin's disease and other malignant lymphomas. In Figure 4–5, rectangles are drawn to indicate equivalent fields for the points of interest. Because the A/P of the equivalent fields at these points are usually not too different, an average value of A/P is often used for the purpose of determining %DD and BSF. Equation 1 may be used to correct for changes in SSD within the field.

CLARKSON'S METHOD

The principle of this method is to separate the primary and scattered components of dose at a point in a phantom. Special functions have been developed to facilitate the computation of scattered dose. These include scatter function, scatter–air ratio (SAR), and scatter–phantom (or scatter–maximum—SMR) ratio. The definition and use of these functions in calculating depth dose have been dis-

			TUMOR DOSE						
					POINT NO.				
TREATMENT NO.	DMAX ANT	DMAX POST	CA 1	M MED 2	Thrd 3	NECK 4	S CLAV 5	U AX 6	L AX 7
1	147		150	147	142	169	173	157	157
2		187	300	294	284	338	346	314	314
3	374		450	442	426	507	519	470	471
4		374	600	589	568	676	692	627	629
5	562		750	736	710	845	865	784	786
6		562	900	883	851	1014	1038	941	943
7	749		1050	1030	993	1183	1211	1098	1100
8		749	1200	1177	1135	1352	1385	1254	1257
9	936		1350	1325	1277	1520	1558	1411	1414
10		936	1500	1472	1419	1699	1731	1568	1571
11	1123		1650	1619	1561	1858	1904	1725	1729
12		1123	1800	1766	1703	2027	2077	1881	1886
13	1310		1950	1913	1845	2196	2250	2038	2043
14		1310	2100	2060	1987	2365	2423	2195	2200
15	1498		2250	2208	2129	2534	2596	2352	2357
16		1498	2400	2355	2271	2703	2769	2509	2514
17	1685		2550	2502	2412	2872	2942	2665	2671
18		1685	2700	2649	2554	3041	3115	2822	2829
19	1872		2850	2796	2696	3210	3288	2979	2986
20		1972	3000	2943	2838	3379	3461	3136	3143
21	2059		3150	3091	2980	3548	3634	3293	3300
22		2059	3300	3238	3122	3717	3807	3449	3457
23	2247		3450	3385	3264	3886	3981	3606	3614
24		2247	3600	3532	3406	4055	4154	3763	3771
25	2434		3750	3679	3548	4224	4327	3920	3928
26		2434	3900	3826	3690	4392	4500	4077	4086 R+
27	2621		4050	3974	3832	4561	4673	4233	4243
28		2621	4200	4121	3974	4730	4846	4390	4400
29	2808		4350	4268	4115	4899	5019	4547	4557 L+
30		2808	4500	4415	4257	5068	5132	4704	4714
31	2995		4650	4562	4399	5237	5365	4860	4871
32		2995	4800	4709	4541	5406	5538	5017	5028
33	3183		4950	4857	4683	5575	5711	5174	5186
34		3183	5100	5004	4825	5744	5894	5331	5343
35	3370		5250	5151	4967	5913	6057	5488	5500

Fig. 4–4. Computer printout showing daily cumulative tumor (midline) dose from anterior and post mantle fields, at selected points of interest. As soon as an area has received a prescribed dose, it is shielded during subsequent treatments.

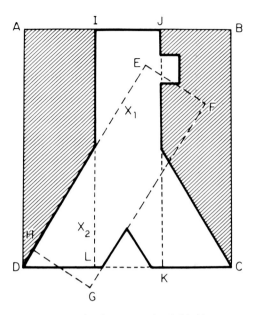

Fig. 4–5. Example of an inverted Y field. The approximate equivalent fields at points 1 and 2 are IJKL and EFGH, respectively.

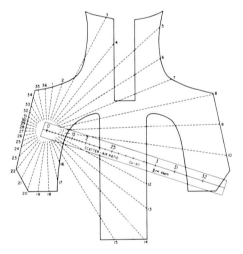

Fig. 4–6. Diagram illustrating Clarkson technique of obtaining averge scatter–air ratio from equal sectors centering on a point of dose calculation. (From Cundiff et al.: Dosimetry Workshop. Hodgkin's Disease, Chicago, 1970.)

cussed in detail in the literature.[1,7,11,13,19,20] Clarkson's method was elaborated by Johns and Cunningham.[13] Its manual use for mantle field calculations has been described by Cundiff et al.[7]

The method is rather tedious for manual

calculations and unless a computer is programmed to perform the method, it is not practical for routine patient calculations. A brief description of the computer method will be given here to illustrate the principle. As seen in Figure 4–6, the computer divides the field into elementary sectors using the coordinates of the field contour and the point-of-dose calculation. The radii of the sectors are calculated mathematically. The scatter–air ratio (SAR) values for the sectors are assigned by interpolation of the SAR(r,d) table for circular fields stored in the computer. Here r is radius and d is depth. The values are summated to give average scatter-air ratio ($\overline{SAR}(r,d)$) for the field at the given point at depth.

The computed $\overline{SAR}(r,d)$ is converted to average tissue-air ratio ($\overline{TAR}(r,d)$) by equation

$$\overline{TAR}(r,d) = TAR(0,d) + \overline{SAR}(r,d) \quad (2)$$

where TAR (0,d) is the TAR for 0×0 field (i.e.,

$$TAR(0,d) = e^{-\mu(d' - d_m)},$$

where μ is the linear attenuation coefficient, d' is the depth of point Q of calculation along the line joining Q with the source, and d_m is the depth of maximum electronic buildup).

The %DD at Q may be referred relative to the maximum dose (D_{max}) on the central axis at depth d_m. Let f_1 be the nominal SSD.

$$\%DD = 100 \times \{K \times TAR(0,d) + \overline{SAR}(r,d) \}$$

$$\times \left(\frac{F_1 + d_m}{F_1 + g + d} \right)^2 /BSF_o \quad (3)$$

where K, d and g are defined earlier in Equation 1. BSF_o is the backscatter factor that is defined as $\overline{TAR}(r,d_m)$ on central axis. It is, therefore, necessary that the first point of computation be the central axis at which the BSF_o is calculated and used in Equation 3. If the central axis passes through a shielded area, another point in the open portion, where output or dose rate in "free space" is known, may be chosen for the computation of BSF_o. Percent depth doses at other points will then be referred to the D_{max} at this point.

Extension to the Tissue–Maximum Ratio Concept

The TAR and SAR functions have been successfully used for ^{60}Co gamma rays. For higher energies, the tissue–maximum ratio (TMR) concept was introduced by Holt et al.[11] Application of TMR and SMR is similar to TAR and SAR except that the term BSF is no longer used and instead phantom-scatter-correction-factor S_p at depth d_m is used.[20]

Measurement of Dosimetric Parameters

Scatter–Air Ratio or Scatter–Maximum Ratio Table

A table of SARs or SMRs is required for Clarkson-type calculations. For ^{60}Co these data are available in reference 13. Accurately measured data has to be available for other energies. In addition, a table of TARs or TMRs for 0×0 field is necessary for primary-dose values in the Clarkson formulation.

Primary Beam Profile

The parameter K in equation 2 is a measure of primary-dose variation within the field in a plane perpendicular to the central axis. It is an off-axis ratio of dose rate in free space and can be readily measured in air with an ion chamber with a build-up cap. The data may be obtained for a typical unblocked field and normalized with respect to field width as shown in Figure 4–2. The data presented in this form are insensitive to variations in the overall field dimensions.

Field Contour

The outline of the irregular field may be obtained from the port film with shielded areas marked by actual blocks or lead markers. Field contour points are selected so that if they are joined by straight lines, the generated contour closely approximates the actual contour. The coordinates (x,y) of these points are introduced into the computer. The format in which these coordinates are entered depends on the specific computer program.

Points of Interest. The points of calculation are selected depending upon the region of dosimetric interest. For consistency, these points may be standardized by anatomic landmarks (Fig. 4–7). The coordinates (x,y) of these points are introduced into the computer as discussed above.

Source-to-Film Distance. The field contour taken from the port film is to be reduced because of magnification. The computer program appropriately reduces the length of the computer sector radii at any depth by using the film-magnification factor.

Change in SSD. The change in nominal SSD within the field (represented by g in equations 1 and 3) is to be measured on the patients for each point of dose calculation. Special devices have been developed to make such measurements on a routine basis.

Thickness. Body thickness is one of the most important parameters that influences dose distribution in parallel-opposed fields. This should be accurately measured at the established points of interest. Calipers that accurately measure body thickness must be used. Half thickness at a given point is used for the computation of midline depth dose.

It is convenient to design a data form to record dosimetric parameters for both computer and manual methods of calculation (Fig. 4–7).

Output Calibrations. In calculating

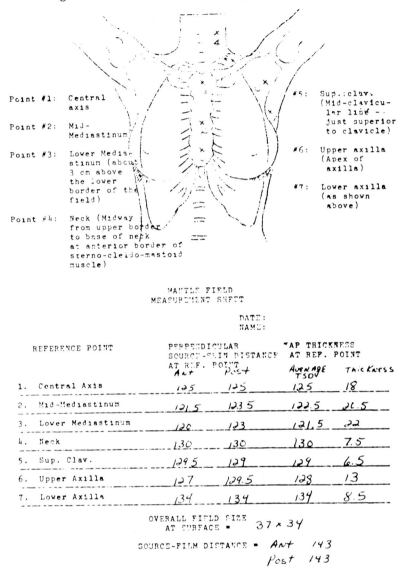

Point #1:   Central
            axis

Point #2:   Mid-
            Mediastinum

Point #3:   Lower Media-
            stinum (about
            3 cm above
            the lower
            border of the
            field)

Point #4:   Neck (Midway
            from upper border
            to base of neck
            at anterior border of
            sterno-cleido-mastoid
            muscle)

#5:   Sup.:clav.
      (Mid-clavicu-
      lar line -
      just superior
      to clavicle)

#6:   Upper axilla
      (Apex of
      axilla)

#7:   Lower axilla
      (as shown
      above)

MANTLE FIELD
MEASUREMENT SHEET

DATE:
NAME:

REFERENCE POINT	PERPENDICULAR SOURCE-SKIN DISTANCE AT REF. POINT		AP THICKNESS AT REF. POINT	
	Ant	Post	Average TSov	Thickness
1. Central Axis	125	125	125	18
2. Mid-Mediastinum	121.5	123.5	122.5	21.5
3. Lower Mediastinum	120	123	121.5	22
4. Neck	130	130	130	7.5
5. Sup. Clav.	129.5	129	129	6.5
6. Upper Axilla	127	129.5	128	13
7. Lower Axilla	134	134	134	8.5

OVERALL FIELD SIZE AT SURFACE = 37 × 34

SOURCE-FILM DISTANCE = Ant 143
                       Post 143

Fig. 4–7. Patient data form for recording dosimetric parameters. For consistency, the points of interest are standardized by anatomic land marks.

treatment time, the dose rate in free space or the field-size-dependence factor in air at the dose reference point should correspond to the overall, or unblocked field. The presence of secondary blocking alters the exposure rate only slightly (usually less than 1%) except at a point close to the edge of the block shadow where the exposure rate may increase or decrease because of scattering from the blocks or attenuation of collimator scatter reaching that point.

This has been discussed in the literature.[7,14,17]

Negative-Field Method

The concept of negative field has been described in the literature[14,15,25] for partially blocked fields. In this method, the dose at any point at a given depth is equal to the dose from the overall field minus the dose expected if the entire field were blocked, leaving the shielded volume

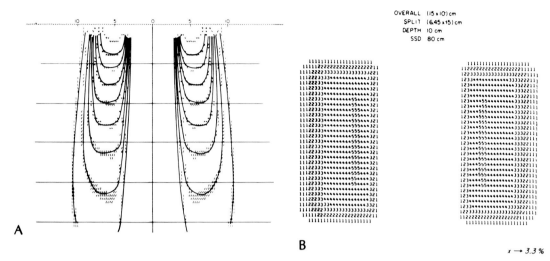

Fig. 4–8. Isodose printout of a split field: *A)* distribution in the principal plane containing beam axis; *B)* cross sectional distribution at depth.[15]

open. In other words, the blocked portion of the field with the associated primary and scattered dose is a negative field and its contribution is subtracted from the overall-field dose distribution. Usual computer techniques may be used to determine dose at a point (x,y,z) for the rectangular fields—overall and negative.

The negative-field method is a fast method of obtaining isodose curves in a partially blocked field. Its main limitation is that both the overall and the blocked fields have to be approximated to a rectangle. If the method is extended to more complex shaped blocks, it loses its simplicity and its main advantage, speed. It is recommended for isodose distribution in split fields, spinal shields, and other cases where blocks can be approximated to be rectangular in shape. Figure 4–8 shows dose distribution in a split field determined by negative-field method.

Computer Programs

Computer programs have been written[8,15,17] for the irregular field dosimetry. Most minicomputers used for radiotherapy treatment planning have programs based on Clarkson's principle and Cun-

ningham's computer algorithm.[8] Fortran listings of programs that I have written are described in references 8 and 22 and are available upon request. One of these programs, based on Clarkson's technique, has been adopted to the Artronix PC-12 treatment-planning computer.

REFERENCES

1. American Association of Physicists in Medicine: Dosimetry Workshop, Hodgkin's Disease. Chicago, American Association of Physicists in Medicine, 1970.
2. Anderson, R.E., D'Angio, G.J., and Khan, F.M.: Dosimetry of irregularly shaped radiation therapy fields. Part I. Radiology 92:1092, 1969.
3. Anderson, R.E., D'Angio, G.J., and Khan, F.M.: Dosimetry of irregularly shaped radiation therapy fields. Part II. Radiology 92:1094, 1969.
4. Beck, G.G., McGonnagle, W.G., and Sullivan, C.A.: Use of a styrofoam block to make tissue-equivalent compensators. Radiology 100:694, 1971.
5. Boge, J.R., Edland, R.W., and Matthes, D.C.: Tissue compensators for megavoltage radiotherapy fabricated from hollowed styrofoam filled with wax. Radiology 111:193, 1974.
6. Clarkson, J.R.: A note on depth doses in fields of irregular shape. Brit. J. Radiology 14:265, 1941.
7. Cundiff, J.H., Cunningham, J.R., Golden, R. et al.: The calculation of dose in the radiation treatment of Hodgkin's disease. In Dosimetry Workshop, Hodgkin's Disease. Chicago, American Association of Physicists in Medicine, 1970.
8. Cunningham, J.R., Shrivastava, P.N., Wilkinson,

J.M.: Computer calculation of dose within an irregularly shaped beam. *In* Dosimetry Workshop, Hodgkin's Disease. Chicago, American Association of Physicists in Medicine, 1970.

9. Faw, F.L., Johnson, R.E., Warren, C.A. et al.: A standard set of individualized compensating filters for mantle field radiotherapy of Hodgkin's disease. Amer. J. Roentgenol. *111*:376, 1971.
10. Hendee, W.R.: Medical Radiation Physics. Chicago, Year Book Medical Publishers, 1970, p. 236.
11. Holt, J.G., Laughlin, J.S., Moroney, J.P.; The extension of the concept of tissue–air ratios (TAR) to high energy x-ray beams. Radiology *96*:437, 1970.
12. Hospital Physicists' Association: Depth dose tables for use in radiotherapy. Brit. J. Radiol. Suppl. 11, 1978.
13. John, H.E., and Cunningham, J.R.: The Physics of Radiology, 3rd ed. Springfield, Illinois, Charles C Thomas, 1969.
14. Khan, F.M.: Dose Distribution Problems in Cobalt Teletherapy. Ph.D. Thesis, University of Minnesota, 1969.
15. Khan, F.M.: Computer dosimetry of partially blocked fields in cobalt teletherapy. Radiology *97*:405, 1970.
16. Khan, F.M., Levitt, S.H., Moore, V.C., and Jones, T.K.: Dosimetric considerations in "sanctuary" radiotherapy of acute lymphoblastic leukemia in children. Radiology *105*:665, 1972.
17. Khan, F.M., Levitt, S.H., Moore, V.C., and Jones, T.K.: Computer and approximation methods of calculating depth dose in irregularly shaped fields. Radiology *106*:433, 1973.
18. Khan, F.M., Moore, V.C., Burns, D.J.: The construction of compensators for cobalt teletherapy. Radiology *96*:187, 1970.
19. Khan, F.M., Moore, V.C., Sato, S.: Depth dose and scatter analysis of 10 MV x-rays. Radiology *102*:165, 1972.
20. Khan, F.M., Sewchand, W., Lee, J., and Williamson, J.F.: Revision of tissue-maximum ratio and scatter-maximum ratio concepts for cobalt 60 and higher energy x-ray beams. Med. Phys. 7(3):230, 1980.
21. Meurk, M.L., Green, J.P., Nussbaum, H. et al.: Phantom dosimetry study of shaped cobalt-60 fields in the treatment of Hodgkin's disease. Radiology *91*:554, 1968.
22. Page, V., Gardner, A., Karzmark, C.J.: Physical and dosimetric aspects of the radiotherapy of malignant lymphomas. I. The mantle technique. II. The inverted Y technique. Radiology *96*:609, 1970.
23. Sampiere, V., Almond, P.R., Shalek, R.J.: Radiation measurements and dosimetric practices. *In* Textbook of Radiotherapy, 2nd ed. Edited by G.H. Fletcher. Philadelphia, Lea & Febiger, 1973, p. 7.
24. Sterling, T.D., Perry, H., Katz, L.: Derivation of mathematical expression for the percent depth dose surface of cobalt 60 beams and visualization of multiple field dose distributions. Brit. J. Radiol. *37*:544, 1964.
25. Sundbom, L.: Method of dose planning on application of shielding filters in cobalt 60 teletherapy. Acta Radiol. (Ther.) 3:210, 1965.
26. Svahn-Tapper, G.: Dosimetric studies of mantle fields in cobalt 60 therapy of malignant lymphomas. Acta Radiol. (Ther.) 9:190, 1970.

Chapter 5

INTERSTITIAL IRRADIATION TECHNIQUES

Luis Delclos

Interstitial irradiation, the implantation of radioactive sources within and around a tumor, has the unique advantage of continuously delivering a high dose within a short time to a well-circumscribed area without excessive irradiation to the surrounding structures. In the last decade there has been a renaissance of this modality of radiation treatment due to the perfection of afterloading techniques and the availability of new radioactive materials.

The main advantages of afterloading are the increased flexibility of implant design and the reduction of radiation exposure levels, resulting in more accurate placement of needles and guides. The reduction of radiation exposure has been somewhat overemphasized. Although it is true for moderate and large implants, it does not necessarily apply to small implants. In small implants of the oral cavity, for example, it has been shown that the exposure sustained by an experienced interstitial radiation therapist is the same whether he is applying radium needles or afterloaded iridium guides.[24] A small permanent stock of selected radium or cesium needles for implantation of small lesions of the oral cavity may be very useful.

RADIOACTIVE MATERIAL SELECTION

To meet all clinical situations, a variety of gamma-ray sources must be available.

Table 5–1 shows the main isotopes, including radium, currently used as interstitial irradiators. The permanent stock of radium needles available at The University of Texas at M.D. Anderson Hospital and Tumor Institute at Houston is listed in Table 5–2. Radium needles are used, either alone or in combination with external beams, to treat lesions of the tongue and the floor of the mouth. Large tumors of these areas are implanted with iridium wires.

Gold grains are selected for permanent implants in less accessible areas that necessitate the use of narrow instruments (e.g., a suspension laryngoscope) and for tumors that require surgical exposure at laparotomy or thoracotomy. Gold grains are also useful for tumors that occur in the thin mucosa that covers the bone, as in the retromolar trigone and the oropharyngeal area.

Afterloaded iridium wires are used in all other sites. The wires are thin and can be cut to the desired length. Although iridium has a relatively short half-life, this is not a problem because of the short time needed for interstitial applications. It is necessary to calibrate the wires often, which involves a fairly elaborate bookkeeping system.

Figure 5–1 shows the physical characteristics of the three radioactive materials used for interstitial irradiation at M.D. Anderson Hospital.

TABLE 5–1. Radium and Its Substitutes

	Half-Life	Energy of Gamma Ray (MeV)	Γ Factor (R/hr/mc at 1 cm)	Half-Value Layer (cm Pb)
Cesium-137	30 y	0.662	3.26	0.65
Cobalt-60	5.26 y	1.17, 1.33	13.0	1.2
Gold-198	2.7 d	0.412	2.32	0.33
Iodine-125	60.2 d	0.027–0.035	1.23	0.003
Iridium-192	74.2 d	0.136–1.07	5.0	0.3
Radium-226	1600 y	0.047–2.45	8.25	1.3
Radon-222	3.823 d	0.047–2.45	8.35	1.3
Tantalum-182	115.1 d	0.03–1.3	6.13	1.2

(From Delclos, L.: *In* Topical Reviews in Radiotherapy and Oncology-2. Edited by T.J. Deeley. London, John Wright & Sons, 1982.)

TABLE 5–2. Radium Needles Stock

THE UNIVERSITY OF TEXAS
M.D. ANDERSON HOSPITAL AND TUMOR INSTITUTE

No. in Stock	Milligrams	Milligrams (Corrected to 0.5 mm Pt filter)	Linear Activity (mg/cm)	Active Length (mm)	Total Length (mm)	Actual Wall Thickness (mm)
15	3.00	2.91	0.66	45	58	0.65
10	2.66	2.58	0.66	40	50	0.65
12	2.33	2.28	0.66	35	45	0.60
16	2.00	1.96	0.66	30	42	0.60
10	1.33	1.33	0.66	20	32	0.50
9	1.00	1.00	0.66	15	25	0.50
48	1.50	1.45	0.33	45	58	0.65
12	1.33	1.29	0.33	40	50	0.65
12	1.16	1.14	0.33	35	45	0.60
41	1.00	0.98	0.33	30	42	0.60
20	0.66	0.66	0.33	20	32	0.50
10	0.50	0.50	0.33	15	25	0.50
12	0.75	0.75	0.165	45	59	0.50
12	0.58	0.58	0.165	35	48	0.50
41	2.00	1.94	Dumbbell	45	58	0.65
37	1.50	1.47	Dumbbell	30	42	0.60
18	1.75	1.70	Indian Club	45	58	0.65
12	1.66	1.61	Indian Club	40	50	0.65
12	1.50	1.47	Indian Club	35	45	0.60
20	1.25	1.22	Indian Club	30	42	0.60
12	2.25	2.18	0.50	45	58	0.65
12	2.00	1.94	0.50	40	50	0.65
12	1.75	1.71	0.50	35	45	0.60
10	1.125	1.09	0.25	45	58	0.65
12	1.00	0.97	0.25	40	50	0.65
12	0.875	0.86	0.25	35	45	0.60

(From Delclos, L.: *In* Topical Reviews in Radiotherapy and Oncology-2. Edited by T.J. Deeley. London, John Wright & Sons, 1982.)

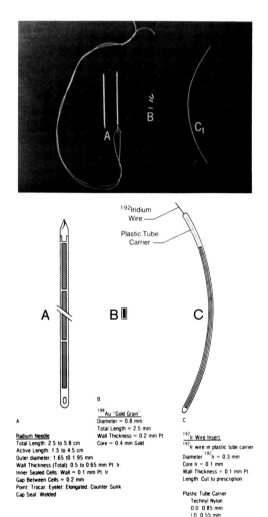

Fig. 5–1. Radioactive materials used for interstitial irradiation at M.D. Anderson Hospital and Tumor Institute. ^{192}Ir wires (C1) and gold grains (B) are compared with a 4.5 cm active length (5.8 cm total length) radium needle. (A) The iridium wire is thinner than the radium needles, is flexible, and can be tailored to any length; its cross section is excellent (750 Barns), and the half-life is acceptable for treatment times between 2 and 8 days. It is the most practical isotope for afterloading removable implants. For safe and easier manipulation, the iridium wire is mounted inside a nylon or Teflon tube carrier (C). The ^{198}Au seeds are small and, therefore, can be inserted in thin mucosa overlying bone and narrow spaces. Although they are used for permanent implants, the short half-life of the gold allows it to deliver most of the dose in the first 5 to 10 days. (Modified from Delclos, L.: Front. Radiat. Ther. Oncol. *12*:42, 1978.)

RADIUM NEEDLES

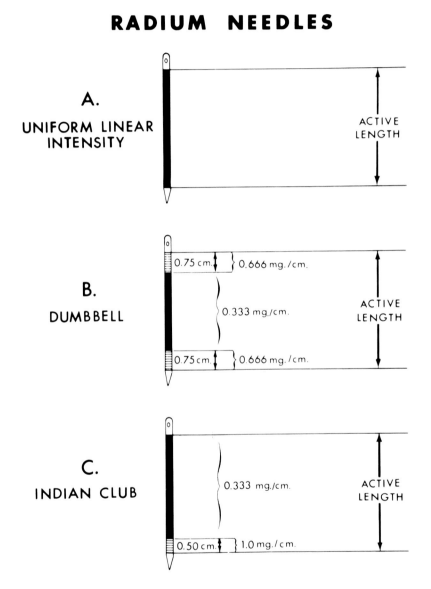

Fig. 5–2. Linear intensity of radium needles. (From Fletcher: *In* Textbook of Radiotherapy, 3rd ed. Edited by G.H. Fletcher. Philadelphia, Lea & Febiger, 1980.)

MATERIALS AND METHODS

Radium Needles

In Figure 5–2 the physical characteristics of a uniform-intensity needle are compared with those of an Indian Club needle and a Dumbbell needle. As longer iridium wires have become available, the necessity for crossing one or both ends has almost disappeared and Dumbbell and Indian Club needles are seldom used. Needles of 0.66 mg and 0.5 mg/cm linear intensity are used for single-plane arrangements and needles of 0.33 mg and 0.25 mg/cm linear intensity are used for multiple-plane or volume implants. The two intensities are combined for complex implants.

I consider the Paterson-Parker system[17] of geometric patterns, rules of distribution, and methods of calculation the basic system from which adaptations and exceptions are made for the individual patient. Since 1961, however, calculations have been done by computer as well as manually. Deviations from the Paterson-Parker method, described in detail in other publications,[4,10] are often used because cancer frequently does not follow geometric patterns. Tumors of the posterolateral border of the tongue or glossopalatine sulcus that extend into the anterior pillar or base of the tongue require the combination of several lengths and strengths of needles in order to cover the tumor with the desired isodose distribution. Figure 5–3 shows a variety of needle-length combinations and patterns for tumors in these areas.

Anesthesia

Although small implants can sometimes be done under local anesthesia, general anesthesia is almost always preferable. Good visualization of the tumor and relaxation of the patient are more possible with general anesthesia. It is frequently impossible to determine the full extent of the tumor in the conscious patient. The patient in the supine position, the position preferred by the anesthesiologist, does not offer the best visualization of the posterior oral cavity and oropharynx. Visualization and application of the radioactive sources are improved when the implant is performed with the patient in Fowler's position or, even better, in the sitting position.

General anesthesia is administered by nasotracheal intubation for implants of the oral cavity and lips. A tracheostomy is done for very extensive lesions requiring large implants and for all tumors requiring implantation of the glossopalatine sulcus, base of the tongue, or vallecula, because the associated edema may cause serious breathing difficulties.

Needle Identification, Suturing, and Removal

Color-coded silk threads are used to identify radium needles of different lengths and strengths. This facilitates both the selection of needles at the time of the implant and the orderly removal of the implant.

The needles must be sutured to the implanted tissues. The various ways to secure the needles to the implanted tissues are shown in Figure 5–4. I prefer to use separate 00 silk or cotton sutures (Fig. 5–5) permanently attached to a ½-circle taper-point needle that is threaded through the loop of the color-coded silk before insertion (see Fig. 5–6B). The scrub nurse hands the already-threaded needle to the operating radiation therapist. To avoid losing the suture during manipulations, the two loose ends of the suture are held together with a small amount of bone-wax.

Needles should be sutured in a systematic way. As shown in Figure 5–6, for a double-plane implant all suturing is done outside the implant. This method simplifies the removal of the needles. Before cutting the needle suture, the head of the needle should be securely held (see Fig. 5–6A) with a radium-needle holder and both the color-coded silk thread and the

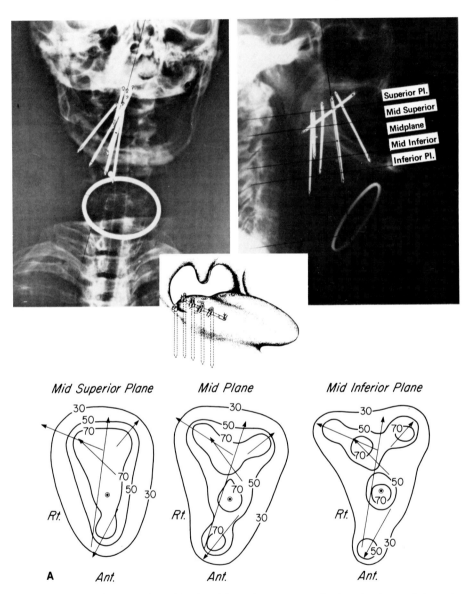

Fig. 5–3. Tumors of the posterolateral border of the oral tongue extending into the glossopalatine sulcus and anterior pillar, or toward the base of the tongue, require additional needles in the areas of extension. This can be achieved efficiently with radium needles of different strengths and lengths.

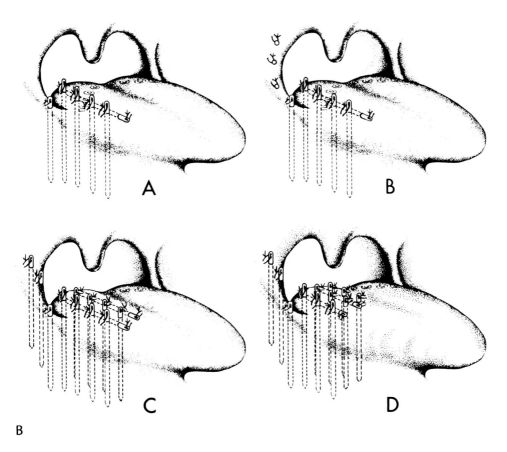

B

Fig. 5–3. *Continued* The implant shown in *A* is of type A or B where one needle was inserted in the glossopalatine sulcus to cover the tumor adequately. The isodoses show good coverage of the glosso-palatine area. This individualized "minitraumatic" implant cannot be done easily with afterloadable modalities. (From Delclos, L.: Front. Radiat. Ther. Oncol. *12*:42, 1978.)

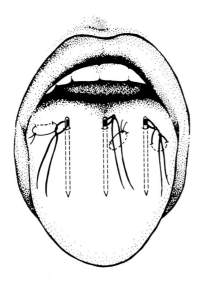

Fig. 5–4. Three ways of stitching radium needles. (From Fletcher, G.H., and MacComb, W.S.: Radiation Therapy in the Management of Cancers of the Oral Cavity and Oropharynx. Springfield, Illinois, Charles C Thomas, 1962.)

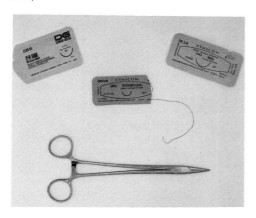

Fig. 5–5. Samples of 00 sutures attached to half-circle needles, frequently used for suturing radium needles and afterloadable stainless steel guides. A long-handled needle holder is recommended when suturing radium needles. (From Delclos, L.: *In* Genitourinary Tumors: Fundamental Principles and Surgical Techniques. Edited by D.E. Johnson and M.A. Boileau. New York, Grune & Stratton, 1982.)

suture should be identified. In spite of the appearance of the threads when the implant has been in place for 3 to 7 days, the difference in the color and thickness of the threads and sutures makes possible an orderly removal of needles.

Small implants of the anterior oral cav-

ity can generally be removed in an adjacent treatment room, but not in the patient's room. It is preferable, and often essential, for implants in the posterior area and for less-than-cooperative patients, to remove the implant in the operating room under good anesthesia where adequate lighting, suction, and one or two assistants are available. Bleeding at the time of needle removal is uncommon but, when it occurs, can be quite dramatic. It may create panic in the patient and in the assisting staff. To accidentally cut the needle thread instead of the suture is not uncommon. Trying to find the uncontrolled needle requires an optimal surgical environment because the task is complex and time-consuming. Radiographic localization of the needle may be required before the needle base can be surgically exposed (Fig. 5–7).

IMPLANT SITES

Posterolateral Tongue Border

Implantation of the posterolateral border of the tongue requires pulling the tongue forward in order to start the implant at the base of the tongue (Fig. 5–8). The first needle is inserted pointing posteroinferiorly (Fig. 5–9A) at about 45 degrees; a lesser angle is used for successive needles (Fig. 5–9B,C). At the end of the implant, when the tongue returns to its normal position, the implant becomes vertical.

Undersurface of Tongue and Floor of Mouth

These lesions are implanted through the tongue. The anterolateral needles emerge from the undersurface of the tongue and are reinserted into the floor of the mouth (Fig. 5–10). The sequence of needle implantation for lesions involving the undersurface of the tongue and the posteroanterior floor of the mouth is shown and described in detail in Figure 5–11.

Most lesions of the oral cavity in patients at M.D. Anderson Hospital are first

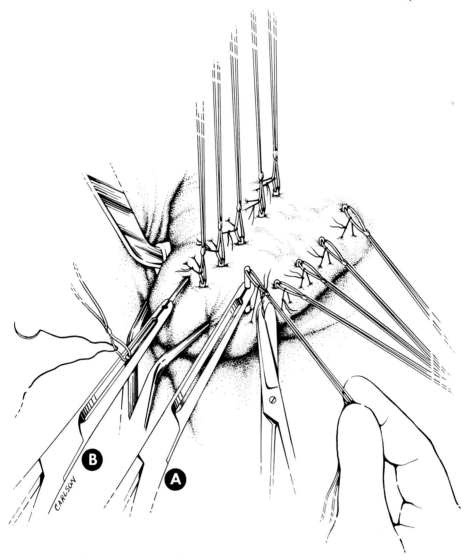

Fig. 5–6. Note the orderly position of the sutures outside the double-plane implant. This simplifies the removal of the needles.

treated with external irradiation. External radiation causes the lesion to flatten or the margins to become less distinct; the original tumor extent should therefore be identified with black, nonabsorbable sutures securely fastened to the tissue (Fig. 5–12). The implant should extend beyond the visible or palpable tumor by at least 1 cm (Fig. 5–13).

Protection of Surrounding Normal Tissues

Whenever possible, the anterolateral needles of an implant of the oral cavity are kept away from the thin mucous membrane that covers the bone in the upper and lower gum as well as away from the periosteum, teeth, and bone. To increase and maintain the distance, a regular fluoride carrier (Fig. 5–14) is thickened on the inside by one to four layers (one layer = 2 mm) to increase the distance so that the unavoidable hot spot around each needle is kept away from the adjacent normal structures (Fig. 5–15).

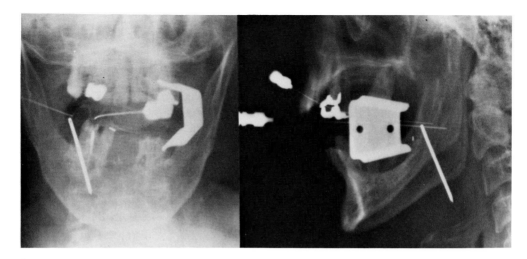

Fig. 5–7. The identification thread and suture of this radium needle were cut accidentally and the needle was buried in the tongue. The needle was localized with anteroposterior and lateral radiographs taken in the operating room. Two spinal needles of different diameters, to aid identification in the radiographs, were implanted in the tongue. The top of the radium needle was about 0.5 cm proximal to the tip of the thin spinal needle. An incision was made at this site and the radium needle was removed with a needle holder. The incision was sutured.

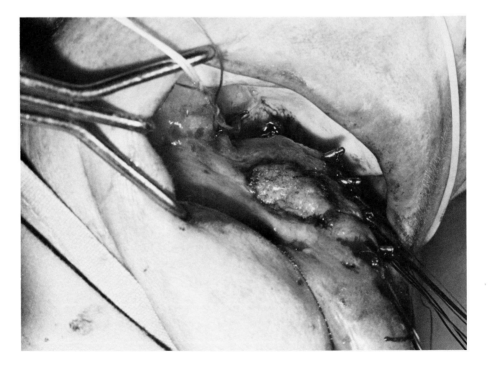

Fig. 5–8. Implanting the posterolateral border of the tongue requires pulling the tongue forward. The first needle is pointed posteroinferiorly; successive needles are inserted at a lesser angle. At completion of the implant, when the tongue is pushed back into normal position, the implant becomes almost vertical (see also Fig. 5–9). (From Delclos: Front. Radiat. Ther. Oncol. *12*:42, 1978.)

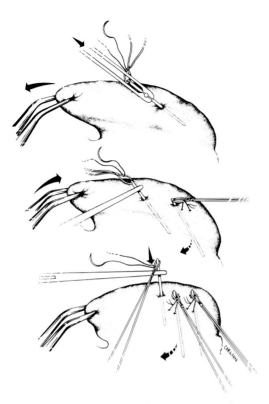

Fig. 5–9. Detail of recommended technique for implants of the posterolateral border of the tongue (see also Fig. 5–8).

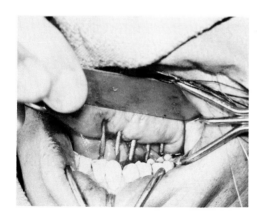

Fig. 5–10. Lesions of the undersurface of the tongue and floor of the mouth are implanted through the tongue. The anterolateral needles emerge from the undersurface of the tongue and are then inserted into the floor of the mouth.

Anchoring the Needles

All the needle identification threads are passed through a ⅓-inch or ½-inch Penrose tube, 8 cm to 10 cm in length, to minimize trauma to the buccal commissure (Fig. 5–16). The identification threads are sutured, not taped, to the skin of the cheek to discourage the patient from pulling them out during recovery from anesthesia or during sleep.

Feeding the Implanted Patient

Although some patients can be allowed to sip a liquid formula through a straw, the majority of patients are fed through a nasogastric tube (see Fig. 5–16). This is a necessity when the lips have been sutured together for implants involving the buccal commissure (Fig. 5–17).

Exposing and Outlining the Tumor

Interstitial irradiation is a surgical procedure requiring good field-exposure. Implants are done in the main operating room with anesthesia, scrub and circulating nurses, good lighting, and suction. At least one and sometimes two assistants are needed. When needles are being implanted in the oral-cavity area, one of the assistants retracts the lips (Fig 5–18) and the other pulls or depresses the tongue while the operating radiation therapist performs the implant.

The oral cavity can be kept dry with adequate preanesthesia medication, including Scopolamine, and suction. Although it is desirable to outline the tumor (Fig. 5–19) with gentian violet, Castellani's paint, or one of the available surgical markers (Fig. 5–20), this is not always possible. A metric ruler should always be available on the implanting tray.

Instrument Trays

Figure 5–21 shows the instruments employed for most implants of the oral cavity. Laryngopharyngeal implants require, in addition, a suspension laryngoscope. The

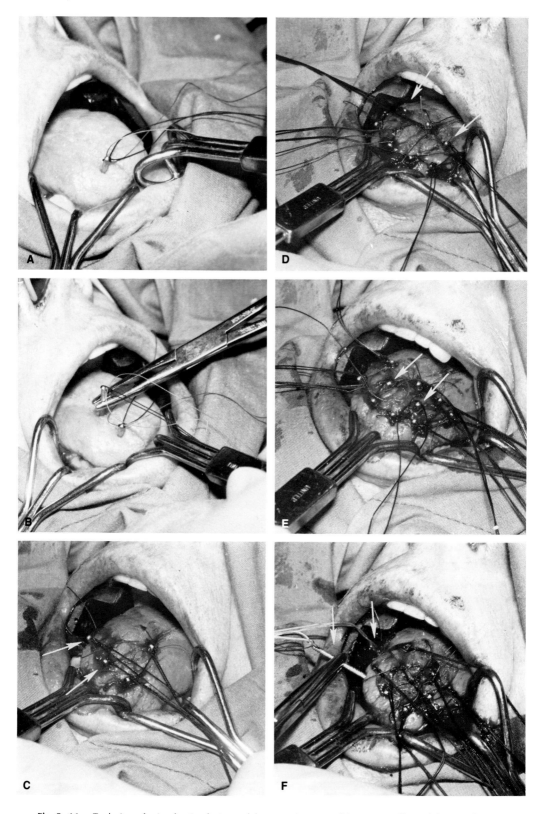

Fig. 5–11. Technique for implanting lesions of the posterior area of the anterior floor of the mouth, not fixed to the periosteum, and also for lesions of the undersurface of the tongue: A central anterior needle (A) is inserted first. To determine the angle of the implant, the first needle is inserted in front of the tumor, parallel to but away from the inner table of the jaw. A second needle (B) is placed posterior to the tumor, parallel to the first (anterior) needle to cover the posterior extent of the tumor. The remaining anterior (C) and posterior needles (D) are then implanted. The central needles (E) and finally the crossing needles (F) are then inserted.

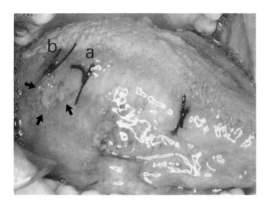

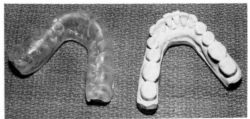

Fig. 5–12. Black silk sutures are placed anteriorly and posteriorly to outline the tumor edges. In this particular case, the patient developed an area of tumoritis after a few treatments with external irradiation. The tumoritis (arrows) was posterior to the posterior suture *(a)*. Biopsy was positive. A new suture *(b)* was placed further back. Underestimation of tumor extent, especially posteriorly, is not uncommon.

Fig. 5–14. A fluoride carrier can be used to keep the radioactive needles or wires away from the lower or upper jaw. To the carrier, 2 mm thick, add 1 to 4 more layers, making the carrier 4–8 mm thick. This further increases the distance between the needles and the normal tissues. (From Delclos, L.: *In* Topical Reviews in Radiotherapy and Oncology-2. Edited by T.J. Deeley. London, John Wright & Sons, 1982.)

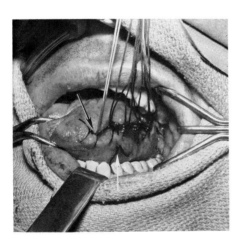

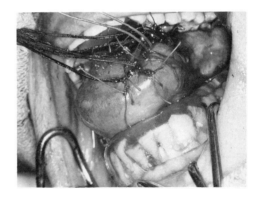

Fig. 5–13. The last needle (black arrow) for a single-plane implant of the left lateral border of the tongue is inserted at least 1 cm in front of the anterior outlining suture (white arrow).

Fig. 5–15. Thick fluoride carrier (3 thicknesses = 4 mm) in place. Note that the tongue is pushed away from the lower teeth and jaw. (From Delclos, L.: *In* Topical Reviews in Radiotherapy and Oncology-2. Edited by T.J. Deeley. London, John Wright & Sons, 1982.)

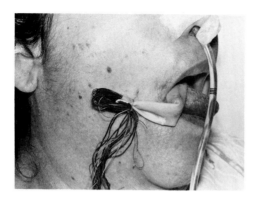

Fig. 5–16. The identification threads of the radium needles are placed inside a ⅔″ or ½″ Penrose tube and then sutured (not taped) to the skin. The patient is fed through a nasogastric tube.

same basic tray is employed for radium, iridium, or gold-grain implants. Figure 5–22 shows the instruments employed for most implants of the vagina. A simplified tray is used for implants of the anal area.

Figure 5–23 shows the instruments employed for radium-needle and iridium-wire removal. All instruments should be long-handled for the protection of the radiation therapist, and trainees should be initiated in their use. The index finger of the operator's opposite hand guides the needles or the wires during the implant procedures (Fig. 5–24).

AFTERLOADING METHODS FOR INTERSTITIAL GAMMA-RAY THERAPY

Afterloading modalities were employed as early as 1904 by Abbe.[1] The flexible carrier method was designed and first used with radon seeds by Hames in 1937,[11] and later by Morton et al.,[19] who used cobalt sources. Interstitial afterloading was systematized for practical application by Henschke et al.[14]

The use of iridium wires, and later iridium seeds in plastic tubing, was introduced by Henschke and initiated in 1959 at M. D. Anderson Hospital by Suit.[24] Because of difficulties encountered with stock and record keeping, only selected patients were treated with this technique. At M. D. Anderson Hospital in the last

decade there has been a gradual switch to the use of afterloading iridium for implanting procedures except for small and medium-size tumors of the tongue and floor of the mouth, for which intracavitary radium has been found to be as practical as afterloaded iridium. Trends in the use of iridium, radium, and gold grains for tumors in various sites were presented in a recent publication.[6]

Since the early 1960s, Pierquin[22] and Chassagne,[23] in France, have popularized Henschke techniques with personal modifications, and have contributed the use of "hairpins" for afterloading with thicker iridium wires (0.5-mm diameter), mainly for lesions of the oral cavity and oropharynx. In addition, there are several reports[2,3,12–15,18,20,21] in the literature describing techniques and instrumentation for the use of afterloading interstitial therapy modalities, using radium and other isotopes such as tantalum wires and ^{125}I seeds. Radium needles have been used in Teflon or nylon tubing and Medicut intravenous cannulae in an ingenious afterloadable manner. Iridium wires or seeds, mounted in plastic tubing, can be applied more flexibly, can be made any length, and therefore can be tailored to any individual clinical situation.

Methods of Afterloading

Delayed Afterloading With [192]Ir Wires or Ribbons (Removable Implants)

Removable implants are implants in which the radioactive sources are removed after they have delivered the selected dose. These implants are performed either with stainless steel needles or flexible Teflon or nylon guides.

Stainless Steel Needles (Figs. 5–25 and 5-26). Stainless steel tubing of gauge 16 (1.6 mm in outer diameter) is cut into the desired length. The distal end of the tubing is beveled at a 30° or 45° angle and is crimped, but not closed, to hold the afterloaded iridium insert in place, still allow-

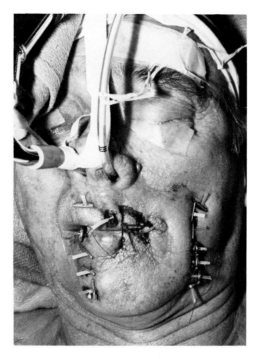

Fig. 5–17. To implant lesions of the buccal commissure, the lips are sutured together in order to obtain an acceptable geometrical implant pattern. A nasogastric tube is placed before the implant. Nasotracheal intubation is a requirement for all implants of the oral cavity. Massive implants of the oral cavity and lesions involving the base of the tongue, glossopalatine sulcus, and oropharyngeal areas require a tracheostomy.

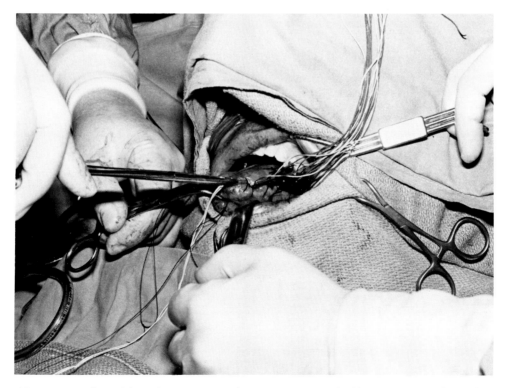

Fig. 5–18. Implants of the oral cavity require at least one assistant, preferably two, to expose adequately the areas to be implanted.

69

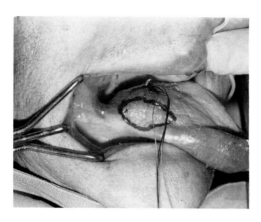

Fig. 5–19. The tumor should be outlined with gentian violet, Castellani's paint, or a surgical marker (see Fig. 5–20).

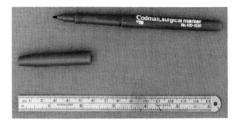

Fig. 5–20. Sample of surgical marker. A metric ruler should always be available.

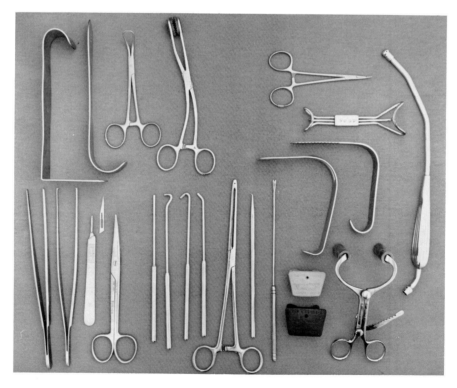

Fig. 5–21. Instrument tray for oral cavity *(from left to right):* Byford double-ended retractor (2); Flexsteel ribbon retractors (2); Large Towel forceps (1); Young tongue forceps (1); Mosquito forceps (12); Cheek retractors (2); Weder and Andrews tongue depressors (2 of each); Suction tubes—one large Yankaver type, one small Frazier type (not shown); Dressing and tissue forceps (1 each); #11 blades and handle; Straight and curved pointed scissors; Radium needle pushers (different angles); Radium needle holder; Radium needle extractor; Jacobsen "Y" suture pusher; McKesson mouth prop (child and several adult sizes); Mouth gag (Sluder-Jansen).

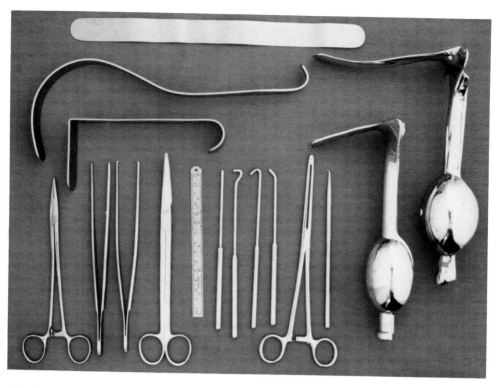

Fig. 5–22. Instrument tray for vaginal implant *(from left to right):* Flexsteel ribbon retractor 1″ and 2″ wide (2); Deaver retractors (2); Heaney (or Kristeller) retractors (2); Auvard weighted retractor 3″ to 4″ long (Crisp & Gosevek weighted retractor should also be available on demand); Long dressing forceps (8″); Long tissue forceps (8″); Long scissors (straight & curved, pointed); Ruler (in cm); Radium needle pushers (different angles); Radium needle inserting forceps (straight and 90° grooves); Radium needle-suture extractor. (From Delclos, L.: *In* Genitourinary Tumors: Fundamental Principles and Surgical Techniques. Edited by D.E. Johnson and M.A. Boileau. New York, Grune & Stratton, 1982.)

ing repositioning should a major vessel or the urinary bladder be entered. A nylon or Teflon ball is fitted snugly at the proximal end. To this Teflon ball, which is a further development by Paine[21] of the glass ball used by Hames,[11] is added a hole to thread the suture and a lead bit for x-ray localization. Figure 5–27 systematically shows the procedures followed for insertion and afterloading of the iridium guides. This type of rigid guide is used in tumors approachable from one side only (e.g., in tumors of the collumela and nasal septum, female urethra, and anal margin). This technique can also be used to treat involved nodes in the neck, the parotid gland, the scrotum, and for a boost to primary breast cancer.

Flexible Guides (Fig. 5–28). The use of Teflon or nylon tubes of gauge 16, preferably with one end closed and the other tapered, or both ends tapered, first requires the insertion of a stainless steel guide of the same diameter through the tumor. Figures 5–29 and 5–30 systematically show the procedure followed for the insertion, afterloading, and removal of the iridium and guides.[7] This type of technique is used when a tumor can be transfixed from either of two sides, (e.g., lower and upper lip, buccal mucosa, breast or neck masses).

Afterloading with both stainless steel needles and flexible guides can be done after the patient is back on the ward. Radiation exposure is thereby eliminated from the operating and recovery rooms.

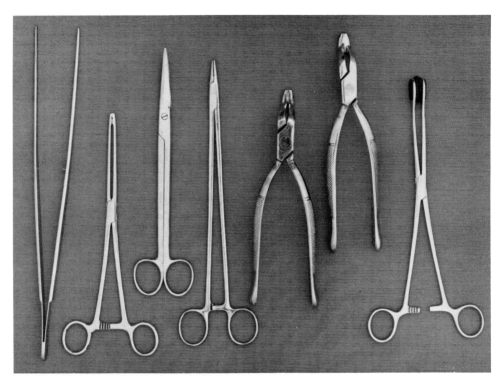

Fig. 5–23. Instrument tray for needle removal (*from left to right*—all instruments should be long-handled): 10–12″ handling forceps (2), needle-inserting forceps (1); long straight and curved pointed scissors (one of each 10–12″); long (Thoracic) needle holder (10–12″); custom-designed closing and opening forceps; applicator holding forceps with rubber jaws (1).

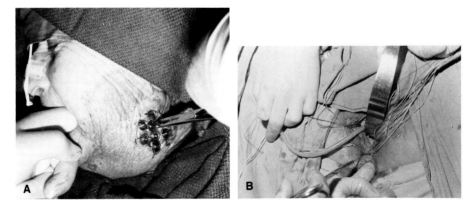

Fig. 5–24. The index finger of the opposite hand is vital to determine the length of the needles or stainless steel guides to be used in implants of the *(A)* oral cavity or *(B)* vagina, anal margin, and prostate.

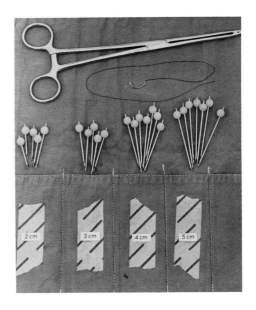

Fig. 5–25. Stainless-steel needles are manufactured to any desired length; a Teflon or nylon button with a hole for suturing and a lead pellet for radiographic identification is incorporated at the ball. The distal end is crimped to position the ^{192}Ir insert and to prevent it from dropping out. The needles are inserted with a standard needle-inserting forceps (Radium Chemical Company, 161 East 42nd Street, New York, New York 10017), and sutured into place with a 00 suture. The Teflon ball, which causes less trauma, substitutes for the metal flange used in earlier years. (From Delclos, L.: *In* Textbook of Radiotherapy, 3rd ed. Edited by G.H. Fletcher. Philadelphia, Lea & Febiger, 1980.)

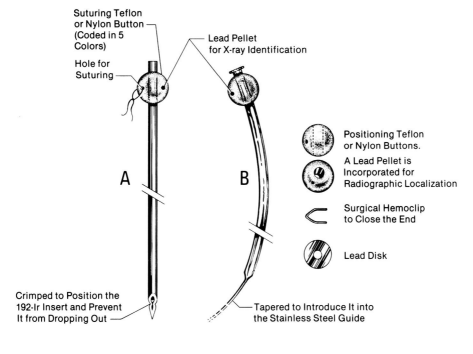

A	B
Stainless Steel needle	**Plastic Tube**
Total Length: Made to prescription	Plastic Tube: Nylon (or Teflon)
Outer Diameter = 1.6 mm (16 Gauge)	O.D. = 1.6 mm (16 Gauge)
Inside Diameter = 1.2 mm	I.D. = 1.2 mm
Point: Crimped to position ^{192}Ir insert	Nylon or Teflon Button at both ends
End: Suturing Nylon or Teflon Button	

Fig. 5–26. Diagram of: (A) stainless-steel afterloadable needle of the newer model with plastic Teflon or nylon buttons. The needles are made of any desired length. (B) Teflon or nylon tube, closed-end variety, used for the through-and-through technique. A stainless-steel guide of the same outside diameter is inserted first. (From Delclos, L.: *In* Genitourinary Tumors: Fundamental Principles and Surgical Techniques. Edited by D.E. Johnson and M.A. Boileau. New York, Grune & Stratton, 1982.)

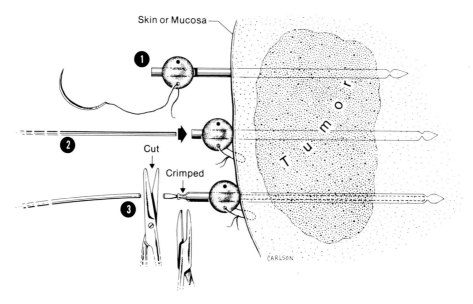

Fig. 5–27. One-End Technique. For Tumors Approached from One Side: *(1)* insertion of empty stainless-steel needle with nylon button. The needle is sutured to the skin or mucosa through a hole in the nylon button; *(2)* the iridium wire mounted in plastic tube carrier (we call it "insert") is introduced into the stainless-steel needle; *(3)* the open end is crimped to close it. The plastic tube carrier is cut, leaving about 0.5 cm protruding to facilitate removal of the iridium wire when indicated. To remove it we can either cut the suture and remove the needle with the iridium inside, then deposit it in the leaded carrier for transportation and further manipulation in the laboratory, or uncrimp the end of the stainless steel needle with a specially designed uncrimper and pull out the plastic tube carrier with the iridium insert inside. (From Delclos, L.: *In* Textbook of Radiotherapy, 3rd ed. Edited by G.H. Fletcher. Philadelphia, Lea & Febiger, 1980.)

Immediate Afterloading with Gold Grains (Permanent Implants)

This technique is used in treating adenocarcinoma of the prostate or recurrent pelvic tumors. Stainless steel needles are inserted into the prostate after the prostate has been exposed through a suprapubic approach (Fig. 5–31).[5] The index finger of the opposite hand is introduced through the anus to palpate the prostate. When the needles are inserted, the finger feels the tip of the guides before they enter the rectum and, therefore, eliminates the risk of a high dose to the rectum or fistulae formation. There is no exposure to the finger because the needles are empty. After the needles have been completely inserted, the finger is removed and the radioactive gold seeds are introduced by connecting the slim gold-grain implanter to each of the needles (Fig. 5–32).[8] A similar procedure is used to implant recurrent pelvic masses.

Slim Multiple Gold-Grain Implanter

The slim gold-grain implanter in adaptable lengths (Figs. 5–33 and 5–34) was designed to implant areas accessible only through long, narrow, examining instruments, such as a suspension laryngoscope (Fig. 5–35). The implanter is loaded with the same 14-grain magazine designed for and supplied with the Royal Marsden "guns."

SPECIAL PRECAUTIONS FOR LESIONS OF THE VAGINA, VULVA, AND ANAL CANAL

The indications for and techniques of interstitial therapy for carcinomas of the vagina, vulva, and anal canal have been described elsewhere.[9] These areas are vul-

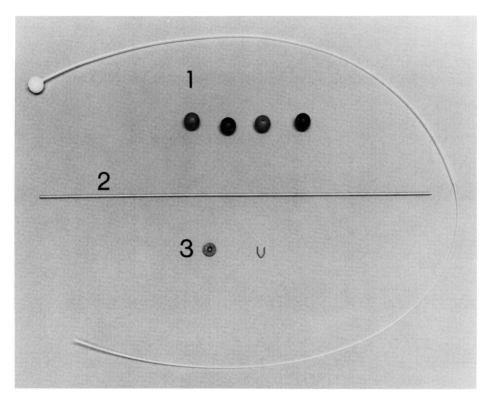

Fig. 5–28. Teflon tube *(1)* with one end closed and the other tapered to introduce it into the stainless-steel guides *(2)* necessary for this type of implant. A Teflon or nylon button is fitted snugly at the closed end. The buttons are available in 5 colors for identification at the time of the afterloading in multiple or volume implants. *(3)* Lead disc or hemoclips are used to close the other end of the nylon tube. (From Delclos, L.: *In* Textbook of Radiotherapy, 3rd ed. Edited by G.H. Fletcher. Philadelphia, Lea & Febiger, 1980.)

nerable to severe radiation complications because of the intolerance of the surrounding tissues to radiation and because they are closely exposed to the constant irritation of perspiration, urine, and feces; it is therefore important to minimize the irradiation to the surrounding normal areas. A 23% local necrosis rate in patients treated in Manchester and about the same percentage in those treated at the Foundation Curie have been reported.

The most important consideration is selecting a lesion suitable for treatment by an implant. Implants should be restricted to lesions of the anal canal requiring implantation of no more than half the circumference of the anal canal. The same rule should apply to lesions of the vagina.

The remaining normal tissues should be kept away from the implanted area. For lesions of the vagina, an empty dome cylinder is used (Fig. 5–36). Two rolls of gauze are placed between the labia (Fig. 5–37). Additional sponges are placed on top of and between the thighs, so that when the legs are brought down from the lithotomy position in which the implant is done, the inside surfaces of the thighs are separated as much as possible from the radioactive source.

The same placement of gauze and sponges applies to lesions of the anal canal. The anal canal is kept distended with a custom-designed rectal plug (Figs. 5–38 and 5–39). This reduces the dose to the opposite side of the canal to less than 15%

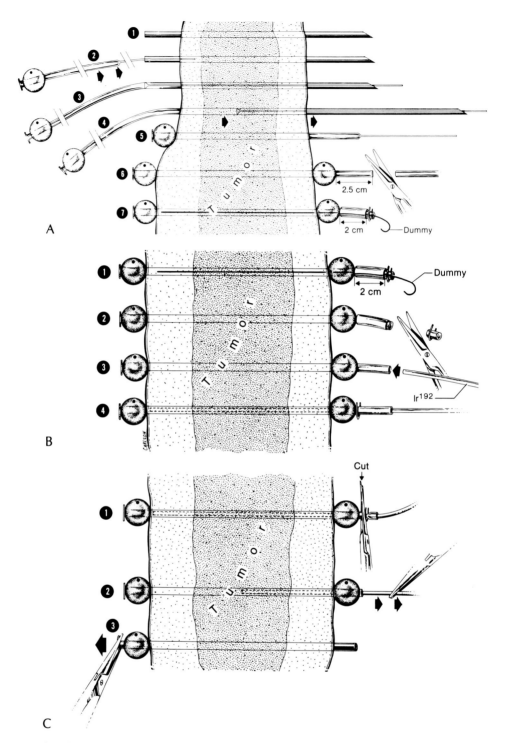

Fig. 5–29. Through-and-through technique for tumors approachable from two sides. *(A)* To insert: [1] insert the stainless-steel guide; [2] the leader (tapered end) of the nylon implant tube is introduced and [3] passed down the guide until the plastic tube is in contact with the end of the stainless-steel guide; [4] both the stainless-steel guide and the tapered end (leader) of the nylon implant tube are pulled through the other end; [5] when the stainless-steel guide is out, the nylon tube is pulled until the closed-end nylon implant tube with the nylon button is in contact with the surface; [6] another nylon button is inserted at the opposite end of the nylon implant tube—the nylon tube is cut at about 2.5 cm from the nylon button surface; [7] a larger nylon tube 2 cm in length is placed on top of the protruding end of the nylon tube. A dummy wire is placed inside, protruding 1 cm, for localization. A hemoclip is placed at the end to prevent the nylon tube from slipping out during manipulation.

(B) To load: [1] the dummy wire is removed; [2] the nylon end of the implant tube is cut with the hemoclip; [3] the ^{192}Ir wire in plastic tube carrier (insert) is inserted into the nylon implant tube; [4] a hemoclip is placed near the nylon button, to close the nylon tube.

(C) To remove: [1] The nylon implant tube is cut; [2] the inner ^{192}Ir wire in the plastic tube carrier (insert) is removed; [3] the outer plastic tube is pulled from the other side. (Modified from Delclos, L.: *In* Textbook of Radiotherapy, 3rd ed. Edited by G.H. Fletcher. Philadelphia, Lea & Febiger, 1980.)

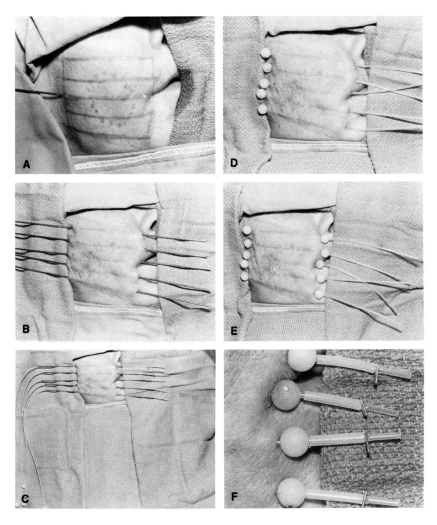

Fig. 5–30. *(A)* The first stainless-steel guide is inserted into the center of the tumor. Note that the tumor is outlined with dots and that the implant design is drawn on the skin. *(B)* All the stainless-steel guides are inserted above and below the central guide, about 1 cm apart for small implants and up to 1½ cm for larger implants. *(C)* The tapered end of the Teflon, or nylon, tubing is inserted into all the stainless-steel guides. Note the Teflon ball with lead insert at the closed end of the nylon tube. *(D)* The stainless-steel guides are pulled from the implanted area through the outer end together with the tubing until all the Teflon balls are in contact with the skin. *(E)* A second Teflon ball is placed at the other end. *(F)* The Teflon tube is cut at about 2½ cm from the second Teflon ball. A larger Teflon tube (2 cm in length) is placed on top of the protruding end of the Teflon tube. An 18–20 gauge stainless-steel wire is placed inside for x-ray localization. The wire is held in place temporarily with a medium size hemoclip. (From Delclos, L.: *In* Topical Reviews in Radiotherapy and Oncology-2. Edited by T.J. Deeley. London, John Wright & Sons, 1982.)

of the minimum tumor dose at the implanted area. In addition, Ivalon or gauze is placed in the intragluteal space (Fig. 5–40).

Although a colostomy may be avoided with diligent care of the implanted area, this is not always practical. It may be necessary to precede the implant with a tem-porary diverting colostomy, regardless of tumor size or lack of bowel constriction.

Open-Bladder Implants for Lesions of the Female Urethra

An open-bladder implant is necessary for lesions occupying the proximal portion or the entire length of the female ure-

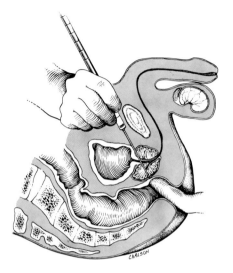

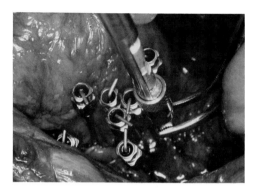

Fig. 5–31.   Implants of the prostate are done through a suprapubic exposure of the prostate. A finger is inserted into the rectum to prevent the needles from entering the rectum.[5] (From Chan, R.C. and Gutierrez, A.E.: Carcinoma of the prostate. Cancer *37*:2749, 1976.)

Fig. 5–32.   Implants of the prostate are generally done through trocars that are inserted first. After all trocars have been inserted into the tumor, the gold-grain implanter is connected to the trocars. A clamp is used to hold the trocar while connecting the Luer-Lok top, to prevent dislodgement of the trocar. The seeds are ejected at 1 cm intervals by withdrawing the implanter and the trocar together. Because both the body of the implanter and the trocar are calibrated, a point of reference can be found for depth-measuring purposes as the implanter is withdrawn either at the tumor surface or at the edge of an abdominal retractor.[8] (From Delclos, L. and Moore, E.B.: A slim [198]gold-grain implanter loaded with standard Royal Marsden 14-grain magazines. Cancer *43*:1023, 1979.)

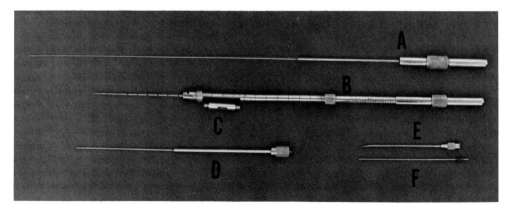

Fig. 5–33.   The slim [198]Au-grain implanter: *(A)* Long plunger to be used with extension needle *(D)*. *(B)* Unloaded implanter with regular plunger in place and standard needle for direct implants connected to the distal end of the body of the implanter by means of a holder threaded to the body. The holder has a Luer-Lok tip so that it can be attached to trocars. The body of the implanter, standard needle, and trocars are calibrated in centimeters. In the body there is a 14-grain scale. *(C)* Standard Royal Marsden 14-grain magazine. *(D)* Extension needle. *(E)* Trocar (standard) with Luer-Lok base. *(F)* Guide for use with trocars. (From Delclos, L. and Moore, E.B.: A slim [198]gold-grain implanter loaded with standard Royal Marsden 14-grain magazines. Cancer *43*:1022, 1979.)

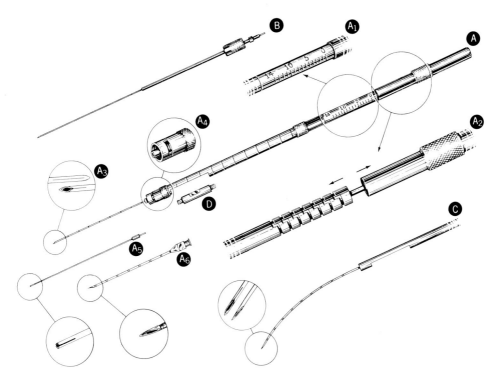

Fig. 5–34. *(A)* Assembled but unloaded gold-grain implanter: [A₁] 14-gold grain scale inscribed in the body; [A₂] the plunger is slightly pulled out to show the spiral staircase-like groove along which a pin inside of the plunger will advance the plunger every half a revolution (180°), pushing one seed at a time through the end of the needle, guide, or extension needle; [A₃] the tip of the needle is split and narrowed to prevent the seeds from falling off; [A₄] needle and guide holder with Luer-Lok tip adapter to connect guide to afterloadable trocars. [A₅] split and narrowed round-tipped guide; [A₆] trocar with Luer-Lok base for connection to Luer-Lok tip adapter. The body, standard needles, and trocars are calibrated in centimeters. *(B)* Extension needle for use along narrow examining instruments. *(C)* A gold-grain implanter is also available with a curved, calibrated needle for direct implantation. The tip is also split and narrowed. *(D)* A standard Royal Marsden 14-gold grain magazine. (From Delclos, L. and Moore, E.B.: A slim ¹⁹⁸gold-grain implanter loaded with standard Royal Marsden 14-grain magazines. Cancer *43*:1022, 1979.)

thra. This procedure also allows direct visualization of possible tumor extension into the bladder. If the tumor has extended, the implant procedure is stopped and external irradiation is used.

After the bladder has been opened through a suprapubic cystostomy (Fig. 5–41), the index and middle fingers are inserted with one on each side of the Foley catheter balloon. The radiotherapist inserts the needles into the urethra and the vesicovaginal septum with the other hand. The needles are guided with the fingers that are on either side of the Foley catheter balloon.

Tumors of the Rectovaginal Septum

When implanting needles or stainless-steel guides for tumors of the posterior vaginal wall, the rectal ampulla is kept distended with a 30-ml Foley catheter to minimize radiation to the opposite rectal wall (Fig. 5–42).

Protection in the Operating Room

There is no need for protection in the operating room for the majority of implants because afterloading is done when the patient returns to the ward. Radium- and cesium-needle implants, gold-grain implants, and immediate afterloading with gold grains and iridium wires require specific protective procedures.

An operating room work bench with shielding (Fig. 5–43) is placed in one corner of the room so that, during the final

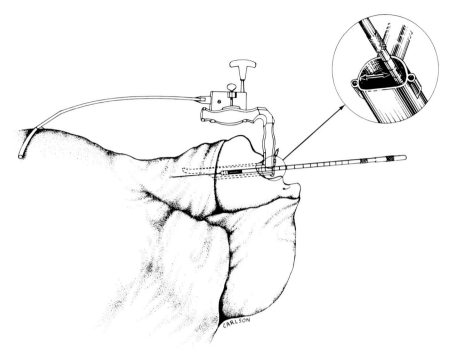

Fig. 5–35. Diagram of the slim gold-grain implanter as used along a suspension laryngoscope. The insert shows that with the gold-grain implanter within the suspension laryngoscope, there is enough space not only to visualize the area to be implanted, but also to introduce, for instance, a suction tip. The depth scale at the outside of the implanter body is read with the edge of the suspension laryngoscope as point of reference. The largest possible section suspension laryngoscope should be used, as it affords a better view and permits free access for additional instrumentation. (From Delclos, L. and Moore, E.B.: A slim [198]gold-grain implanter loaded with standard Royal Marsden 14-grain magazines. Cancer *43*:1022, 1979.)

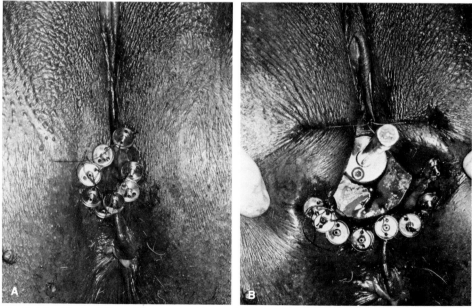

Fig. 5–36. Afterloadable stainless-steel guides implanted to the posterior vaginal wall. *(A)* Without the dome cylinder the vaginal implant collapses into a small circle creating a hot spot. *(B)* The empty dome cylinder distends the vagina, moving the anterior vaginal wall away from the implant, and maintains the needles in a slightly single-curved-plane implant. (From Delclos, L.: *In* Topical Reviews in Radiotherapy and Oncology-2. Edited by T.J. Deeley. London, John Wright & Sons, 1982.)

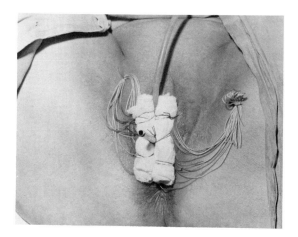

Fig. 5–37. Every effort should be made to keep normal tissues away from the implanted radioactive material. For implants of the vaginal walls, in addition to the empty vaginal cylinder, two rolled sponges are placed between the labia majora. Sponges (not seen in this picture) are added on top to separate the thighs.

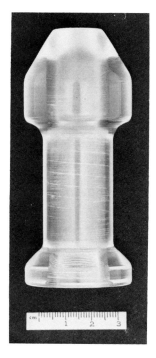

Fig. 5–38. For implants of the anal canal we use a hollow rectal plug that reduces the dose to the opposite side of the implant (see also Fig. 5–39). Several sizes are available.

preparation of radium needles, gold grains, or iridium wires, no one except the nurse or technician preparing them is exposed to radiation. To minimize exposure, the work bench is designed with a frontal working area with an L-shaped lead screen to protect the trunk, lower extremities, and medial aspect of the arms. In addition, a leaded-glass screen reduces exposure to the eyes.

Behind the barrier there is a lead well to store the remaining radioactive material while the individual needle, wire, or gold grains are prepared for insertion into the patient. The bench is covered with sterile drapes. The radioactive sources are immediately placed in the storage well of the work bench when they are brought into the operating room.

Sterilization of the radioactive sources is done by soaking the needles in a germicidal solution such as Cydex. Gold-grain magazines and iridium wires are sterilized by gas.

The operating surgeon, the assistant, and the anesthesiologist work behind individual lead barriers (Fig. 5–44). Exposure to the eyes and hands can only be reduced

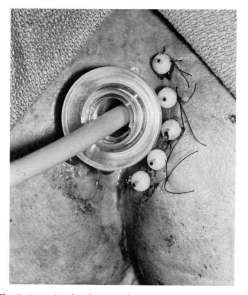

Fig. 5–39. Single-plane implant of the anal canal using stainless-steel needles with Teflon balls. Note the rectal plug in place. In addition, the patient has a Foley catheter inserted into the rectum to keep the rectum distended. The catheter retractor is only recommended for implants done with long guides. (From Delclos, L.: *In* Topical Reviews in Radiotherapy and Oncology-2. Edited by T.J. Deeley. London, John Wright & Sons, 1982.)

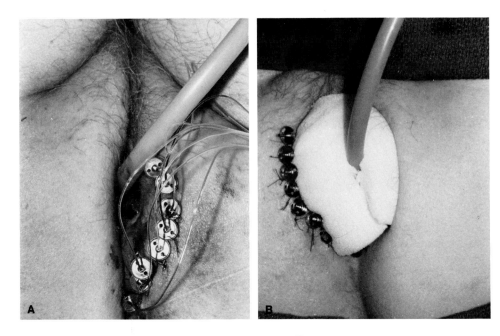

Fig. 5–40. *(A)* Single-plane implant for a tumor of the anal margin. In spite of the rectal plug the distal end of the implant would touch the opposite gluteal skin. *(B)* The distance can be increased with an additional piece of Ivalon, sponges, or lamino pads. (From Delclos, L.: *In* Topical Reviews in Radiotherapy and Oncology-2. Edited by T.J. Deeley. London, John Wright & Sons, 1982.)

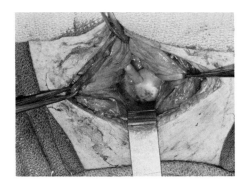

Fig. 5–41. A suprapubic cystostomy allows the placement of the index and middle finger around the balloon of the Foley catheter to guide the stainless steel guides, or needles, along the vesicovaginal septum and bladder trigone. This minimizes the possibility of a needle entering the urinary bladder. (From Delclos, L.: *In* Topical Reviews in Radiotherapy and Oncology-2. Edited by T.J. Deeley. London, John Wright & Sons, 1982.)

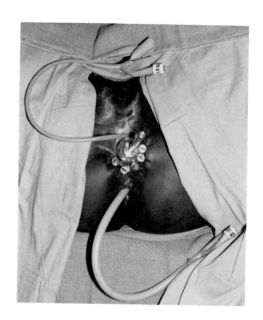

Fig. 5–42. For lesions of the posterior vaginal septum, a 5-cm Foley catheter is inserted into the urinary bladder, a dome cylinder of adequate size is placed in the vagina to keep it distended, and a 30-ml Foley catheter is inserted into the rectum to keep the lower rectum distended. (From Delclos, L.: *In* Topical Reviews in Radiotherapy and Oncology-2. Edited by T.J. Deeley. London, John Wright & Sons, 1982.)

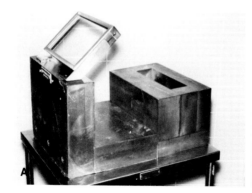
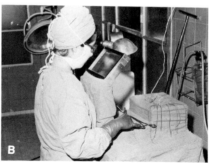

Fig. 5–43. Operating room work bench. *(A)* uncovered, and *(B)* covered. (From Van Roosenbeek, E. and Delclos, L.: The Radioactive Patient: Care, Precautions, and Procedures in Diagnosis and Therapy. Flushing, New York, Medical Examination Publishing Company, 1975.)

by distance and the dexterity gained through experience. All radioactive sources should be handled with long instruments. Because most procedures are afterloading modalities, exposure to the fingers during manipulation is minimal.

The details of protective procedures used during the preparation and transportation of radioactive materials, and the regulations governing them, have been described in detail by Van Roosenbeek and Delclos.[25]

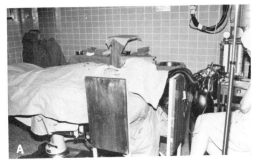
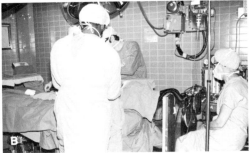

Fig. 5–44. For oral cavity implants with radium needles, shields are placed at each side of the head and also between patient and anesthetist. *(A)* Uncovered shields. *(B)* The radiotherapist and assistant behind the covered shields. (From Delclos, L.: *In* Topical Reviews in Radiotherapy and Oncology-2. Edited by T.J. Deeley. London, John Wright & Sons, 1982.)

REFERENCES

1. Abbe, R.: Radium in surgery. Arch. Roentgen. Rad. 14:277, 1910.
2. Allt, W.E.C., and Hunt, J.W.: Experience with radioactive tantalum wire as a source for interstitial therapy. Radiology 80:581, 1963.
3. Bier, R., Small, R.C., Leake, D.L., and Howard, J.H.: An afterloading technique for radium needles in the treatment of carcinoma of the oral cavity. Radiology 108:711, 1973.
4. Bloedorn, F.G.: Application of the Paterson–Parker system in interstitial radium therapy. Am. J. Roentgenol. 75:457, 1956.
5. Chan, R.C., and Gutierrez, A.E.: Carcinoma of the prostate. Cancer 37:2749, 1976.
6. Delclos, L.: Are interstitial radium applications passe? Front. Radiat. Ther. Oncol. 12:42, 1978.
7. Delclos, L.: Afterloading method for interstitial gamma-ray therapy. *In* Textbook of Radiotherapy, 3rd ed. Edited by G.H. Fletcher. Philadelphia, Lea & Febiger, 1980.
8. Delclos, L., and Moore, E.B.: A slim 198 gold-grain implanter loaded with standard Royal Marsden 14-grain magazines. Cancer 43:1021, 1979.
9. Fletcher, G.H.: *In* Textbook of Radiotherapy, 3rd ed. Edited by G.H. Fletcher. Philadelphia, Lea & Febiger, 1980.
10. Fletcher, G.H., and MaComb, W.S.: Radiation Therapy in the Management of Cancers of the Oral Cavity and Oropharynx. Springfild, Illinois, Charles C Thomas, 1962.
11. Hames, F.: A new method in the use of radon gold seeds. Am. J. Surg. 38:235, 1937.
12. Henschke, U.K.: Artificial radioisotopes in nylon ribbons for implantation in neoplasms. International Conferences on the Peaceful Uses of Atomic Energy. New York, United Nations, 1956.
13. Henschke, U.K.: Interstitial implantation with radioisotopes. *In* Therapeutic Use of Artificial Radioisotopes. Edited by P.F. Hahan. New York, John Wiley & Sons, 1956.
14. Hensche, U.K., James, A.G., and Myers, W.G.: Radiogold seeds for cancer therapy. Nucleonics 11:46, 1953.
15. Hilaris, B.S.: Handbook of Interstitial Brachytherapy. Acton, Publishing Sciences Group, 1975.
16. Hodt, H.J., Sinclair, W.K., and Smithers, D.W.: A gun for interstitial implantation of radioactive gold grains. Br. J. Radiol. 25:419, 1952.
17. Meredith, W.J.: Radium Dosage: The Manchester System. Edinburgh, E. & S Livingstone, 1949.
18. Morphis, O.L.: Teflon tube method of radium implantation. Am. J. Roentgenol. 83:455, 1960.
19. Morton, J.L., Callendine, G.W., Jr., and Myers, W.G.: Radioactive cobalt-60 in plastic tubing for interstitial radiation therapy. Radiology 56:553, 1951.
20. Mowatt, K.S., and Stevens, K.A.: Afterloading: A contribution to the protection problem. J. Fac. Radiol. 8:28, 1956.
21. Paine, C.H.: Modern afterloading methods for interstitial radiotherapy. Clin. Radiol. 23:263, 1972.
22. Pierquin, B.: En Precis de Curietherapie; Plesiocurietherapie. Paris, Masson & Cie, 1964.
23. Pierquin, B., Chassagne, D., Baillet, F., and Castro, J.R.: The place of implantation in tongue and floor of mouth cancer. JAMA 215:961, 1971.
24. Suit, H.D., Shalek, R.J., Moore, E.B., and Andrews, J.R.: Afterloading technique with rigid needles in interstitial radiation therapy. Radiology 76:431, 1961.
25. Van Roosenbeek, E. and Delclos, L.: The Radioactive Patient: Care, Precautions and Procedures in Diagnosis and Therapy. Flushing, New York, Medical Examination Publishing Co. 1975.

Chapter 6

INTERSTITIAL IRIDIUM TEMPLATE TECHNIQUES

Roger A. Potish
Jeffrey F. Williamson

Interstitial brachytherapy can be defined as the use of encapsulated radionuclides implanted in malignant tissues.[9] Over the past 8 decades, its popularity has waxed and waned. Despite dramatic advances in the technology of external-beam therapy, the benefits of interstitial therapy have outweighed its conspicuous drawbacks: the necessity of minor surgery, greater personnel radiation exposure, and substantial technical difficulties.[11] Although the biologic basis of the success of brachytherapy remains uncertain, one obvious advantage is the ability to administer sizable doses of radiation directly to a tumor with a corresponding rapid dose falloff in adjacent normal tissues.[8] There are two additional differences between brachytherapy and teletherapy: the dose rate of brachytherapy is lower and is continuous, and an identical physical dose can be given in a matter of days rather than weeks.

The modern era of brachytherapy began 30 years ago with the development of artificial radionuclides and afterloading capabilities.[9] A few years ago, Syed and Feder introduced the "transperineal parametrial butterfly" template implantation technique with [192]Ir.[4,19] This has added another useful tool in the treatment of malignant disease. Clinical experience with this system is limited, and this chapter reviews its use at the University of Minnesota Hospitals.

[192]IR

[192]Ir is an ideal radionuclide for interstitial therapy.[17] It is commercially available in convenient lengths and activities. It can be manufacturered so thin that flexible plastic encapsulation of sources allows afterloading to be accomplished with ease. Iridium is available in 3 mm × 0.5 mm seeds that are encapsulated in nylon ribbons; there is a spacing of 1 cm between the centers of adjacent seeds. Its average photon energy of 0.38 MV is sufficiently high that differential energy absorption between tissues of varying composition is minimal. Radiation protection is aided by its relatively low first half-value layer (HVL) of 2.2 mm and second HVL of 2.8 mm in lead. Its half-life of 74 days is long enough that activity varies by only a few percent during the duration of an average implant.

THE SYED/NEBLETT TEMPLATES

A variety of Syed/Neblett templates are available from Alpha Omega Services, Inc. (16220 Gundry Avenue, Paramount, Cali-

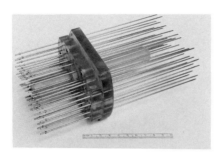

Fig. 6–1. The Syed/Neblett Gyn #2 template is shown with its full complement of 44 afterloading needles and 2-cm diameter vaginal cylinder. The template is 108 mm by 70 mm in greatest dimensions, and the diameter of the central hole is 21 mm. If desired, an afterloading uterine tandem may be inserted through a hole in the center of the plastic vaginal cylinder.

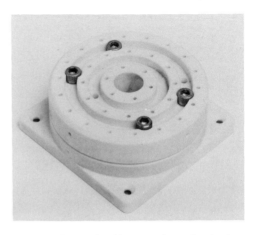

Fig. 6–3. The Syed/Neblett Rectal template is shown here without its needles. Its overall dimensions are 70 mm by 70 mm, with a central hole diameter of 12 mm. Because it can be placed over the perineal area as well as the rectal area, it can also be used for treatment of vulvar or vaginal lesions.

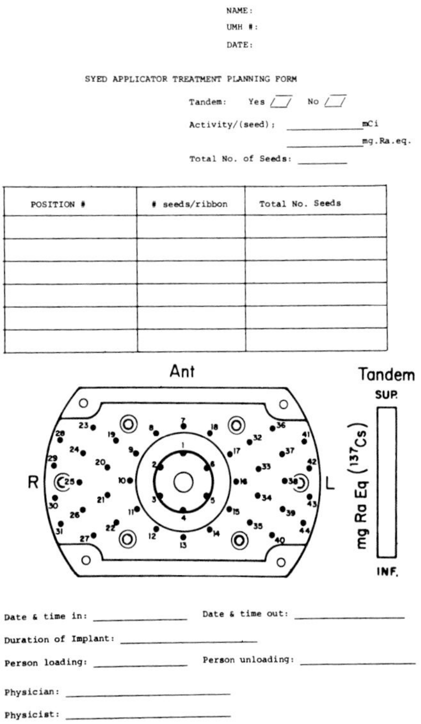

Fig. 6–2. The Gyn #2 treatment planning form used at the University of Minnesota is useful for recording the positions of the needles that are inserted through the template. It is also valuable for preliminary planning of the implant because it is drawn with a magnification factor of unity.

fornia 90723). The majority of our implants have been performed with "Gyn #2" templates (Fig. 6–1). This template is fabricated from two lucite plates joined by six machine screws that tighten to grasp as many as 38 afterloading, hollow, stainless-steel needles. An additional 6 needles fit into grooves of a 2-cm diameter plastic vaginal cylinder that is placed inside an opening in the middle of the template. These 44 needles are arranged in concentric circles or arcs with a spacing of 1 cm between adjacent needles (Fig. 6–2). A 4 cm × 10 cm area can be implanted in a "butterfly" distribution.[4] The 17-gauge needles supplied by the company are 15 cm and 20 cm long, but we have shortened some of them to 11 cm to treat shallow regions more conveniently. There is also an opening in the vaginal cylinder for placement of a tandem.

The rectal template is similar to Gyn #2 (Fig. 6–3). The two plates contain three concentric rings with a total of 36 needles with 1-cm spacing (Fig. 6–4). Cylindrical volumes with diameters of 2, 4, or 6 cm can be implanted. Four machine screws fix the needles at the chosen depth. A rectal tube can be placed in the central hole

NAME:

UMH #:

DATE:

SYED APPLICATOR TREATMENT PLANNING FORM

Total No. of Seeds:_____   Tandem: Yes /__/   No /__/

Total Activity: _____ mCi   Activity/(seed): _____ mCi

_____ mg.Ra.eq.   _____ mg.Ra.eq.

Type of Applicator: _____

Position #	# seeds/ribbon	Total No. Seeds

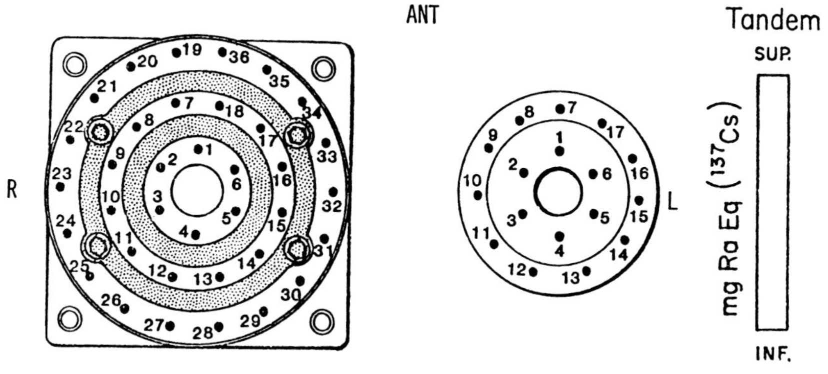

ANT   Tandem

Fig. 6–4. The University of Minnesota treatment planning form shows the Rectal template on the left and the Urethral template on the right.

Date & time in: _____   Date & time out: _____

Duration of Implant: _____

Person loading: _____   Person unloading: _____

Physician: _____

Physicist: _____

if necessary but the hole can be left open if the template is placed on an area of the vulva or perineum in such a way that it does not cover the anus.

The urethral template has two concentric rings with a total of 17 needles with the same 1-cm spacing as the rectal template (Figs. 6–4, 6–5). A cylindrical volume with either a 2-cm or a 4-cm diameter is implanted with this template. This is a single plate with no machine screws. A Foley urethral catheter is inserted through

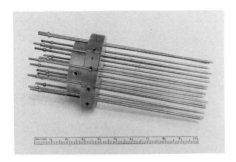

Fig. 6–5. The Syed/Neblett Urethral template has small set screws to fix the 17 afterloading needles. Its diameter is 45 mm, with a central hole diameter of 9 mm.

the central opening to drain the urinary bladder when a template is placed for a urethral tumor.

DOSE AND VOLUME CONSIDERATION

As clinical radiotherapy completes its ninth decade, time, dose, and volume factors continue to defy understanding. The interactions of total dose, dose rate, and total volume are impossible to decipher with the existing clinical data. Radiation biology has added some qualitative and quantitative data, but the clinical experience of various investigators and institutions is the best guide for a specific technique.

An excellent review of volume and time factors in interstitial therapy has been provided by Barkley and Fletcher.[1] At dose rates between 30 and 100 rad per hour, total dose was believed to be the critical factor, with dose-rate effects of only secondary importance. However, dose rate was thought to be important by Ellis, who proposed a "dose-factor F" for correcting total dose as a function of dose rate.[3] His factor ranged from 1.033 at 30 rad per hour to 0.672 at 100 rad per hour, a change of magnitude of 1.54 (1.033/.672). At the University of Minnesota, iridium is ordered in activities that will achieve a dose rate of 35 to 55 rad per hour. This is comparable to the classic dose rate of 42 rad per hour of an ideal Paterson-Parker implant (7000 rad in 7 days)[3] The Ellis F factor changes

only by 1.16 (1.001/.864) between 35 and 55 rad per hour.

Volume factors are even more difficult to quantitate. With the circular template, the largest implantable cross-sectional area is 28 cm², whereas the "butterfly" template can have a maximum cross-sectional area of 40 cm². The depth of most applications varies from 5 cm to 10 cm; total volume is generally less than 400 cm³. At the Univesity of Minnesota, we make no volume or dose-rate corrections. Large tumors are treated primarily with external beam, and the effects of dose rate and volume are minimized because the interstitial therapy is only a small fraction of the total treatment. In establishing tolerance levels, we add the teletherapy and brachytherapy dose contributions, even though this sum is "radiobiologically uninterpretable."[15]

Typical isodose patterns with the three standard iridium templates are shown in

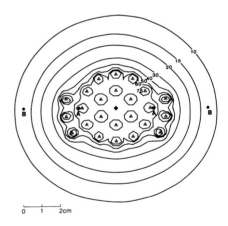

Fig. 6–6 A cross-sectional isodose pattern for a Gyn #2 template application depicts the uniformity of dose rate achieved throughout the implanted volume. The center of the implant is represented by a cross, individual ribbons are represented by triangles in this and subsequent isodose patterns. All isodoses are expressed in rads per hour. This application contained 24 ribbons, 8 iridium seeds per ribbon, and .198 milligram radium equivalents (mg Ra eq) per seed: total activity was 38 mg Ra eq. The 50 rad isodose surrounded all the ribbons, and the 60 rad isodose encompassed the inner two rings. Point A, 2 cm superior and 2 cm lateral to the external cervical os, received 60 rads per hour, while Point B, 3 cm lateral to Point A, received 13 rads per hour.[20] Treatment planning radiographs for this implant may be seen in Figs. 6–16 and 6–17.

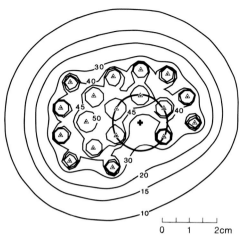

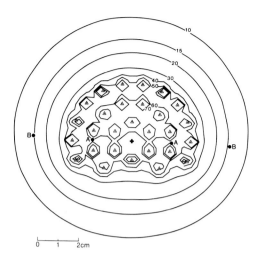

Fig. 6–7. A Gyn #2 template application demonstrates the flexibility of the iridium system in the management of vaginal cancer. The position of the plastic vaginal cylinder is represented by the 2 cm diameter circle. This application contained 18 ribbons, 7 iridium seeds per ribbon, and .174 mg Ra eq per seed: total activity was 22 mg Ra eq. By proper choice of needle placement, the isodoses were made to follow the distribution of the cancer on the lateral and anterior vaginal walls. The rectum and the uninvolved vagina could be excluded from high dose volume. The tumor was covered by the 45 rad isodose, while the anterior rectal wall received less than 30 rads per hour.

Fig. 6–8. Transverse-central plane isodoses are shown for the Rectal template loaded with 28 ribbons, 10 iridium seeds per ribbon, and .171 mg Ra eq per seed, for a total activity of 48 mg Ra eq. Point *A* received 55 rads per hour, with Point *B* achieving 15 rads per hour. The patient had a cervical cancer, but a Fletcher application was impossible because of vaginal stenosis. Ileal bladder had been created to correct a vesicovaginal fistula. The Rectal template was positioned with its center anterior to the middle of the vagina, so that the cervix and the adjacent involved posterior bladder wall could be implanted. The anterior positioning also permitted more rectal sparing.

Figures 6–6 through 6–13. The dose rate is remarkably uniform throughout the implanted volume demarcated by the outer needles, with a rapid falloff thereafter. As illustrated in Figures 6–10 through 6–13, there is relatively little variation in dose rate regardless of whether the calculation plane is taken through or between rows of needles. Except for "hot spots" immediately next to the seeds, the dose rate varies by only 5 to 10 rad per hour through the implanted volume.

INDICATIONS

Feder, Syed, and Neblett utilized their iridium-template system to improve the homogeneity of pelvic intracavitary therapy, particularly in patients whose anatomy was unsatisfactory for placement of conventional tandem and colpostat systems.[4] A uterine tandem was inserted centrally and afterloaded with cesium or radium, while the parametrial areas were

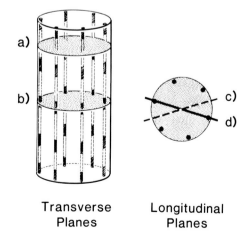

Transverse Planes   **Longitudinal Planes**

Fig. 6–9. Diagram illustrating the locations of isodose calculation planes described in Figs. 6–10 through 6–14. Planes *a* and *c* depict transverse and longitudinal calculation planes positioned midway between adjacent pairs of seeds and ribbons, whereas planes *b* and *d* intersect the central seeds and ribbons of the implant.

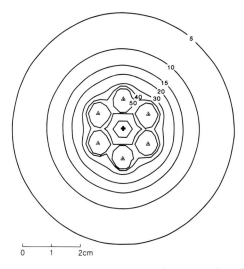

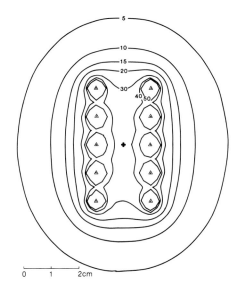

Fig. 6–10.   A cancer of the distal urethra was implanted by the Urethral template, with 6 ribbons, 5 iridium seeds per ribbon, and .328 mg Ra eq per seed. Total activity was 10 mg Ra eq. This cross section was taken through the seeds.

Fig. 6–12.   Isodose curves in the longitudinal plane containing the central ribbons of the implant shown in Fig. 6–10.

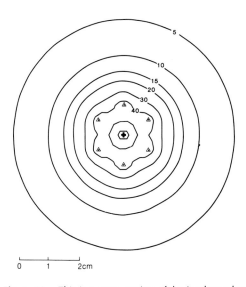

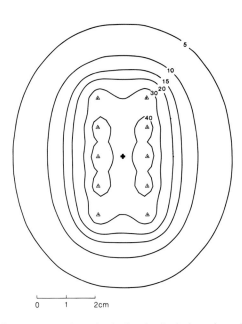

Fig. 6–11.   This is a cross section of the implant taken 5 mm away from the plane of Fig. 6–10. It lies midway between adjacent seeds. The 5- to 30-rad isodoses were virtually identical, and even the 40 rad isodoses were displaced relatively little from each other. The 50 rad isodose did not appear in this plane.

Fig. 6–13.   Isodoses in the longitudinal plane through the implant of Fig. 6–10, positioned midway between the seeds, demonstrating the correspondence of the 5- to 30-rad isodoses with those of Fig. 6–12.

treated primarily with iridium. With loading of both the tandem and the template, representative dose rates were 40 to 80 rad per hour in the lateral parametria and 80 to 120 rad per hour in the medial parametria. Total dose, including external beam, to the lateral parametrial (Point B) area was 6800 to 8000 rad.

At the Univesity of Minnesota, tolerance doses of 8000 to 8500 rad at Point A and 6000 rad at Point B are standard when external-beam therapy is combined with two Fletcher afterloading cesium applications. When external beam alone is administered, a 7000-rad shrinking-field technique is used, with field size progressively reduced to 10 cm × 10 cm.[7] We have not yet accepted the Syed tolerance levels nor replaced the Fletcher system with templates because we are waiting for the accumulation of more clinical data. We use the template system without the central tandem in the treatment of cervical cancer only when placement of a standard Fletcher tandem is impossible because of vaginal stenosis or inability to locate the cervical os. The isodose patterns are quite different from a conventional intracavitary application, and tolerance levels have not yet been established with certainty.

Our most frequent use of the template system is for primary or metastatic cancers of the vaginal area. In addition, the urethral template is efficacious in therapy of distal urethral cancers. Our cesium and radium needle implants have almost been replaced by the template system. The wide range of available iridium-seed activities and ribbon lengths offers great flexibility. The vaginal cylinder and the plastic template maintain parallel and equal spacing between adjacent needles. Because the system is afterloaded, personnel exposure is minimized.

Our dose recommendations for vaginal carcinomas are identical to those of the M.D. Anderson Hospital: 4000 to 5000 rad of external beam therapy to the pelvis are followed by a single implant delivering another 3000 to 2000 rad.[21] The proportions of external beam and interstitial dose are determined by the tumor volume, with relatively more external-beam therapy and less interstitial therapy for larger lesions. Fleming et al. have recommended that 5000 rad of external beam be administered (with a midline block after 4000 rad), followed by a 2-week rest period, followed by another 4500 to 5000 rad given interstitially in two sessions with another 2-week rest period interspersed.[5] Recommendations for management of cancers of the female urethra are presented elsewhere.[6,10]

The template system has a number of disadvantages. Because of the equal spacing of the template holes, it may be difficult to avoid bladder penetration. The needles can perforate the small intestine. It is virtually impossible to implant the posterior vagina with a sufficient margin

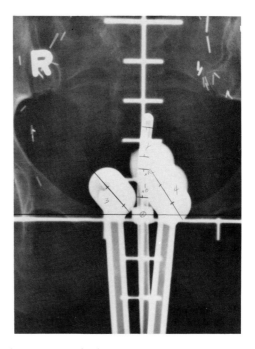

Fig. 6–14. A Fletcher cesium application was performed on a woman with cervical cancer who also had a Gyn #2 iridium application (Figs. 6–16 and 6–17). The anterior-posterior treatment-planning radiograph is shown. Note the position of the cervical collar, which was sutured to the cervix.

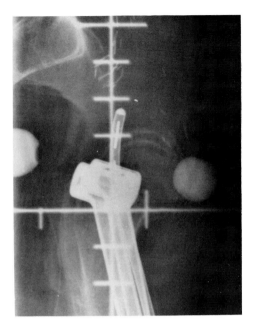

Fig. 6–15. A lateral treatment planning radiograph of the application of Fig. 6–13 shows considerable displacement between the sacrum and the tandem.

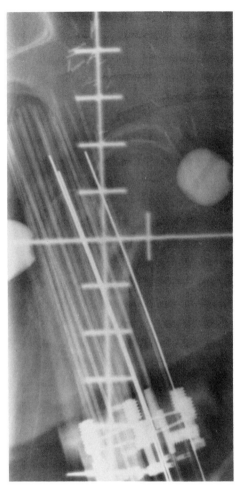

Fig. 6–17. A lateral treatment planning radiograph shows the iridium system to be angled more posteriorly and closer to the sacrum, relative to the cesium application of Fig. 6–15.

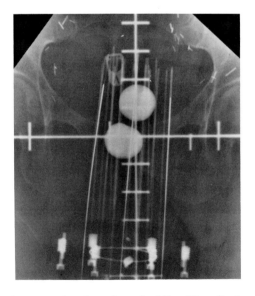

Fig. 6–16. Anterior radiograph of Gyn #2 application on the patient described in Figs. 6–14 and 6–15. The iridium needles were both lateral and superior to the cesium system.

without entering the rectum. Visualization and palpation are quite restricted during and after template placement. Both anteriorly and laterally, the implant may be bounded by the pelvic bones. Because the template is flush with the perineum and the vaginal cylinder is parallel to the vagina, the direction of implantation is fixed. Thus, the templates, while useful in certain situations, cannot completely replace conventional interstitial, intracavitary, or external beam therapy.

Anatomic considerations play an important role in the choice of interstitial and

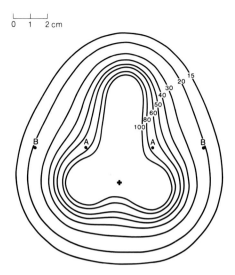

0 1 2 cm

Fig. 6–18. This is an anterior-posterior isodose distribution of a standard Fletcher cesium application with a conventional loading of 9.8–9.8–14.3 mg Ra eq in the tandem and an 18.8 mg Ra eq source in each colpostat. As may be seen by comparison with Figs. 6–6 and 6–8, the isodose patterns differ markedly.

intracavitary therapy. Figures 6–14 and 6–15 show a typical Fletcher cesium application, while Figures 6–16 and 6–17 depict a Gyn #2 iridium application in the same patient. The iridium application is distributed more laterally and superiorly, which is advantageous to the parametrial areas. The template system, however, radiates a greater rectal length. The Fletcher tandem is curved anteriorly, whereas the Gyn #2 system follows the vaginal axis, which is tilted more posteriorly. Differences in the pattern of radiation distributions must be kept in mind: tolerance levels are not necessarily synonymous with the two systems. Although similar ratios of Point A dose to Point B dose may be obtained, the three-dimensional isodoses are quite different (Figs. 6–6, 6–18).

TECHNIQUE OF INSERTION

All template insertions[4,5,19] are performed under general anesthesia with members of the radiation-therapy and gynecologic-oncology staffs in attendance. A meticulous pelvic and rectal examina-

tion is mandatory to assess the tumor volume because visualization and palpation are limited during placement of the template. Next, the perineal area is sterilely prepared and draped while the patient is in the dorsal lithotomy position. A Foley urethral catheter is inserted into the bladder, and the bulb is filled with 5 ml of Hypaque. The bladder is not drained at this time so that inadvertent bladder entry may be noted by the passage of urine through the hollow afterloading needles, which have a hole in the distal end. Bladder entry may occasionally be demonstrated by deflation of the Foley bulb from a needle puncture.

A guide needle is inserted into the deepest portion of the tumor to establish the depth to be implanted. The location of this guide is checked by vaginal and rectal examinations, with appropriate glove changes following rectal examination. The template is then inserted over the guide needle with maintenance of proper depth. Needles are then placed through the template into the relevant volume with the aid of obturators (Fig. 6–19). Depth may be checked by measuring the distance of the ends of the needles from the template surface and by frequent rectal examinations. The vaginal cylinder is inserted through the central-template opening; needles slide easily down the appropriate grooves. The

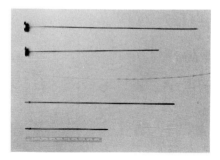

Fig. 6–19. Various accessories for the template system include *(from top to bottom)* an obturator for the afterloading needles, a tungsten obturator for localization films, a ribbon of "dummy" seeds, a 20 cm needle, an 11 cm needle, and a 10 cm ruler. Not shown is the guide needle.

order of needle insertion varies from patient to patient. The first should always be inserted in the deepest portion of the tumor. Subsequent needles are then placed anteriorly because unintentional bladder entry is not unusual. If a needle enters the bladder, it is removed. The posterior area is next implanted. Rectal entry can be demonstrated by rectal examination. If a needle has penetrated the rectal mucosa, it is removed. The remainder of the needles are then inserted at the appropriate sites. If significant bleeding is encountered, the relevant needle is withdrawn. The implant may be limited laterally by the pelvic bones. All needles are inserted to the same depth.

The machine screws are tightened to secure the template needles, and the vaginal cylinder is similarly fixed. Four sutures are placed in the perineal area adjacent to the corners of the template. The skin loops are left loose because there will be swelling around them later. They are tied. The ends of the sutures are then placed through holes in the corners of the template and tied with a second knot. Cotton or gauze packing is placed laterally around the template to help protect the medial thigh areas from necrosis caused by pressure. A rectal Foley catheter is placed, with Hypaque in its bulb to facilitate radiographic localization. After simulation radiographs have been obtained, the patient is returned to her room, where the iridium is quickly af-

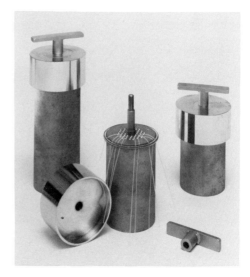

Fig. 6–21. Iridium containers or "pigs" can be used to carry the iridium to the patient's room. The iridium containers are transported inside a lead cart for additional shielding. (Photograph courtesy of Radiation Products Design, Inc., 17500 Wright County Road 19, R.R. 3, Box 132-F, Buffalo, MN 53313.)

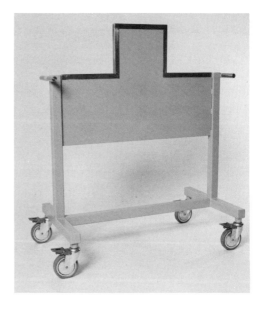

Fig. 6–22. Fixed rolling radiation one-inch-thick lead radiation shields are valuable in reducing radiation exposure to personnel. (Photograph courtesy of Radiation Products Design, Inc.)

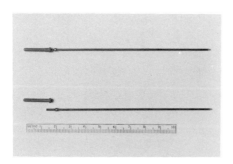

Fig. 6–20. A 17-gauge afterloading needle and a flexible plastic "blue tip" cap for sealing the template needles are shown, both separately and as an assembled unit.

terloaded while standing behind a steel or lead shield (Figs. 6–20, 6–21, 6–22). Strict radiation protection guidelines are followed, with no visitors allowed in the room when the iridium is in place. The patient must rest in bed, though she may move her legs and turn from side to side with the assistance of a nurse. When the patient is lying on her side, a pillow is inserted between her knees so that the legs do not press on the needle ends extending beyond the template surface.

Oral or intramuscular narcotics are administered shortly before removal of the template, but the amount of pain during removal is surprisingly small. The four sutures are cut, and then the template, vaginal cylinder, needles, and iridium are quickly removed as a single unit. Gentle pressure applied for a few minutes stops any oozing at the sites of needle entry through the perineum and vagina. The patient and her room are surveyed for any residual radioactivity. The iridium is extracted from the needles in the radiation-therapy department where it is possible to work behind shielding. The patient is usually discharged within 1 day after removal of the template.

Although we have observed no chronic radiation damage yet, our number of patients and length of follow-up are limited. Prophylactic antibiotics have not been routinely administered. No infections have occurred, except in one woman who developed a small abscess at the site of a posterior suture. Only one patient has required a transfusion for bleeding secondary to the procedure. One woman developed a pressure necrosis on the medial thigh areas from the template, but this healed with conservative management. Another patient developed transient lower extremity pain and paresthesias, possibly from nerve trauma. Overall, acute toxicity has been relatively slight. As with any new technique, complications can be expected to decline as clinical experience increases.

PHYSICAL CONSIDERATIONS

The use of encapsulated iridium seeds as interstitial brachytherapy sources presents a number of practical challenges to the radiological physicist. Among these are quality control, calibration, and treatment planning. Each of these aspects are briefly discussed below with emphasis on their applications to template implants.

Calibration and Quality Control

The intensity of sealed gamma-ray brachytherapy sources is currently specified in terms of exposure rate at a distance of 1 meter from and perpendicular to the long axis of the source at its center and is usually expressed in R cm^2/hr or mR m^2/hr.[14] Since 1979, the National Bureau of Standards (NBS) has calibrated ^{192}Ir seeds against the national exposure rate standard according to this specification.[12]

Even though vendor calibration of iridium seeds is consistent with NBS exposure rate standards, they often state source intensity in units of activity (Curies or Becquerels) or equivalent mass of radium (mg Ra eq) based on assumed values of the exposure-rate constant, Γ. Care must be taken to use the same value of Γ as assumed by the source vendor to convert intensity given in mg Ra eq or mCi to exposure rate rather than the Γ values recommended by the current literature. For example, our source vendor (Alpha Omega Services, Inc.) specifies iridium-seed intensity in mg Ra eq. Thus, to compute exposure rate, $\dot{X}(r)$, at a distance of r cm from the source, a value of 8.25 R cm^2/mg–hr should be used:

$$X(r) = \frac{(\text{mg Ra eq}) \times 8.25}{r^2} \qquad (1)$$

These values can easily be converted to dose rates in tissue by applying the appropriate Roentgen-to-rad conversion factor and tissue attenuation and build-up factors.[13]

At the University of Minnesota, the vendor calibration is verified by using the nuclear medicine dose calibrator illustrated in Fig. 6–23.[2] Six or seven ribbons, drawn randomly from the shipment, are conveniently 'read out' using a special jig that positions the source along the axis of the well. The readings are then converted to exposure rate per seed after correction for source elongation. Readings are also taken with a [226]Ra standard source to insure that the calibrator response has not changed through time. The average value of the assayed seeds generally agrees within ±4% with the Alpha-Omega calibration although individual ribbons may deviate from the average value by as much as 12%.

The dose calibrator is not a suitable primary instrument for performing relative exposure measurements: its response depends significantly upon source energy, filtration, and position in the well.[22] The instrument must be calibrated empirically using an exposure calibrated seed having the same physical construction as the seeds to be assayed. Such calibrated standards can be obtained from NBS. An in-house exposure-rate calibration of iridium may also be performed, using a suitably calibrated external-beam chamber.

While calibration is performed, all ribbons should be examined to insure that no seeds are missing or irregularly spaced and that none of the nylon ribbons are fractured or frayed. It is useful to place the ribbons in the transport pig (see Fig. 6–21) several hours before afterloading. This straightens them and improves ease of handling.

Treatment Planning

Computer-generated isodose curves are used as the basis of dose prescription for all template implants. The primary calculation plane, perpendicular to the needle axes, is chosen so as to bisect the implanted volume. Additional planes can be chosen to examine other sites of the treatment volume.

The usual method of generating iridium-isodose curves is based upon reconstructing the seed coordinates in three-dimensional space by individually identifying the image of every seed on each of two radiographs.[17] The radiographs are exposed using either orthogonal or stereo-shift geometry. Because the template implants may contain several hundred seeds and up to 44 needles, identification of the lateral and anterior-posterior images of each source is very tedious, time-consuming, and prone to error, as Figures 6–16 and 6–17 illustrate. Identification of corresponding images on stereo-shift radiographs is not significantly easier. We have also found the latter imaging technique to be very sensitive to patient-motion errors and small errors in entering the data from the radiograph into the computer, often

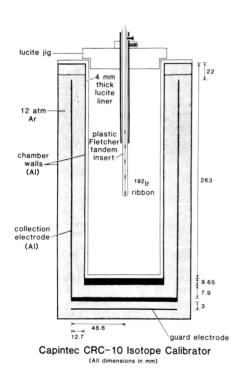

Capintec CRC–10 Isotope Calibrator
(All dimensions in mm)

Fig. 6–23. Cutaway view of the Capintec CRC-10 dose calibrator illustrating the special jig used to position iridium ribbons along the source axis during routine calibration. All dimensions are in mm. (From Williamson, J.F. et al.: Methods for routine calibration of brachytherapy sources. Radiology *142*:512, 1982.)

resulting in a distorted picture of the source geometry.[18] Once the seed coordinates have been obtained, the dose contribution from each seed to any point of interest in the implant is calculated by treating it as an isotropic-point source (Equation 1).

To avoid these difficulties, we have evolved a simple, rapid, and sufficiently accurate method of approximating the central-plane dose distribution for template implants. Several simplifying assumptions are made:

1. Because the iridium ribbons are encased in rigid, stainless-steel needles, we assume each ribbon is described by a straight line.
2. Because all needles are held in a rigid

configuration by the template, their relative positions in any plane transverse to the needles are assumed to be given by the coordinates of the needle holes in the template.

3. Each ribbon, consisting of 3-mm long seeds, spaced at 1-cm intervals, is approximated by an unfiltered line source consisting of continuously distributed radioactivity.

Figures 6–24 and 6–25 compare isodose curves calculated on the basis of the unfiltered linear-source model with those derived from the more realistic isotropic-

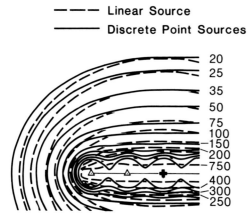

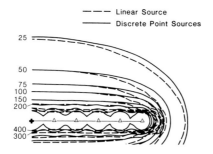

Fig. 6–24. Comparison of isodose curves generated using the point source and linear source models for a 4 cm long iridium ribbon containing 5 seeds.

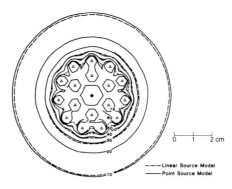

Fig. 6–26. Comparison of urethral template isodose curves derived from the point source and linear source models where the calculation plane contains all central seeds. Both rings of the template were loaded with 4 cm long ribbon having an intensity of 0.25 mg Ra eq per seed.

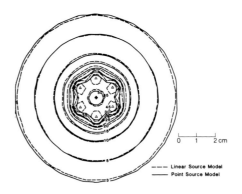

Fig. 6–25. Comparison of linear source and point source isodose curves for an iridium ribbon consisting of 11 seeds.

Fig. 6–27. Comparison of point source and linear source isodoses for the urethral template with the calculation plane positioned midway between the third and fourth seeds. Only the inner ring was loaded, again with 4 cm long ribbons of 0.25 mg Ra eq per seed.

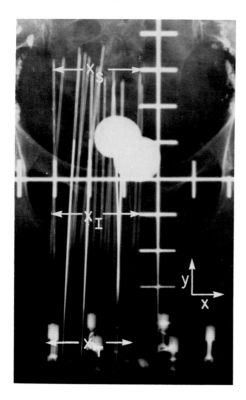

Fig. 6–28. Anterior isocentric radiograph illustrating the coordinate system used in reconstructing the source positions and the measurements necessary to correct for distortion of implant shape. The center of the coordinate system is located at the level of the template at its center.

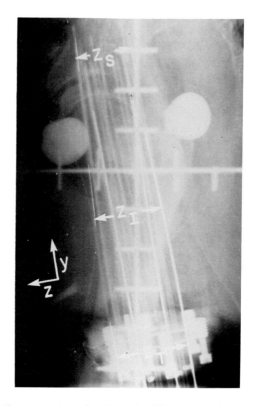

Fig. 6–29. Lateral radiograph of the same application as Fig. 6–28.

point source model for ribbons containing 5 and 11 seeds respectively. The two sets of isodose curves match within 0.5 mm in the transverse plane that bisects the ribbons and that contains the central seeds from 0.5 cm to 3 cm from the ribbon. When the transverse calculation plane lies midway between two seeds, the linear source isodoses are displaced outward, relative to the seed isodoses, by 1 mm to 1.5 mm for points near the ribbon axis. Although larger discrepancies occur near the ends of the ribbons, the linear-source model is an excellent approximation of iridium-ribbon isodoses provided that the transverse calculation plane is positioned at least 1 cm from the ribbon end.

Figure 6–26 compares linear-source and point-source isodose curves for the Syed urethral template loaded with 4-cm long

iridium ribbons where the calculation plane intersects the central seed of each ribbon. The two sets of curves are nearly indistinguishable. Even in the worst possible case (Fig. 6–27), where the calculation plane is located midway between adjacent seeds, the linear-source and point-source models agree within 5% to 7%. Because it is impossible to insert all needles to exactly the same depth, it is highly unlikely that this "worst case" would arise in clinical practice.

Obtaining Isodose Curves

Localization Radiographs. After the patient has recovered from anesthesia, she is transported to the simulator room. Prior to exposing localization films, several 'dummy' ribbons of the appropriate length are inserted into the applicator to facilitate visualization of the caudad and cephalad boundaries of the implanted region. If the patient is obese, tungsten obturators are inserted into strategically located peripheral needles so that the dimensions of the implant are clearly delineated on the radiographs.

Orthogonal isocentric anterior-posterior and lateral radiographs are then exposed with the isocenter located at the center of the implanted volume. Typical examples are shown in Figures 6–16, 6–17, 6–28, and 6–29, which show the Hypaque-filled Foley catheter bulbs used to visualize the bladder and rectum. Both the needle tips and the template must be visualized.

Corrections for Distortion of Implant Shape. Because of the presence of bony structures and critical organs near the implanted volume, the needles are often not exactly perpendicular to the template, causing the cross-sectional area of the implant to vary along the needle axes. The lateral radiograph of Figure 6–29 shows that the cephalad end of the implant is significantly smaller than the anterior-posterior width at the template level. According to the Quimby volume-implant tables, a change of 10% in one of the linear dimensions of the implant results in dosimetry errors of 5% to 7%.[16] Changes of 5% to 15% in anterior-posterior or lateral dimensions are typical.

Whenever the anterior-posterior or lateral dimensions deviate from the template dimensions by at least 5%, the coordinates of the template needle holes used to define the relative needle positions are modified. Corrections are made by comparing the lateral (x-axis) and anterior-posterior (z-axis) dimensions at the needle tips and most inferior seed position with the corresponding dimensions on the template. Referring to Figures 6–28 and 6–29, the distances (x_S, x_I, x_T) and (z_S, z_I, z_T) are measured from the radiographs. If the axis of the implant is not parallel to the central axis of the lateral radiograph, correction for the variation of the anterior-posterior magnification factor may be necessary.

Then, given the coordinates (x_i, z_i) of the ith needle in the template plane relative to its center, the tip and end coordinates (x_i, y_i, z_i) of each n seed ribbon may be computed as follows:

$$\left[\left(\frac{x_S}{x_T}\right) \cdot x_i, \; \frac{(n-1)}{2}, \; \left(\frac{z_S}{z_T}\right) \cdot z_i \right] \quad \text{Cephalad}$$

$$(2)$$

$$\left[\left(\frac{x_I}{x_T}\right) \cdot x_i, \; \frac{-(n-1)}{2}, \; \left(\frac{z_I}{z_T}\right) \cdot z_i \right] \quad \text{Caudad}$$

Computer Generation of Isodose Curves. At the University of Minnesota, the linear-source program (QISODO) of the TP-11 treatment-planning system is used to generate template isodose curves. For an implant consisting of n seeds/ribbon, the quantity $(n - 1)$ cm is entered for active and physical lengths, and a source filtration of 0.01 mm platinum is used. Where M is the seed strength in mg Ra eq decayed to the estimated midpoint of the implant, the quantity $(n \times M)$ is entered as source strength. Then the computed coordinates (Equation 2) are entered into the computer at unit magnification using the keyboard. Bladder and rectal coordinates may be entered as points of interest using coordinates measured from the radiographs.

Clinical examples of isodose curves are shown in Figures 6–6 through 6–8 and 6–10 through 6–13. For implants using more than 25 needles, seed strengths of 0.19 ot 0.25 mg Ra eq are required to obtain dose rates of 40 to 60 rad per hour at the periphery of the implanted volume. For implants using only 6 needles, seed strengths of .25 to .40 mg Ra eq are necessary to achieve dose rates of 35 to 55 rad per hour. Close collaboration between the physician and physicist is necessary to ensure that a satisfactory dose is obtained.

The Syed/Neblett Iridium system offers a useful resource in the management of gynecologic malignancies. Although its indications are currently limited, its full potential has not yet been realized. Brachytherapy continues to occupy an important niche in clinical radiotherapy, and its role will grow with technologic advances.

REFERENCES

1. Barkley, H.T., Jr. and Fletcher, G.H.: Volume and time factors in interstitial gamma-ray therapy. Am. J. Roentgenol. *126*:163, 1976.
2. Cobb, P.D. and Bjarngard, B.E.: Calibration of brachytherapy Iridium-192 sources. Am. J. Roentgenol. *120*:211, 1974.
3. Ellis, F.: Radiation effect and tolerance. *In* Handbook of Interstitial Brachytherapy. Edited by B.S. Hilaris. Acton, Publishing Sciences Group, 1975, pp. 45–52.
4. Feder, B.H., Syed, A.M.N., and Neblett, D.: Treatment of extensive carcinoma of the cervix with the "transperineal parametrial butterfly": A preliminary report on the revival of Waterman's approach. Int. J. Radiat. Oncol. Biol. Phys. *4*:735, 1978.
5. Fleming, P., Syed, A.M.N., Neblett, D. et al.: Description of an afterloading ^{192}Ir interstitial-intracavitary technique in the treatment of carcinoma of the vagina. Obstet. Gynecol. *55*:525, 1980.
6. Fletcher, G.H., Delclos, L., Wharton, J.T., and Rutledge, F.N.: Tumors of the vagina and female urethra. *In* Textbook of Radiotherapy, 3rd ed. Edited by G.H. Fletcher. Philadelphia, Lea & Febiger, 1980, pp. 812–828.
7. Fletcher, G.H. and Hamberger, A.D,: Squamous cell carcinoma of the uterine cervix: Treatment technique according to size of the cervical lesion and extension. *In* Textbook of Radiotherapy, 3rd ed. Edited by G.H. Fletcher. Philadelphia, Lea & Febiger, 1980, pp. 720–773.
8. Hall, E.J.: The promise of low dose rate: Has it been realized? Int. J. Radiat. Oncol. Biol. Phys. *4*:749, 1978.
9. Hilaris, B.S.: Historical review. *In* Handbook of Interstitial Brachytherapy. Edited by B.S. Hilaris. Acton, Publishing Sciences Group, 1975, pp. xiii–xvi.
10. Hilaris, B.S. and Batata, M.A.: Cancer of the female urethra. *In* Handbook of Interstitial Brachytherapy. Edited by B.S. Hilaris. Acton, Publishing Sciences Group, 1975, pp. 235–239.
11. Hilaris, B.S. and Henschke, U.K.: General principles and techniques of interstitial therapy. *In* Handbook of Interstitial Brachytherapy. Edited by B.S. Hilaris. Acton, Publishing Sciences Group, 1975, pp. 61–85.
12. Loftus, T.P. and Weaver, J.T.: Standardization of Iridium-192 gamma-ray sources in terms of exposure. J. Res. Nat. Bur. Stand. (U.S.) *80*:19, 1979.
13. Meisberger, L.L., Keller, R.J., and Shalek, R.J.: The effective attenuation in water of the gamma-rays of Gold 198, Iridium 192, Cesium 137, Radium 226, and Cobalt 60. Radiology *90*:953, 1968.
14. National Council on Radiation Protection and Measurements: NCRP Report No. 41: Specification of gamma-ray brachytherapy sources. Washington, D.C.: NCRP, 1974, pp. 1–24.
15. Pierquin, B., Chassagne, D.J., Chahbasian, C.M., and Wilson, J.F.: Brachytherapy. St. Louis, Warren H. Green, 1978, pp. 157–191.
16. Quimby, E.H. and Castro, V.: The calculation of dosage in interstitial radium therapy. AJR *70*:739, 1953.
17. Shalek, R.J. and Stovall, M.: Dosimetry in implant therapy. *In* Radiation Dosimetry, 2nd ed., Vol III. Edited by F.H. Attix and E. Tachilin. New York, Academic Press, 1969, pp. 743–807.
18. Sharma, S.C., Williamson, J.F., and Cytacki, E.: Dosimetric analysis of stereo and orthogonal reconstruction of interstitial implants. Int. J. Radiat. Oncol. Biol. Phys. 1982 (in press).
19. Syed, A.M.N. and Feder, B.H.: Technique of afterloading interstitial implants. Radiol. Clin. *46*:458, 1977.
20. Tod, M. and Meredith, W.J.: Treatment of cancer of the cervix uteri—a revised "Manchester Method". Br. J. Radiol. *26*:252, 1953.
21. Wharton, J.T., Fletcher, G.H., and Delclos, L.: Invasive tumors of the vagina: Clinical features and management. *In* Gynecologic Oncology: Fundamental Principles and Clinical Practice, Vol. 1. Edited by M. Coppleson. Edinburgh, Churchill Livingstone, 1981, pp. 345–359.
22. Williamson, J.F., Khan, F.M., Sharma, S.C., and Fullerton, G.D.: Methods for routine calibration of brachytherapy sources. Radiology *142*:511, 1982.

Chapter 7

COMPUTERIZED TOMOGRAPHY IN RADIATION THERAPY TREATMENT PLANNING

Carlos A. Perez
James A. Purdy
Donald R. Ragan

Over the past 75 years, radiation therapy has evolved from empirical methods and technical uncertainties to great accuracy in delivering higher doses of irradiation to a tumor. The ultimate goal of radiation therapy is to combine the highest possible uncomplicated local and regional tumor control with an acceptable post-treatment quality of life and as few anatomic, physiologic, and psychologic disturbances as possible for the patient.

Herring[7] discussed the theoretical aspects of dose-response curves for tumor control and normal tissue damage. He based his considerations on the precision with which the dose of irradiation and the volume treated are defined, and postulated that with an imprecise treatment system, it is possible to have a high incidence of necrosis associated with relatively low tumor control. The radiotherapist, in an effort to reduce the complication rate, may lower the doses, thereby further decreasing the probability of tumor control.

Several reports in the recent past have correlated the doses of irradiation with tumor control in carcinoma of the oral tongue, base of the tongue, floor of the mouth, tonsil, larynx, vagina, and in some of the lymphomas (e.g., Hodgkin's disease). A close correlation exists between dose of irradiation and major complications in most organs. Fletcher[4] indicated that the tolerance of the normal tissues is related to the dose of irradiation, volume irradiated, nature and function of the organ within that volume, and the stage of the cancer being treated.

It is apparent that, in order to improve the quality of radiation therapy, better treatment planning must be developed. This involves a variety of factors: (1) clinical evaluation of the tumor extent and definition of the critical volume to be irradiated; (2) determination of the dose of irradiation that will provide high tumor control with minimal damage to surrounding normal tissues; (3) simulation and localization of treatment portals by radiographic techniques; and (4) elaborate dosimetric techniques for treatment verification, adequate immobilization and repositioning techniques.

One of the obstacles to optimal treatment planning in the past was the inability to accurately outline the tumor extent and the relationship of this volume to adjacent radiation-sensitive normal structures. Computerized tomography (CT) has greatly enhanced our ability to better define the contour of the patient, the extent of the tumor, and the location of normal organs. Several investigators have noted that the CT numbers correlate fairly well with the electron density of the absorber, which is the pertinent parameter for inhomogeneity correction used in current treatment-planning programs. Some computer software allows for the direct interfacing of the CT number matrix with a treatment-planning computer. Some computer programs also use multiplanar treatment-planning computations that approach a three-dimensional representation of the volume treated and the distribution of the radiation dose.

CT scanning is of value in a number of patients with tumors in the central nervous system (brain), thorax, retroperitoneal structures, or pelvis. These patients are usually treated with high-energy photons. It is predictable that CT scanning may play an even greater role in treatment planning with electron beams and high-linear-energy transfer particles. Because of the physical properties of these radiations, the definition of the tumor volume and the site at which the highest dose of irradiation is delivered are far more critical than with high-energy photons.

At present there is a need to evaluate the impact of CT scanning in radiation-therapy treatment planning and to accurately define those patients in whom the use of this sophisticated technology results in improved radiation distribution. The incorporation of CT information in treatment planning allows for optimization of dose while demanding better patient immobilization and repositioning techniques to insure the optimal delivery of irradiation to critical volumes.

Inaccuracies in treatment planning and delivery result from patient movement during scanning and treatment, daily variations in the source–surface distance (SSD), patient weight loss without a change in the treatment plan, timer or dose-monitoring imprecisions, inaccuracy in machine calibrations, nonlinearities and artifacts of the CT scanner, and inaccuracies of the tissue-air ratios (TAR).[5,6] Other factors that may affect the biologic effectiveness of radiotherapy include the number of fields treated daily, the number of fractions per week, interruption of the therapy without increasing the total dose.

It must be stressed that the skills of the clinician can never be totally replaced by technologic advances in diagnostic techniques, computer software, or technical aspects of radiotherapy. The ultimate responsibility for the selection and execution of radiation-therapy techniques, as well as for its consequences, rests with the radiation oncologist; no computer calculations or physics procedures can compensate for the radiation therapist's errors in judgment, misunderstanding of physical concepts, or unsatisfactory planning and delivery of radiation therapy.

TECHNICAL ASPECTS OF COMPUTERIZED TOMOGRAPHY

The CT scan consists of the reconstruction by computer on a tomographic plane of a patient's anatomy developed from multiple x-ray attenuation measurements made around the subject. The CT image is formed by using a mathematical technique known as reconstruction from projections. The data for the reconstruction process are obtained by mounting an x-ray source and an array of x-ray detectors in diametrical opposition on a gantry and moving them synchronously about the patient's body until many sets of transmission data in different directions have been measured.

The data thus obtained are processed by the computer and image reconstruction begins. Simply stated, the reconstruction consists of calculating the linear attenuation coefficient for each picture or pixel, and assigning a corresponding CT number to it (Fig. 7–1).

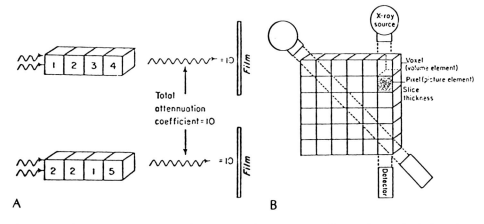

Fig. 7–1. Schematic representations of integration of attenuation coefficients from individual pixels to generate CT image.

The CT scan is composed of many individual volume elements, each with its own characteristic attenuation properties. These volume elements are reduced to a two-dimensional array of pixels. The computer displays this array of pixels on a video display monitor using varying shades of gray to represent the CT numbers. The CT numbers associated with the various tissues are related to the linear attenuation coefficient, μ, by the equation

$$\text{CT number} = \frac{K(\mu\text{tissue} - \mu\text{water})}{\mu\text{water}}$$

where K is a magnifying constant typically chosen to be either 500 (EMI number) or 1000 (Hounsfield number). It is the linear attenuation coefficient that is measured by a CT scan.

For a full discussion on reconstruction algorithms the reader is referred to the article by Brooks.[1] A discussion of the Algebraic Reconstruction Technique (ART) is presented here for illustrative purposes. In this method the *picture* is presented as a two-dimensional array of numbers, each representing the linear attenuation coefficient of an individual pixel; a *ray* is a narrow strip of the picture at a certain angle. The *ray sum* is the sum of the individual linear attenuation coefficients lying along that ray. This method assigns an initial set of linear attenuation coefficients to the two-dimensional picture to be reconstructed, calculates the ray sum along a one-dimensional projection of the initial picture, compares the calculated ray sum with the measured ray sum (transmission data) stored in the computer, and computes the difference and equally divides it among the pixels along the way. This procedure is repeated for all rays from all angles until a representative picture is constructed.

The validity of the final CT image depends on many other aspects of the scanner other than the reconstructs algorithms. These include: 1) nature of the x-ray source; 2) the collimation system; 3) the detectors; 4) the number of x-ray transmission measurements made; 5) the scan motion of the system about the subject; 6) the details of the picture-construction technique; and 7) the method of data display and interpretation.

APPLICATION OF COMPUTERIZED TOMOGRAPHY TO RADIATION THERAPY

CT contributes to the treatment-planning process in at least six areas: patient-contour definition, tumor localization, normal-structure localization, inhomogeneities, three-dimensional reconstruction, and evaluation of tumor status (Table 7–1).

Patient Contour

A CT scan provides patient-contour information that may be more accurate than conventional techniques (e.g., wire, plaster cast). The use of a curve couch or bolus to obtain the scan can result in some surface compression, which distorts the external contour. A more subtle distortion can occur in regard to patient positioning. Due to the small scan-ring size on many scanners, it is not always possible to duplicate the therapy setup; the position of some portion of the body may not be the same as during treatment. The small ring size also results in side-cutoff in many patients (i.e., shoulders, pelvis).

Tumor Location

Tumor localization for therapy treatment planning is determined by clinical examination, orthogonal radiographs, nuclear medicine studies, and ultrasound. It now appears that CT is complementary to these processes. We are now able to differentiate tumors from normal structures in the brain, the mediastinum, the retroperitoneal space, and the pelvis.

Normal-Structure Localization

In current treatment-planning procedures, this information is usually obtained from orthogonal radiographs, conventional transverse tomography, standard

TABLE 7–1. Applications of CT Scanning to Treatment Planning

1. Definition of patient contour
2. Determination of tumor extent
3. Localization of normal structures
4. Definition of tissue inhomogeneities
5. Correlation of multilevel anatomical sections with multiplanar isodose distributions
6. Assistance in dose optimization

anatomic displays available from atlases, or ultrasound scanning. Each of these methods is time-consuming and suffers from such limitations as inaccuracies and the need for special viewing devices. The usefulness of ultrasound is limited in the human thorax, the very region where dose perturbations caused by inhomogeneities may be the greatest. Normal-structure localization with CT is vastly superior to all the aforementioned methods.

Inhomogeneities

Three inhomogeneities are generally encountered in radiation therapy: air cavities, fat, and bone. All of these alter the distribution of irradiation in tissues. To correct fully for these inhomogeneities, it is necessary to know their size, shape, and position as well as their electron density and atomic number. The possibility now exists that CT numbers (which are related to the linear attenuation coefficients for x-rays of diagnostic energies) may be correlated with the electron density of the corresponding tissues (Fig. 7–2).[12,13] This is important because for the radiation used in therapy (all modalities, ^{60}Co through 25 MV x-rays) the Compton scattering is the dominant mode of interaction and the absorption and scattering of photons in tissue therefore depends primarily upon the electron density.

A dosimetric study to determine the accuracy of dose computations based on a CT-interfaced-therapy treatment-planning system has been carried out.[14] This system uses the matrix of CT numbers (160 × 160) generated by a diagnostic CT scan in computing the dose distribution in the plan of the scan. The array of CT numbers was used to do a pixel-by-pixel correction for tissue inhomogeneities. The results of these calculations were compared with experimental measurements using thermoluminescence dosimetry. These results showed that, for beams of simple geometry, the simple conventional inhomogeneity correction (i.e., outlining the inho-

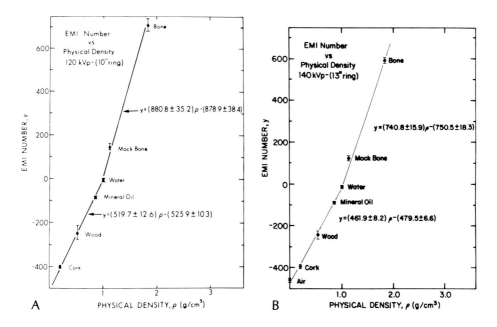

Fig. 7–2.   Draft with EMI numbers *(A)* and electron density *(B)*.

mogeneity and assigning a density) is in agreement with the more sophisticated pixel-by-pixel calculations as long as the geometric outline of the various inhomogeneities and their densities were accurately put into the computer for the conventional method of calculation (Fig. 7–3 and Table 7–2). Assignment of appropriate electron densities poses a problem because such values are normally not readily available and may vary significantly from patient to patient. The pixel calculations that require the CT-scan information seem to have a distinct advantage over conventional calculation as far as these problems are concerned. From a practical point of view, it is a very convenient method of treatment planning; however, this system is more expensive and the cost factor must be considered in the implementation of such a system for routine clinical use.

In an experiment evaluating the effect of tissue inhomogeneity corrections, Sontag et al.[18] showed that if no corrections for changes in the electron density of the patient's structures were considered in the computations, differences as high as 30%

in the dose calculation were noted, with an average difference between measured and computed doses of 9.9%. Using the equivalent TAR method for inhomogeneity corrections with an outline of the lung provided by cross-sectional anatomy text, the average dose difference decreased to 7.6%. When using the equivalent TAR method, the correct patient outline, and the density of the lung, however, the average dose difference was reduced to 1.6%.[19] This difference approached the limits of accuracy of the lithium-fluoride dosimetry that was used for the direct measurements (Figures 7–4 and 7–5).

The experiments were repeated with 25 MV x-rays.[18] With this energy, the average precision for the lithium-fluoride dosimetry was 2.7% and there was a greater effect of the electron buildup and interface over a distance of several centimeters. The change in dose-per-centimeter inhomogeneity can be much greater in this region than in areas where full electronic equilibrium is established. The equivalent TAR method accounts for this effect in the buildup region; however, the calculated

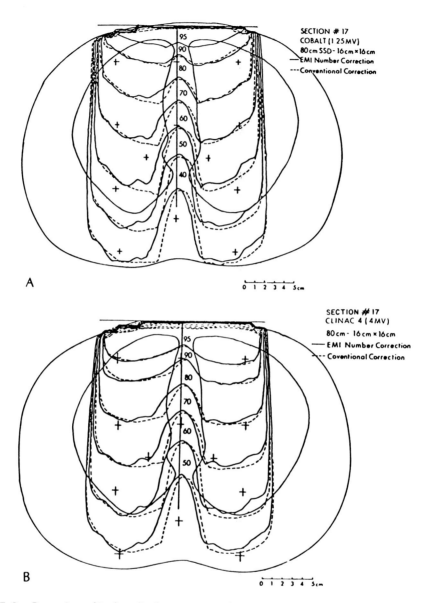

Fig. 7–3. Comparison of isodose distribution corrected *(A)* and uncorrected *(B)* for inhomogeneities.

doses were still in error by 6% to 8%. At these higher energies, most of the scatter of radiation is forward and has an energy similar to that of the primary beam. The lateral extent of the inhomogeneity volumes thus becomes less critical in those computations. In these experiments, the internal structures were delineated with a spatial resolution of about 5 mm and a relative electron density accuracy of about 2%. The dose calculated by the equivalent TAR method under these conditions has an average accuracy of better than 2% for ^{60}Co and 3% for 25 MV photons. We concluded that the most severe errors in computing the dose distribution with high-energy photons are caused by inaccurate delineation of the geometric outlines of tissue inhomogeneities. Less severe errors in dose calculations are due to the use of

TABLE 7–2.   Average Error and Standard Deviation*

Method of Computation	^{60}Co		4 MV		25 MV	
	RAD-8	PC-12	RAD-8	PC-12	RAD-8	PC-12
No inhomogeneity correction	$-12.9 \pm 12.7\%$	$-12.1 \pm 12.7\%$	$-11.0 \pm 12.6\%$	$-11.8 \pm 12.1\%$	$-4.2 \pm 6.7\%$	$-3.7 \pm 5.7\%$
Conventional inhomogeneity correction	$+0.7 \pm 2.8\%$	$+1.8 \pm 2.6\%$	$+1.0 \pm 4.3\%$	$+1.7 \pm 3.6\%$	$+3.3 \pm 2.7\%$	$+1.6 \pm 4.1\%$
Pixel by pixel inhomogeneity correction	$-0.4 \pm 1.8\%$	—	$0 \pm 3.4\%$	—	$+2.5 \pm 3.2\%$	—

*Summary of average errors and standard deviations of computed doses relative to measured values for irradiations with three types of beam in the thoracic region. The average errors were obtained by averaging the errors at various locations of the TL dosimeters.

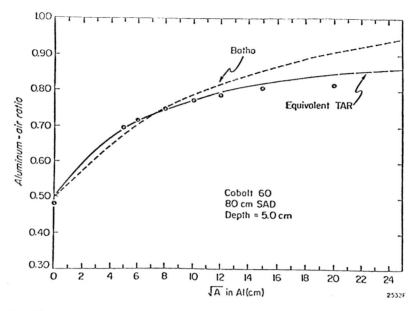

Fig. 7–4. "Aluminum–air ratio" plotted against the side lengths of square beams. The solid circles represent measurements made in an aluminum phantom, the solid line is calculated by scaling depth and field of tissue–air ratios by the electron density (2.33) of aluminum. The dashed line is caclulated using the power law tissue–air ratio method. (From Sontag et al.: Radiology *129*:787, 1978.)

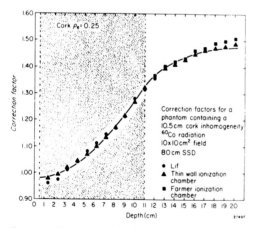

Fig. 7–5. Comparison of calculation and measurement for a phantom containing a large insert of cork. First there was 0.5 cm of polystyrene then 10.5 cm of cork followed by over 30 cm of polystyrene. The calculation is by the effective tissue–air ratio method. (From Sontag et al.: Radiology *129*:787, 1978.)

inaccurate relative electron density for the inhomogeneity, provided its outline is accurate.

Three-Dimensional Reconstruction

The ability of CT to present the physician with multiplanar sections allows a conceptual three-dimensional representation of the tumor, the surrounding internal structures, and the external contour of the patient. A major step will have been made toward developing a true volumetric treatment-planning system when more sophisticated computer software and display systems are developed.

We recommend that CT scans be used for treatment planning whenever possible. Centers intending to purchase a CT scanner for the sole purpose of dose calculations, however, are strongly advised to consider simpler, more economical methods which include the enlargement of the CT scan to life-size by photographic methods and the tracing of patient contours, tissue inhomogeneities, and tumor volume from the magnified image. These outlines can be entered into the present treatment-planning systems with an appropriate transducer; the electron-density values that correspond to the various regions can be assigned by the computer in the conventional manner.[5,6]

Evaluation of Tumor Status

CT scans are extremely useful in the initial diagnostic workup of the patient not only in determining the extent of the tumor, but also in other areas of involvement. They provide information that may influence tumor management (e.g., criteria for resectability, indications for combined irradiation, chemotherapy, and/or surgical resection—Table 7–3). During therapy, CT scans may be useful in evaluating the response of a lesion to the treatment. They can also help the physician decide among the possible modifications that may be introduced in the irradiation techniques (e.g., reduced fields for boosts, planning brachytherapy).

CT may be invaluable in the follow-up of patients. It can be used to quantitatively document the response of a tumor to therapy and for the early detection of tumor persistence or recurrence. Documentation on the effects of irradiation or other agents in normal tissues may also become available.

In patients irradiated for brain tumors studies by Marks[8] demonstrated the capability of CT to document both short- and long-term radiation effects. Although the etiology of the diseases suitable for whole-body CT workups is significantly different from central-nervous-system (CNS) tumors, similar studies should be rewarding for many other lesions.

One of the more exciting uses of CT is the documentation of the location of recurrences (infield, extrafield, or marginal). The physician often wants to know whether the recurrence is on the previous tumor margin. Although CT scanning is not a cost-effective screening tool for patient follow-up, comparison of past and present CT scans upon recurrence can provide invaluable information about the efficacy of current treatment techniques.

An area that has not been adequately explored is that of using CT information to correlate the morphologic characteristics of the tumor and the response to therapy. Areas of avascular tumor necrosis that are known to be more difficult to control by irradiation may have a different electron density than surrounding tissues. The composition of the stroma of the tumor may be an important factor in the tumor's response to irradiation or cytotoxic agents. The spatial relationship of the tumor to surrounding sensitive normal structures may be crucial in determining the factors that affect the incidence of complications following therapy.[10]

CURRENT PROBLEMS WITH COMPUTERIZED TOMOGRAPHY IN TREATMENT PLANNING

The use of CT in treatment planning is not without technical problems. Some of these have been partially corrected in the recent past and others need further refinement.

The curved couch that was customarily used for early diagnostic CT scans deforms the patient's external anatomy. It is therefore necessary to use a "filler" to provide a flat surface on which the patient lies; however, this decreases the amount of space available in the ring and excludes large patients from examination. In some areas (e.g., the thorax, the abdomen, the pelvis) the lateral portion of the contours are lost. In volumes with no tissue inhomogeneity, the problem may be corrected when doing the treatment plan; however, it remains an unresolved problem in the thorax.

An extremely important technical detail is the performance of CT scans in exactly

TABLE 7–3.   Application of Computed Tomography to Tumor Status

1. Pretherapy staging
2. Correlation of morphology with tumor histology and clinical course
3. Resectability criteria
4. Morphology after surgery
5. Regression after therapy
6. Detection of persistence or recurrence

the same position in which the patient will be treated. This increases the accuracy of treatment planning.

The transfer of the tissue densities to the treatment-planning computer can be carried out by photographic means; an enlargement stand can be used to produce the necessary outline of the patient's contour, the tumor volume, and the location of normal structures. The direct transfer of the density matrix (EMI numbers) from the diagnostic CT scanners to the treatment-planning computer is a more sophisticated method. A tape or floppy-disk drive is needed for this method.

According to Geise and McCullough,[5] the need to interface a treatment-planning computer to provide access to the CT numbers (which can be individually converted to relative electron densities) is of questionable value for megavoltage-photon beams at the present time. They recognize that, with the excellent detail in cross-sectional anatomy provided by the CT scan, the present methods used for correction of dose distribution for inhomogeneities may be replaced by other, more accurate approaches. They concluded that the use of CT numbers for treatment planning must include a method of normalizing the variability of machine operation[9] from scan to scan and the variations in CT numbers that may result when performed in sequential scans due to differences in subject size. A user-oriented control program that calibrates the contrast scale over a large range of electron densities is needed. The image improprieties of each CT scan must be documented, as indicated by McCullough et al.[9] When such a system becomes available it may be a major contribution to the improvement of the accuracy of treatment planning in radiation therapy. A need for such a system must be carefully established before undertaking extensive development of a CT-scanner treatment-planning computer that interfaces with costly hardware.

The vast majority of treatment-planning calculations available are two-dimensional, even if performed in more than one plane. Current computer software does not allow for three-dimensional treatment-planning dose calculations or display of isodose distributions. Payne et al.[12] carried out multiple ^{60}Co phantom transmission measurements to generate attenuation coefficients that are used in dose computations to provide more accurate three-dimensional isodose distributions.

The increased information provided by the diagnostic CT scans must be used to obtain optimal dose distribution of the irradiation in the target volume and the surrounding normal tissues. At the present time the dose optimization is accomplished through trial and error. Optimization programs such as that developed by Redpath,[16] which, under limited conditions, can compute doses with up to six beams with greater capabilities, are needed in making better use of the additional CT information.

It should be stressed that sophisticated treatment planning should be followed by extremely accurate treatment delivery, patient repositioning, and verification techniques (Figs. 7–6, 7–7, and 7–8).

EVALUATION

There is little doubt that CT scanners contribute significantly to the diagnosis of CNS tumors. It is also true that CT has had a major impact in the area of tumor localization in many anatomic sites. There are some lesions, such as mediastinal, retroperitoneal, and pancreatic tumors, that can only be effectively outlined through the use of CT. There is, however, no clear definition as to when CT scans are indicated, nor are there many conventional tests that could be replaced by CT scanning.

According to Stewart et al.[22] the incorporation of CT in treatment planning will have an impact in several areas of radiation therapy:

> A It will improve clinical assessment of tumor extent and location

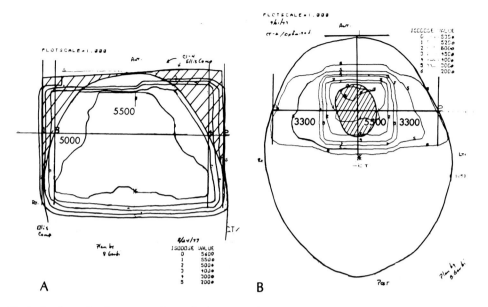

Fig. 7–6. Example of treatment plan with conventional information *(A)* and CT scan *(B)* in patient with pituitary tumor.

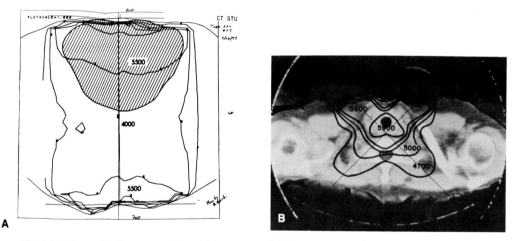

Fig. 7–7. Example of treatment plan with conventional information *(A)* and CT scan *(B)* in patient with anaplastic carcinoma of superior mediastinum.

of adjacent critical normal structures.

B It will provide a systematic approach to the accuracy of radiation dose distribution by introducing a three-dimensional volumetric approach to treatment planning.

C It will provide more reliable information (through more accurate

computations) on the maximum tolerated doses of irradiation by normal tissues.

D It will focus attention on the accurate reproducibility of treatment conditions with daily fractionated irradiation to deliver the planned dose to the patient.

It is critical that efficacy studies be performed under controlled conditions to as-

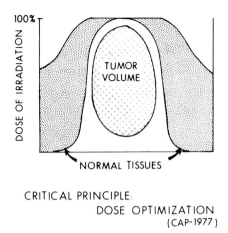

CRITICAL PRINCIPLE:
DOSE OPTIMIZATION
(CAP-1977)

Fig. 7–8. Use of CT information in treatment planning.

sess the impact of CT treatment planning on tumor control, complications, and survival of patients treated with irradiation.

Even if not interfaced directly with a treatment-planning system, CT provides more accurate tumor and normal-structure localization. Initial reports[15,21] indicate significant differences in accuracy between CT scans and estimates based on conventional treatment-planning techniques. Differences in structure localization of between 1 cm and 3 cm were not uncommon.

Munzenrider et al.[11] studied 75 patients with primary tumors in the head and neck, the breast or chest wall, the thorax, or the pelvis who had CT scans done for treatment-planning purposes. They reported that the planned treatment volume was unchanged in 41 of the patients (55%), larger in 16 (21%), and smaller in 18 (24%). The CT scan showed that the initial tumor coverage, analyzed with the added CT-scan information, was clearly inadequate in 15 patients (20%), marginal in 20 (27%), and adequate in 40 (53%). They concluded that CT-scan information was critical for treatment planning in 41 patients (55%), helpful in 23 (31%), and unnecessary in 11 (14%). Frequently, however, these discrepancies did not motivate an improvement in treatment plan.

We felt that the added CT information was extremely helpful in treatment planning in 16 of 25 patients (64%) with abdominal lesions, and in 14 of 21 patients (67%) with primary bronchogenic carcinoma treated with radiation therapy. We thought that the CT data had relatively little effect in the treatment planning of patients with head and neck cancer or pelvic neoplasias. In the breast and in postoperative radiation of the chest wall, CT scans were thought to be useful in determining the location or the status of the internal mammary lymph nodes. In our experience this information may be of some use when the patients are treated with electrons; it is not necessary when photons are used for irradiation of the lymph-node-bearing areas. In addition, no significant information is gained with the CT scans if the breast or the chest wall is treated with tangential portals.

Sheedy et al.[17] and Stanley et al.[20] concluded that CT scanning was especially helpful in the diagnosis of suspected lesions in the retroperitoneal space (e.g., lymph nodes, pancreas, kidney, liver).

In a similar report by Ragan et al.[15] 25 out of 45 patients had modifications in

TABLE 7–4. Treatment Plan Optimization with CT

	Optimization		
	Yes	**No**	**Total**
CNS	3	3	6
Head & Neck	3	5	8
Breast	0	4	4
Lung*	3	0	3
Gynecologic	5	1	6
Prostate	3	2	5
Abdomen (NOS)	6	2	8
Lymphoma	2	3	5
TOTAL	25	20	45

*Lung patients benefited not only from improved localization of tumor but also from improved inhomogeneity corrections upon treatment planning with CT information.

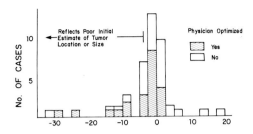

Fig. 7–9. Phase I–Phase II nonuniformity graph.

treatment volume and dose distribution on the basis of CT information (Table 7–4). In this study, an attempt was made to quantify the contribution that CT information would make to treatment planning. A strong correlation between local efficiency and nonuniformity of dose[2] and physician estimation of the quality of treatment plan was documented. Large discrepancies were found to exist between the uniformity prescribed by the physician using a conventional treatment-planning workup versus the uniformity measured taking advantage of CT information (Fig. 7–9). This in turn correlated with the physician's desire to improve the patient's treatment plan. There is, therefore, a strong indication that discrepancy exists between structure localization in conventional patient workups and reality and that the physicians are both willing and able to take advantage of the improved CT information in order to optimize patient treatment.

In addition to the use of treatment plans for patient treatment, much of the use of treatment-planning systems is for dosimetric documentation. Because the documentation is only as good as the initial estimate of tumor location and patient structure by the physician, significant advantage can be gained in clinical research by the addition of CT documentation of patient structure. This may be an asset in both research and legal problems arising from complications of treatment.

COST

Along with the potential benefit of CT scanning for radiation oncology, there is a concomitant cost. If contouring and external patient definition ($10–$20) were to be replaced by CT scan ($100–$200), there would be a 10-fold increase in cost. Computer-assisted treatment-planning systems that use CT information can cost two or three times as much as conventional treatment systems. At the present time, it would be difficult to justify a CT scanner devoted entirely to treatment planning unless it were in a very large radiation therapy center. Time-sharing with diagnostic applications should provide enough usage to reduce the cost of the examinations. It is not known how many slices should be obtained in order to generate the necessary information for planning; it is probable that 1 cm intervals are adequate. A careful analysis of operational cost of CT scans has been published by Evens and Jost.[3] Initial cost of installation and projected operational cost are shown in Tables 7–5 and 7–6.

As shown by Stewart et al.,[22] the increased accuracy in treatment planning provided by CT may result in significantly higher local and regional tumor control. This will be reflected in substantial sav-

TABLE 7–5. Whole-Body CT Scanner Cost Data

	All units
Equipment cost ($)	526,000
Years depreciated	5
Accelerated depreciation	4/52
Space allocation (ft²)	694
Remodeling cost ($)	55,500
Space cost ($/ft²/yr)	13.52
Technologists (FTE)	2.0
Other personnel	1.0
Contrast cost ($)/patient	6.83
Other supply cost ($)/patient	12.66

(From Evens, R.G., Jost, R.G.: Radiology 127, 1978.)

TABLE 7–6.   Whole-Body CT Effect of Patient Volume on Technical Costs

Costs	Patient/Week			
	25	30	40	50
Fixed	217,183	217,183	217,183	217,183
Variable	22,230	26,676	35,568	44,460
Indirect	119,707	121,930	126,376	130,822
Total	359,120	365,789	379,127	392,465
Cost/patient ($)	276.25	234.48	182.27	150.95

(From Evens, R.G., Jost, R.G.: Radiology 127, 1978.)

ings in the cost of caring for cancer patients.

NEEDS OF COMPUTERIZED TOMOGRAPHY SCANNERS IN RADIATION THERAPY

As outlined in the report by Stewart et al.,[22] current radiation therapy units must have features beyond their purely diagnostic capabilities, in order to optimize the information provided by CT scans in radiation therapy

The position information must be transferred to the radiation-therapy unit.

The reconstructed data should be available in numerical form and readily transferable to the dose-calculation computer.

Multiple scans of a patient should be made to generate three-dimensional reconstructions in multiple plans.

Scans should be reproducible under various physical conditions (correlation of EMI or Hounsfield units and electron density).

Special criteria for the design of the CT scanner should be kept in mind to improve the operation of the unit, to obtain multiple sections, to provide adequate coverage and special resolution of volumes used in radiation therapy, and to display the CT data in any plane or combinations of planes required for treatment planning.

There are specific areas that demand intensive research concerning the applications of CT in cancer management and treatment planning in the future:

1. Development of treatment-planning algorithms to accommodate the additional information about patient contour, inhomogeneities, and multiple-plane definition of tumor and normal structures.

2. Correction for perturbation of dose of photons and electrons by tissue inhomogeneities. This should later be expanded to high LET particles.

3. Incorporation of beam modifiers with moving photon and electron beams and correlation with three-dimensional treatment planning.

4. Development of effective three-dimensional treatment-planning and display techniques.

5. Patient-position verification techniques during treatment planning and radiation treatment, to insure that the planned dose is actually delivered to the patient.

6. Evaluation of tumor response after irradiation, chemotherapy, or surgical resection as well as early detection of recurrences.

7. Evaluation of the effects of therapy on normal tissues.

Computerized tomography represents a new dimension in the definition of the patient's contours, tumor, and organ structures. This provides a greater degree of accuracy in treatment planning and delivery techniques. There are some technical problems in the application of this new development to routine treatment planning in radiation therapy; however, intensive research and development in the near future should overcome some of these difficulties and significantly improve existing capabilities for treatment planning. A careful assessment of the impact of computerized tomography in the treatment planning and outcome of radiation therapy is necessary before large commitments of funds are made.

REFERENCES

1. Brooks, R.A., DiChiro, G.: Theory of image reconstruction in computed tomography. Radiology *117*:561, 1975.
2. Ellis, F., Oliver, R.: The specification of tumour dose. Br. J. Radiol. *34*:258, 1961.
3. Evens, R.G., Jost, R.G.: Economic analysis of body computed tomography units—including data on utilization. Radiology *127*:151, 1978.
4. Fletcher, G.H., Shukovsky, L.J.: The interplay of radiocurability and tolerance in the irradiation of human cancers. J. Radiol. Electrol. *56*:383, 1975.
5. Geise, R.A., McCullough, E.C.: The use of CT scanners in megavoltage photon-beam therapy planning. Radiology *124*:133, 1977.
6. Hendee, W.R., Ibbott, G.S.: The problem of body inhomogeneities in radiation therapy. Appl. Radiol. *5*:138, 1976.
7. Herring, D.F.: The consequences of dose response curves for tumor control and normal tissue injury on the precision necessary in patient management. Laryngoscope *85*:1112, 1975.
8. Marks, J.E., Gado, M.: Serial computed tomography of primary brain tumors following surgery, irradiation and chemotherapy. Radiology *125*:119, 1977.
9. McCullough, E.C. et al.: Performance evaluation and quality assurance of computed tomography scanners, with illustrations from MEI, ACTA, and Delta scanners. Radiology *120*:173, 1976.
10. Mikael, M.A.: Radiation necrosis of the brain: Correlation between computed tomography, pathology, and dose distribution. J. Comput. Assist. Tomogr. *2*:71,1978.
11. Munzenrider, J.E. et al.: Use of body scanner in radiotherapy treatment planning. Cancer *40*:170, 1977.
12. Payne, W.H., Waggener, R.G., McDavid, W.D., Dennis, M.J.: Treatment planning in cobalt-60 radiotherapy using computerized tomography techniques. Med. Phys. *5*:48, 1978.
13. Phelps, M.E., Gado, M.H., Hoffman, E.J.: Correlation of elective atomic number and electron density with attenuation coefficients measured with polychromatic x-rays. Radiology *117*:585, 1975.
14. Prasad, S.C., Glasgow, G.P., Purdy, J.A.: Dosimetric evaluation of computed tomography treatment planning system. Radiology *130*:777, 1979.
15. Ragan, D.P. et al.: Evaluation of computerized treatment planning utilizing computer assisted tomography. (Abstract) Phys. Med. Biol. *22*:127, 1977.
16. Redpath, A.T., Vickery, B.L., Wright, D.H.: A new technique for radiotherapy planning using quadratic programming. Phys. Med. Biol. *21*:781, 1976.
17. Sheedy II, P.F. et al.: Computed tomography of the body: Initial clinical trial with the EMI prototype. Am. J. Roentgenol. *127*:23, 1976.
18. Sontag, M.R., Battista, J.J., Bronskill, M.J., Cunningham, J.R.: Implications of computed tomography for inhomogeneity corrections in photon beam dose calculations. Radiology *124*:143, 1977.
19. Sontag, M.R., Cunningham, J.R.: The equivalent tissue-air ratio needed for making absorbed dose calculations in a heterogeneous medium. Radiology *129*:787, 1978.
20. Stanley, R.J., Sagel, S.S., Levitt, R.G.: Computed tomography of the body: Early trends in application and accuracy of the method. Am. J. Roentgenol. *127*:53, 1976.
21. Sternick, E.S., Curran, B., Loomis, S.A., Lane, F.W.: The whole-body scanner and the large time sharing computer: Their role in radiotherapy treatment planning. (Abstract) Phys. Med. Biol. *22*:127, 1977.
22. Stewart, J.R., Hicks, J.A., Boone, M.L.M., Simpson, L.D.: Computed tomography in radiation therapy. Int. J. Radiat. Oncol. Biol. Phys. *4*:313, 1978.

Chapter 8

IRRADIATION TECHNIQUES FOR HEAD AND NECK CANCER

James E. Marks

Fransiska Lee

The radiation therapist who treats a patient with head-and-neck cancer has two goals: the uncomplicated destruction of the primary tumor and regional lymphatic metastases, and the preservation of normal tissues and function. For each individual site in the head and neck, the radiotherapist must have an intimate knowledge of the patterns of local and regional tumor spread, the anatomic barriers, and the anatomic relationship between normal structures and the volume to be irradiated. He must then select a field perimeter that adequately encompasses the tumor and its regional lymph nodes, as well as a dose distribution that delivers a potentially tumoricidal dose with relative sparing of normal tissues in the irradiated volume. The optimal field perimeter is large enough to prevent regrowth of tumor at the margins of the irradiated volume and yet limited enough to prevent excessive irradiation of adjacent normal structures. The optimal dose distribution is sufficiently large to prevent tumor recurrence, but not so large as to cause late radiation complications in normal tissues. Achievement of optimal field perimeters and dose distributions for the irradiation of head-and-neck cancers is an art that requires continued practice and revision when fol-

low-up of patients shows excessive recurrence of a tumor within or adjacent to the irradiated volume, or excessive late radiation complications. The goal of this chapter is to illustrate field perimeters and dose distributions used at the Mallinckrodt Institute of Radiology.

PATIENT SETUP

The mechanics of preparing a patient with head-and-neck cancer for irradiation are standardized at Mallinckrodt Institute. These procedures are reviewed here before proceeding to specific field perimeters and dose distributions for individual sites.

Field Perimeter

The patient undergoes a careful physical and radiographic examination to localize the primary tumor. External landmarks are then placed on the patient's skin to define the volume to be irradiated. For some sites, the relationship between the external landmarks and internal anatomy is determined by visual inspection, for others it is determined by radiographic technique. If radiographic technique is used, the following steps are observed: a radiograph is taken of the head-and-neck area, the field perimeter is drawn on the

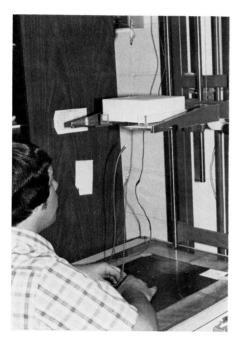

Fig. 8–1. Cutting of styrofoam mold using hot wire apparatus to trace the field perimeter drawn onto a film of the patient.

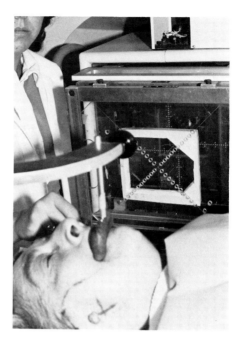

Fig. 8–2. Establishing the relationship between external and internal radiographic anatomy by fluoroscopy on the simulator. A styrofoam pseudoblock is used and external landmarks are traced onto the patient's skin with ink.

film, a Cerrobend block[7] is made (Fig. 8–1), and the block is fluoroscopically adjusted on the simulator to encompass the internal anatomy outlined on the film (Fig. 8–2). Light from the simulator projects through the block onto the patient's skin, thereby defining the field. The margins of the field are outlined in ink on the patient's skin, and the relationship between external landmarks and internal anatomy is determined.

Dose Distribution

An outline of the horizontal contour is made at the level of the primary tumor, and the tumor and normal structures in the irradiated volume are drawn onto the outline. The spatial relationship between the tumor, the normal structures, and the external surface of the patient are determined by physical examination, measurement, radiographs, and computerized tomography (CT) scans. Great care is taken to accurately localize the spinal cord on

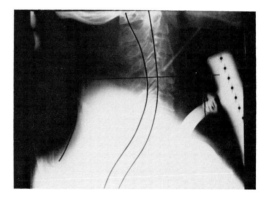

Fig. 8–3. Cross-table lateral radiograph to localize the spinal cord in relation to the anterior and posterior skin surfaces for accurate treatment planning.

the contour outline by taking cross-table-lateral or overhead films on the simulator to determine the position of the spinal cord relative to the anterior and posterior or right and left lateral skin surfaces (Fig. 8–3). Similar care is taken to localize the tumor, parotid glands, temporomandib-

ular joints, mandible, and paranasal sinuses. CT scan is probably the most accurate method of determining the
relationship between external contour,
tumor, and normal structures, but, in the
absence of CT, careful physical examination, measurement, and review of radiographs suffice. The contour, tumor, and
normal structures are traced by a computer
stylus and appear on the computer screen,
which allows the dosimetrist to study various treatment plans and search for an optimal dose distribution. Once determined,
the final dose reconstruction is printed on
paper and given to the radiotherapist who
uses it to execute the irradiation of the
patient.

Limitation of Dose to Normal Structures

To preserve anatomy and function, the
development of techniques that limit dose
to normal structures is emphasized whenever possible. Field perimeters are designed to exclude critical structures when
radiation tolerance is approached; dose
distributions are used that limit the dose
to normal structures within the field perimeter. High-energy x-rays are used to displace the dose centrally, thereby reducing
the dose to superficially located structures. Electrons are used to lateralize the
dose to spare contralateral and sensitive
midline structures. The following is a brief
summary of field perimeters and dose distributions that are used to spare individual
normal structures.

Spinal Cord

The spinal cord is routinely shielded
after a dose of 4000 rad in 4 weeks. Radiographic documentation of the posterior
field margin on the simulator is routinely
done to show that the spinal cord is protected. For nasopharyngeal and oropharyngeal tumors, Cerrobend-block inserts
(Fig. 8–4) are made to shield the cord so
that we may continue to use compensating
filters that have been designed for the
larger fields. An adjustable Cerrobend

block shields the spinal cord for oral-cavity tumors. Electron-beam irradiation is
used to electively or therapeutically irradiate the posterior cervical triangle (Fig.
8–5) so that dose is concentrated superficially to spare the underlying spinal cord.
A 2-cm-wide midline shield on the skin is
routinely used for the anterior low-neck
field (Fig. 8–6); this shield crosses the
junction between the upper lateral fields
and the anterior low-neck field, thereby
reducing the potentially excessive dose to
the spinal cord that might result from overlap of these fields.

Larynx

The larynx is routinely shielded during
the irradiation of nasopharyngeal, oropharyngeal, and oral-cavity tumors. This
is done by constructing the inferior margin
so that it passes beneath the hyoid bone
(see Fig. 8–4) to include the suprahyoid
portion of the epiglottis and to exclude the
vestibule of the supraglottis, arytenoids,
and phonatory larynx. The midline shield
that is used for the anterior low-neck field
shields the larynx as well as the pharynx
and spinal cord. It also significantly reduces arytenoid and endolaryngeal edema
and preserves normal voice quality.

Temporomandibular Joints and Mandible

The temporomandibular joint is necessarily included during the irradiation of
nasopharyngeal, oropharyngeal, parotid,
and temporal bone tumors, but may be excluded for the irradiation of oral-cavity,
laryngeal, and hypopharyngeal tumors.
Much of the body of the mandible can also
be shielded when laryngeal and hypopharyngeal tumors are irradiated. A 2000-
to 3000-rad boost is routinely delivered
with high-energy x-rays for centrally located nasopharyngeal, pharyngeal wall,
and some tonsil tumors in order to cen-
tralize the dose in the region of the tumor
and minimize the dose to the temporomandibular joints and mandible (Fig. 8–7).
A greater proportion of the total dose may

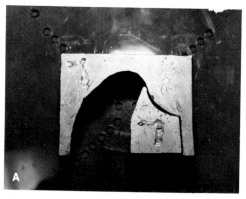

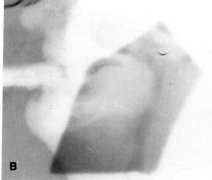

Fig. 8–4. Cerrobend block *(A)* with an insert to protect the spinal cord and a portal film *(B)* documenting that the spinal cord is shielded.

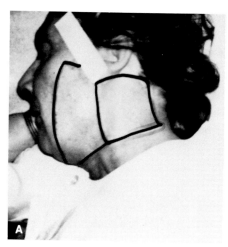

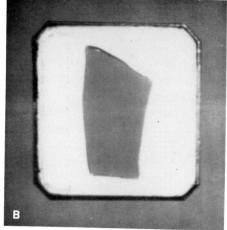

Fig. 8–5. Treatment portal *(A)* and Cerrobend mask *(B)* for electron beam irradiation of the posterior neck.

be delivered using high-energy x-rays for nasopharyngeal tumors than for tonsil tumors because nasopharyngeal tumors are located more centrally than tonsil tumors. Care must be taken not to produce a gradient of dose across a tonsillar fossa lesion when attempting to reduce the dose to the mandible and temporomandibular joint.

To prevent fibrosis of the temporomandibular joint and radiation damage to the mandible (Fig. 8–8), weighting the dose distribution to the side of the lesion using low-energy megavoltage beams (4 MV x-rays and ^{60}Co) should be avoided. Weighting or loading is accomplished whenever

possible by delivering high-energy x-rays to the side of the lesion (Fig. 8–9). To assure homogeneous dose distribution throughout the irradiated volume on a given day, two fields per day are routinely irradiated with 4 MV x-rays and ^{60}Co gamma rays. Only one field per day is irradiated using high-energy x-rays because the maximum dose is deep to superficial structures.

Parotid Glands

Parotid, skin, buccal mucosa, and submaxillary-gland tumors are commonly irradiated with unilateral electron-beam

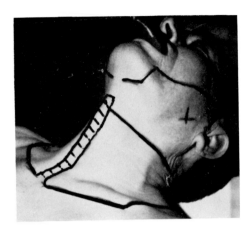

Fig. 8–6. Anterior low-neck field with a central shield that crosses the junction between the upper lateral and low neck fields.

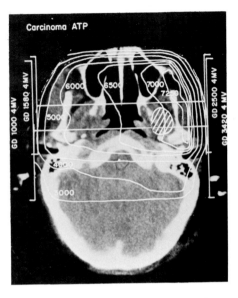

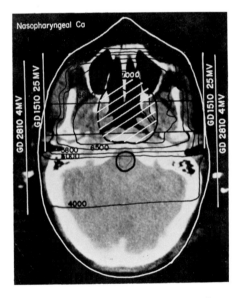

Fig. 8–8. Dose reconstruction and CT scan for carcinoma of the anterior tonsillar pillar. The excessive dose to the temporomandibular joints and mandible that results from weighting the dose distribution to the side of the tumor with 4 MeV x-rays is shown.

Fig. 8–7. Dose reconstruction and CT scan for nasopharyngeal carcinoma showing the use of high-energy x-rays in combination with 4 MeV x-rays to concentrate dose in the central region of tumor with relative sparing of temporomandibular joints.

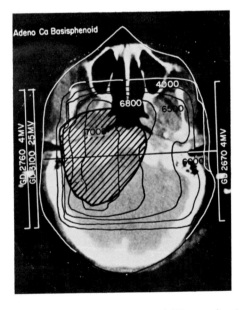

techniques in order to spare the opposite parotid and preserve salivary function.[4] Patients are treated with electron-beam irradiation four times weekly and ^{60}Co irradiation once weekly (Fig. 8–10); the use of ^{60}Co once weekly, in conjunction with electrons, spares skin enough that wet desquamation does not result from doses of 5000 to 6000 rad in 5 to 6 weeks.

Fig. 8–9. Dose reconstruction and CT scan showing concentration of dose in the region of tumor by using high-energy x-rays from the side of the tumor in combination with 4 MeV x-rays.

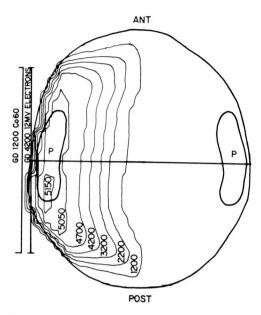

Fig. 8–10. Dose reconstruction showing unilateral technique of irradiating skin and parotid tumors with electron beam and ^{60}Co to spare the opposite parotid (**P**).

High-energy x-rays are used for nasopharyngeal and oropharyngeal tumors in order to spare superficially located parotid glands as well as temporomandibular joints and the mandible.

When irradiating oral-cavity tumors, it is possible to limit the irradiated volume to the tongue with significant sparing of the buccal and retromandibular portions of the parotid. This technique is illustrated in the section on oral-cavity tumors.

Ear

The ear is routinely included in the treatment field for nasopharyngeal cancer because placement of a block to shield the ear can easily shield a portion of the nasopharynx (Fig. 8–11).[5] Some radiotherapists avoid this potential shielding by directing the beam posteriorly, but we believe such complexity in beam direction can only increase technical errors and reduce delivery of dose to the nasopharyngeal tumor. We prefer to treat the resultant external otitis and serous otitis media. The

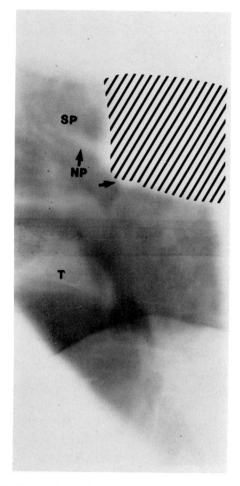

Fig. 8–11. Portal film showing that a block used to shield the ear has nearly shielded the nasopharynx. Arrows point to the vault of the nasopharynx (**NP**). Also shown are the sphenoid bone (**SP**), and the tongue (**T**).

ear can be shielded for most tumors of the oral cavity, larynx, and hypopharynx.

Optic Nerves and Eye

The optic nerves are routinely irradiated with high doses for extensive nasopharyngeal, sphenoid, and ethmoidal-maxillary tumors. An attempt to shield the optic nerve is not made; conventional fractionation of 180 to 200 rad per day is used and the avoidance of excessive doses to these structures is achieved though meticulous treatment planning.

When tumors of the ethmoidal-maxillary region involve the orbit, the eye is

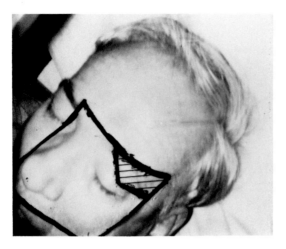

Fig. 8–12. Shielding of the lacrimal gland from the anterior radiation field for a patient with a large tumor of the paranasal sinuses.

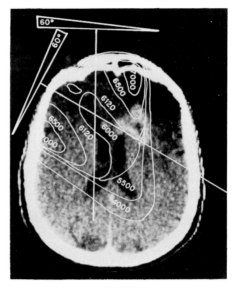

Fig. 8–13. Dose reconstruction superimposed onto a CT scan showing pathologically documented cerebral radionecrosis in a patient who was irradiated for recurrent adenoid cystic carcinoma of the paranasal sinuses.

routinely included. Orbital involvement is usually medial and inferior so that it is possible to shield the upper outer quadrant of the eye for a portion of the treatment (i.e., after 3000 to 4000 rad have been delivered). The medial third of the retina often receives a full dose and is damaged beyond repair. It is impossible to shield the lens; if the patient's tumor is controlled, the lens can later be enucleated.

Lacrimal Gland

Due to its location in the upper outer quadrant of the orbit, the lacrimal gland can frequently be shielded (Fig. 8–12) during the irradiation of a paranasal-sinus tumor; such shielding prevents dry eye, corneal keratitis, and phthisis.

Brain

It is impossible to irradiate ethmoidal-maxillary, sphenoid, and nasopharyngeal tumors without including a portion of the adjacent brain. As much of the brain is included in the treatment volume as is necessary to encompass the tumor. Conventional fractionation of 180 to 200 rad per day is then used. Through meticulous treatment planning, hotspots in the dose distribution that might later cause cerebral

radionecrosis are avoided (Fig. 8–13).[6] For massive, bulky tumors of the maxillary sinus, where possibility of local control is minimal, we limit our dose to 6000 rad or less to reduce the risk of brain necrosis.

Technical Aids

After the field margins are determined, the simulation is performed, and the dose distribution is planned; the destruction of the tumor without complication depends on the accurate delivery of the prescribed radiation dose to the tumor and normal tissues. A number of radiation-treatment aids are indispensable to the accurate delivery of radiation dose.

Cerrobend blocks are used to achieve shaped fields so that tumors close to the central nervous system (CNS) can be irradiated with tumoricidal doses without damage to spinal cord or brain (see Fig. 8–4). *Bite-block* immobilization of patients in the supine position restricts patient movement during irradiation and improves the reproducibility of daily delivery of the radiation dose.[3] A variety of new orthopedic thermal plastic materials,

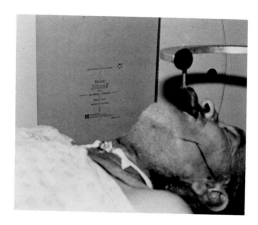

Fig. 8–14. Verification film on the backstop of the treatment machine to image the anatomy irradiated.

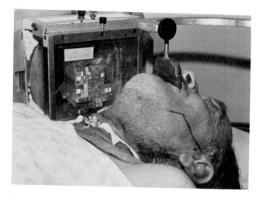

Fig. 8–15. Compensating filter to give a homogeneous dose distribution in the region of the submaxillary triangle.

have recently been used to construct immobilization masks for head-and-neck-cancer patients.[1] *Verification film* (Fig. 8–14) records an image of the anatomy irradiated and can be used to monitor changes in the volume irradiated.[2] Reproducible delivery of the dose to the tumor with sparing of normal tissues is thus assured on a daily basis. *Bolus* over scars to eliminate skin-sparing in the scar tissue and *tissue-equivalent material* in air cavities to eliminate perturbation of dose by air also improves delivery of dose to the tumor. *Compensating filters* and wedges are used to give a homogeneous distribution of dose in regions of variable thickness such as the submaxillary triangle and

neck (Fig. 8–15). Each of these aids is necessary to achieve accurate, homogeneous, and reproducible delivery of the radiation dose to the tumor and structures within the treatment field.

INDIVIDUAL SITES

Oral Cavity

Local Spread

The only barrier to the local spread of oral tongue and floor-of-mouth cancer is the inner table of the mandible. They are otherwise free to invade soft tissues medially, anteriorly, posteriorly, and inferiorly.

Tumors of the oral tongue typically arise from the lateral margin and are often contiguous with the adjacent floor of mouth; in advanced states, tumors that involve the undersurface of the tongue and the floor of mouth (junction tumors) form a painful ulcerated fissure between the tongue and the floor of mouth. As tongue cancers enlarge, they invade musculature and progressively fixate the tongue, thereby limiting protrusion.

Floor-of-mouth cancers are most common in the anterior glossogingival sulcus where they commonly destroy surface anatomy including the sublingual caruncle, the sublingual gland, and the frenulum of the tongue. They often cross the midline to the opposite side of the floor of the mouth and may extend onto the lower gum. In advanced states, they may destroy the mandible, infiltrate and fixate the tongue, and spread directly to the soft tissues of the submentum.

Lymphatic Spread

Lymphatic vessels are abundant in the tongue and the floor of the mouth, and spread of the carcinoma to regional lymph nodes is common. Lymphatic metastases from tongue cancer are usually lateralized to the side of the tumor but lymphatic metastases from floor-of-mouth cancer are more often bilateral because the primary tumor tends to cross the midline. Lymph nodes in the submaxillary triangle and upper cervical chain are the ones most commonly involved by both tumors.

Field margins for oral-cavity tumors	
Margins	Margins include
Anteriorly	Lower lip, if tumor is anterior Mandibular arch with exclusion of lower lip if tumor is more posterior
Superiorly	Superior surface of tongue Glossogingival sulci Mastoid tip
Inferiorly	Submaxillary triangles Hyoid bone

Rationale for Margins

Because of the rich lymphatic vasculature in the tongue and the floor of the mouth and the frequency of metastases to the submaxillary triangles and upper cervical nodes, all are irradiated in contiguity by opposed rectangular fields (Fig. 8–16). The upper lip is excluded by using a cork to keep the mouth open, and the amount of oral-cavity mucosa irradiated is limited by using a tongue blade to depress the tongue. The lower lip is included if the tumor involves the anterior floor of the mouth or the tip of tongue and excluded if the lesion is located more posteriorly. The mastoid tip is included to assure an adequate superior margin for cervical lymph nodes; the inferior margin encompasses the submaxillary triangles. The larynx is excluded whenever possible by placing the inferior margin of the oral cavity fields at the level of the hyoid bone. A midline block for the anterior low-neck field then shields the larynx, prevents arytenoid edema, and preserves voice quality.

For small oral tongue cancers, the posterior margin is limited so that the whole tongue is included, thereby sparing some of the buccal parotid gland and much of the retromandibular parotid glands (Fig. 8–17). Because the risk of contralateral neck metastases is low, the ipsilateral neck and parotid gland are electively irradiated with electron-beam radiation so that the buccal and retromandibular portions of the opposite parotid gland are spared. This technique preserves significant salivary function and leaves the patient with adequate oral moisture.

Tonsil-Faucial Arch

Local Spread

Tumors of the tonsil-faucial arch have no anatomic barriers to their spread other than the ascending ramus of the mandible and the base of the skull; they may spread extensively in the medial, anterior, and in-

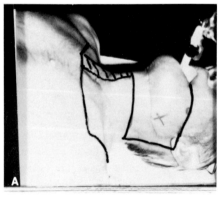
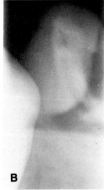
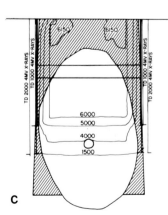

Fig. 8–16. External landmarks *(A)*, portal film *(B)*, and dose reconstruction *(C)* for a patient receiving postoperative radiation after surgery for a large tongue cancer.

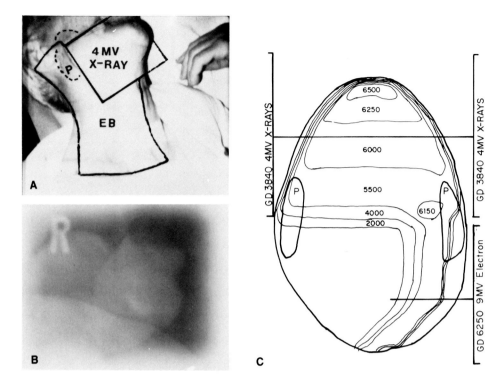

Fig. 8–17. External landmarks *(A)*, portal film *(B)*, and dose reconstruction *(C)* for a patient receiving postoperative irradiation after local excision of a small tongue cancer. The opposite parotid **(P)** is partially spared by limiting the posterior border of the oral cavity fields and using electron beam to irradiate the ipsilateral neck.

ferior directions. Such tumors are localized to a single anatomic structure when small but involve multiple contiguous structures when large. A large tumor, for instance, may involve the tonsillar fossa, pharyngeal wall, anterior tonsillar pillar, soft palate, retromolar trigone, and tongue. The superior portion of the tumor is close to the nasopharynx and, when very advanced, may involve pterygoid muscles and cause trismus. Other tonsillar-faucial-arch tumors simultaneously involve the tonsil and the adjacent tongue and produce a deep ulceration between the mandible and tongue (junction tumor). Still others involve significant portions of the soft palate so that surgical resection and dissolution of the tumor by radiation leave a large palatal defect.

Lymphatic Spread

Tonsil-faucial-arch cancers commonly spread to the upper cervical nodes beneath and anterior to the sternocleidomastoid muscle and to nodes in the submaxillary triangle. Retropharyngeal nodes are also probably involved because they are quite close to the primary tumor, but this involvement can seldom be appreciated by physical examination.

Field margins for tonsil-faucial-arch tumors	
Margins	Margins include
Anteriorly	Midportion of hard palate
	Retromolar trigone
	Posterior half of the oral tongue
	Submaxillary triangles
Superiorly	Nasopharynx
	Base of the skull
Posteriorly	Posterior oropharyngeal wall
	Upper posterior cervical triangles
Inferiorly	Base of tongue
	Suprahyoid epiglottis

Rationale for Margins

Tumors of the tonsil-faucial arch require generous local margins of 2 cm to 3 cm in all directions; the field perimeter usually encompasses the nasopharynx, the oropharynx, and the posterior half of the oral cavity. The size of the field perimeter required to encompass a tumor and its regional lymphatic vessels is directly related to the size of the tumor. In our experience, the anterior margin is the most difficult one to design for adequate irradiation of the tumor. This margin should bulge forward into the oral cavity to encompass the ascending ramus of the mandible on the radiograph with a generous 2 cm to 3 cm margin (Fig. 8–18).

Nasopharynx

Local Spread

Nasopharyngeal cancer commonly spreads beyond the confines of the nasopharyngeal cavity or invades the base of the skull. Polytomography or CT is essential to determine tumor extent.[5] These tumors often spread anteriorly into the nasal cavity, superiorly into the sphenoid sinus, and, less commonly, into the pterygomaxillary space laterally and into the oropharynx inferiorly. When very large, they may invade ethmoids, orbits, and maxillary antra anteriorly, basisphenoid, the floor of the middle cranial fossa, and the cavernous sinus superiorly, and the jugular foramen and upper cervical vertebrae posteriorly.

Lymphatic Spread

Nasopharyngeal cancers commonly spread to retropharyngeal and upper cervical lymph nodes, anterior, beneath and posterior to the sternocleidomastoid muscle. When there is extensive anterior spread into nasal cavity, they may spread to the lymph nodes in the submaxillary triangles.

Field margins for nasopharyngeal tumors		
Margins	Margins include	
	Small tumors	Large tumors
Anteriorly	Posterior half of the nasal cavity	Whole nasal cavity Posterior ethmoids Maxillary antra Posterior orbits
Superiorly	Sphenoid sinus	Sella turcica and sphenoid sinus Floor of the anterior cranial fossa
Posteriorly	Basisphenoid Clivus	Basisphenoid Brain stem Foramen magnum Upper cervical vertebrae
Inferiorly	Hyoid and soft palate	Hyoid and soft palate

Rationale for Margins

Nasopharyngeal tumors exhibit extensive local spread and must be encompassed by generous local margins of 2 cm to 3 cm in all directions. Margins for large tumors are necessarily more extensive and include more of the CNS than small tumors (Fig. 8–19). The brain stem and the cervical spinal cord can generally be shielded after a dose of 4500 rad in 4.5 weeks unless the tumor has spread to the posterior fossa and has destroyed the jugular foramen and upper cervical vertebrae. Field margins depend on tumor extent and must be individualized to encompass the tumor and to spare the adjacent CNS.

Larynx

Local Spread

Ligaments, membranes, cartilaginous framework, and submucosal lymphatic

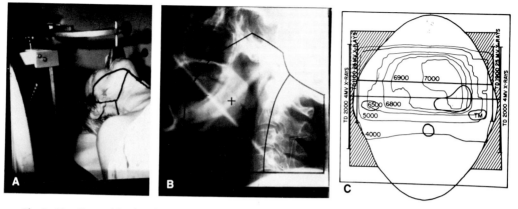

Fig. 8–18. External landmarks *(A)*, simulator film of the anatomy irradiated *(B)*, and dose reconstruction *(C)* for a patient with carcinoma of the tonsil.

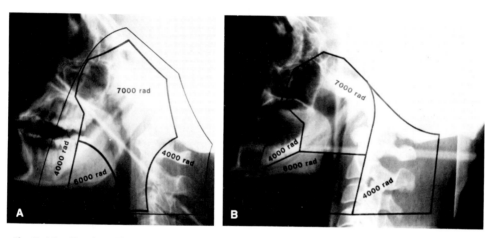

Fig. 8–19. Simulator films showing the anatomy irradiated to various dose levels for patients with *(A)* large nasopharyngeal cancers and *(B)* small nasopharyngeal cancers.

compartmentalization are all effective barriers to the spread of laryngeal cancers.

Unattended, tumors of the vocal cord or glottic larynx progressively infiltrate underlying thyroarytenoid muscle, fixate the vocal cords, and spread superiorly and inferiorly within the paraglottic space to become transglottic; advanced transglottic tumors invade and penetrate thyroid cartilage and cricothyroid membrane into the soft tissues of the neck.

Tumors of the supraglottis are usually contained within the supraglottic compartment because the submucosal lymphatic plexus does not communicate with the ventricle, the true-vocal-cord, or the subglottic region. These tumors commonly penetrate the epiglottis into the pre-epiglottic space but are still contained within the supraglottic compartment by thyrohyoid and hyoepiglottic membranes; in advanced states, supraglottic cancer invades the valleculae and the base of the tongue superiorly and the pyriform sinus laterally.

Lymphatic Spread

Lymphatic density and the incidence of lymphatic metastases to neck nodes is a function of tumor origin. True-vocal-cord cancers seldom metastasize to the neck because lymphatic vessels are relatively lacking; but as these cancers enlarge to become transglottic, neck metastases become more common because the tumor gains access to the more abundant subglottic and supraglottic lymphatic plexi.

Lymphatic density is greater and neck metastases are more common for supraglottic than for glottic cancers. Within the supraglottis, lymphatic density and neck metastases are greater for marginal than for central lesions.

Field margins for laryngeal tumors		
Margins	Margins include	
	True vocal cord	Supraglottis
Anteriorly	Anterior surface of the neck	Anterior surface of the neck
Posteriorly	Arytenoids	Posterior cervical triangle
Superiorly	Infrahyoid epiglottis	Inferior margin of mandible Submaxillary triangle Mastoid tip
Inferiorly	Cricoid cartilage	Clavicles

Rationale for Margins

It is sufficient to irradiate the larynx alone for true-vocal-cord cancers because of the infrequency of neck metastases. The margins specified above are more than adequate for these small tumors; field size ranges from 5 cm × 5 cm to 6 cm × 6 cm. Arytenoids are occasionally shielded in order to reduce edema, but we do not do this because the tumor may be shielded in the process. Arytenoid edema is reduced by limiting the dose to 6000 to 6500 rad in 6 to 6.5 weeks and by using wedges and compensating filters to achieve a homogeneous dose distribution (Fig. 8–20).

For cancers of the supraglottis, the larynx must be irradiated as well as the neck because of the significant incidence of neck metastases. The spinal cord is shielded after 4000 rad and the dose to the posterior cervical triangle is boosted with electrons for those patients with palpable neck nodes. The submaxillary triangles and the upper, middle, and lower neck are electively irradiated to 5000 rad; doses to palpable lymph nodes are therapeutically boosted to 7000 rad (Fig. 8–21).

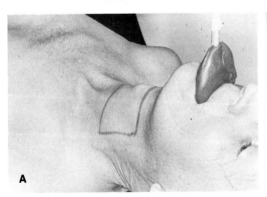
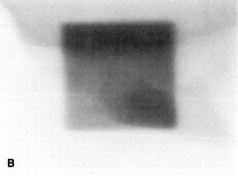

A   **B**

Fig. 8–20. External landmarks *(A)*, and a portal film *(B)* for a patient with carcinoma of the true vocal cord.

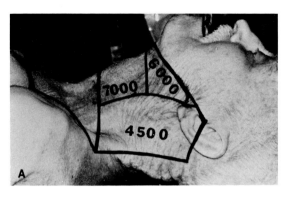 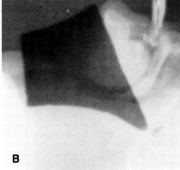

Fig. 8–21. External landmarks *(A)* showing the anatomy irradiated to various dose levels and a portal film *(B)* of a patient with carcinoma of the supraglottic larynx.

Pyriform Sinus

Local Spread

The pyriform sinus has fewer anatomic barriers to restrict spread of the cancer than does the larynx. There are no membranes, ligaments, or submucosal lymphatic compartments in the pyriform sinus, but it is bounded medially by the larynx and laterally by thyroid cartilage. Cancers of the pyriform sinus commonly invade the larynx as well as thyroid and cricoid cartilages. These tumors spread extensively in the submucosa, extend to the pharyngeal wall, postcricoid region, and oropharynx, and occasionally penetrate into the soft tissues of the neck.

Lymphatic Spread

Submucosal lymphatics in the pyriform sinus are abundant and spread to middle, upper, and lower jugular lymph nodes is common.

Field margins for pyriform sinus tumors	
Margins	Margins include
Anteriorly	Larynx
	Pharynx
	Anterior cervical triangle
Posteriorly	Posterior cervical triangle
Superiorly	Lower border of mandible
	Mastoid tip
Inferiorly	Clavicles
	Tracheostoma
	Superior mediastinum (occasionally)

Rationale for Margins

Because of extensive submucosal spread with extension of tumor beyond the pyriform sinus, it is necessary to irradiate the oropharynx above and the cervical esophagus below the target volume. The anterior and posterior cervical triangles must be irradiated because of the significant incidence of ipsilateral and contralateral lymph-node involvement; the tracheostoma should be irradiated to prevent parastomal recurrence; the superior mediastinum should be irradiated when low-neck nodes are present. It is difficult to include the lower neck, the tracheostoma, and the superior mediastinum with lateral opposed fields because the shoulders shield these areas. Three techniques of irradiation have been used in different institutions for carcinomas of the pyriform sinus.

A common technique used by many radiotherapists is lateral opposed upper fields joined with a single anterior low-neck field. Placement of an anterior block at the junction of the upper lateral and low-neck fields shields tumor in the pharynx and may result in pharyngeal recurrence. Failure to place a block at the junction of the fields may result in radiation myelitis due to overlap of the fields and excessive radiation dose to the spinal cord. We feel that some sort of shield at the splice is necessary to prevent radiation myelitis,

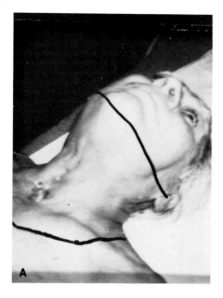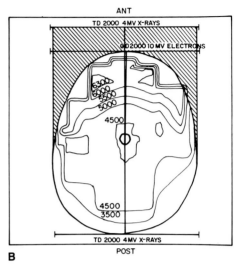

Fig. 8–22. External landmarks *(A)* and dose reconstruction *(B)* for a patient receiving postoperative irradiation for carcinoma of the pyriform sinus.

but prefer not to place it anteriorly, where it will shield the tracheostoma and pharynx.

A second technique, which we have used more recently, is placement of a small spinal-cord shield in the lateral field just posterior to the pharynx at the junction of the upper lateral and low-neck fields. Shielding the spinal cord in this way prevents shielding the pharynx and tracheostoma and avoids the possibility of splice injury to the spinal cord. The disadvantage of placing the block in the lateral upper fields is that some of the lymph nodes in the posterior cervical triangle of the neck are shielded.

A third technique, which we have used in the past, is anterior–posterior photon beams delivered in a dosage of 4000 rad with an anterior electron-beam boost of 2000 rad. This technique is illustrated in Figure 8–22. It successfully irradiates the pharynx, the tracheostoma, and the neck, and prevents the possibility of radiation-splice injury to the spinal cord. A disadvantage is that the dose in the upper part of the neck, just inferior to the mastoid process, may be variable and reduced for the electron-beam portion of the tech-

nique.[8] The anterior–posterior photon technique irradiates the neck circumferentially, unlike the three-field techniques, which spare the nape of the neck. The circumferential irradiation may result in more swelling of the neck tissues than the three-field techniques.

No one technique for irradiating patients with carcinoma of the pyriform sinus is perfect. We most commonly use the second technique, which is a three-field technique that shields the spinal cord laterally and posterior to the pharynx at the junction of the three fields.

Pharyngeal Wall

Local Spread

Pharyngeal-wall cancers lie close to the prevertebral fascia and the spine, which act as barriers to their spread. There are no other barriers and these tumors spread submucosally in many directions. When large, they may involve the tonsillar fossa, the glossopharyngeal sulcus, the pyriform sinus, and the cervical esophagus.

Lymphatic Spread

Pharyngeal lymphatic vessels are relatively abundant; these tumors spread to cervical lymph nodes in approximately half of the patients.

Field margins for pharyngeal wall tumors	
Margins	Margins include
Anteriorly	Base of the tongue Anterior surface of neck
Posteriorly	Posterior cervical triangle
Superiorly	Nasopharynx
Inferiorly	Cervical esophagus Clavicles

Rationale for Margins

Because these tumors spread submucosally beyond the visible borders of the lesion, it is necessary to irradiate 4 cm to 6 cm above and below the visible borders. In case of an oropharyngeal wall cancer, margins must include both the nasopharynx above and the hypopharynx below. Field margins include the base of the tongue but exclude the oral cavity; this limits mucositis. A series of shrinking fields is then constructed; the spinal cord is shielded after 4000 rad are delivered and a boost field is constructed after 6000 rad. Posterior cervical triangles are electively boosted with electrons to 5000 rad.

In the case of hypopharyngeal-wall cancers, it is necessary to irradiate the oropharynx above the level of the palate and the cervical esophagus below with adequate margins. Anterior-oblique beams are necessary to miss the shoulders and ensure adequate inferior margins (Fig. 8–23). This technique fails to adequately irradiate lymph nodes in the posterior cervical triangles, so the patient is usually monitored closely during follow-up for the appearance of lymph nodes; a neck dissection is performed if necessary.

Unknown Primary

Lymphatic Spread

Carcinoma metastatic to middle- or upper-neck nodes with primary tumor un-

detected, despite thorough ear-nose-and-throat (ENT) diagnostic workup, may be treated by high-dose radiation to possible ENT primary sites (e.g., nasopharynx, oropharynx, base of the tongue, pyriform sinus, cervical esophagus, larynx) as well as by bilateral neck irradiation. Supraclavicular-node metastases are usually from infraclavicular primaries, and neck irradiation alone suffices.

Field margins for unknown primary tumors metastatic to cervical lymph nodes	
Margins	Margins include
Anteriorly	Retromolar trigone Posterior tongue Anterior surface of the neck
Superiorly	Nasopharynx Mastoid process
Posteriorly	Posterior cervical triangle Pharyngeal wall
Inferiorly	Hypopharynx Cricoid cartilage

Rationale for Field Margins

Margins and irradiation techniques are similar to those for treatment of nasopharyngeal carcinoma. The difference is that the inferior margin is usually below the cricoid cartilage to ensure coverage of the hypopharynx and larynx (Fig. 8–24).

Paranasal Sinus-Nasal Cavity

Local Spread

The various paranasal sinuses and the nasal cavity are separated by thin, bony, cartilaginous walls that are relatively ineffective barriers to the spread of cancer. These thin, bony partitions are commonly destroyed by the cancer, which then spreads to the adjacent cavity.

Tumors of the maxillary antrum penetrate the lateral and anterior walls into the soft tissues of the cheek, the medial wall into the nasal cavity, and the posterior wall into the pterygomaxillary space. They involve the antral-ethmoid junction superiorly and break through the inferior and

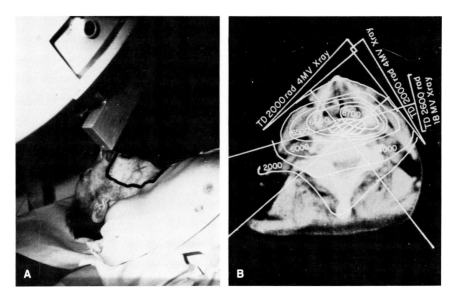

Fig. 8–23. External landmarks *(A)* and dose reconstruction *(B)* superimposed on a CT scan of a patient with a small pharyngeal wall cancer.

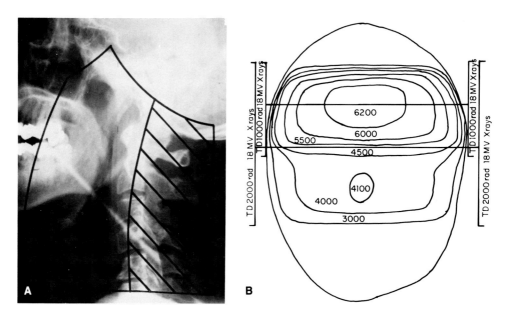

Fig. 8–24. Simulator film *(A)* and dose reconstruction *(B)* for a patient with an unknown primary metastatic to the neck.

medial walls of the orbit. Inferiorly, they invade and destroy the hard palate and the upper alveolus.

Tumors of the nasal cavity perforate the nasal septum and invade adjacent maxillary antra laterally and ethmoids superiorly.

Ethmoid tumors invade the orbits to cause proptosis. They spread posteriorly to the sphenoid sinus and the nasopharynx and inferiorly to the nasal cavity.

Lymphatic Spread

For reasons yet unexplained, lymphatic metastases from tumors of the paranasal sinuses and nasal cavity are relatively uncommon; therefore, treatment portals are seldom designed to include lymph nodes. In the 15% of patients with lymphatic metastases, lymph nodes containing cancer are most commonly noted in the submentum and submaxillary triangles.

Field margins for tumors of the paranasal sinuses	
Margins	Margins include
Anteriorly	Cheek, Nose and Orbit, when involved
Superiorly	Ethmoids Cribriform plate Roof of orbit
Inferiorly	Hard palate Upper alveolus Floor of nose
Posteriorly	Sphenoid Nasopharynx Posterior wall of maxillary antrum

Cork and tongue blade are used to separate the hard palate, which needs to be treated, from the tongue, which does not require treatment. The eyes are kept open during treatment to decrease the corneal dose.

Rationale for Margins

All cavities involved by tumor and any adjacent uninvolved bony septum should be irradiated. For example, when a cancer of the maxillary antrum has destroyed the medial wall of the antrum to involve nasal cavity, the field perimeter should include the antrum, the nasal cavity, and the uninvolved medial wall of the opposite maxillary antrum. The perimeter should also encompass the hard palate, the upper alveolus, the floor of the orbit, and the posterior wall of the antrum.

Dose Distribution

Homogeneous dose distribution is difficult to achieve for paranasal-sinus tumors. A standard wedge-pair technique for maxillary antrum commonly produces a 15% to 20% gradient in dose throughout the volume, with hotspots in the regions of the ethmoids and optic nerves anteromedially and in the temporomandibular joints posterolaterally (see Fig. 8–13). By using anterior 4-MeV and 25-MeV x-ray beams with wedged lateral boost fields posterior to the eyes, the radiotherapist can achieve a relatively homogeneous dose for ethmoidal-maxillary-nasal cavity tumors (Fig. 8–25).[9]

Parotid

Local Spread

Parotid carcinoma may extend from the parotid gland into the soft tissues and muscles of the upper neck, into the skin, the auricle, and the external auditory canal, or into the base of the skull in the space between the styloid process and the posterior border of the ascending ramus of the mandible; parapharyngeal space involvement or mandible involvement may be seen less frequently.

Lymphatic Spread

Parotid cancers spread to the superficial parotid nodes in the preauricular region, the deep parotid nodes, and the submaxillary and upper cervical nodes. Lymph-node involvement is unusual for adenoid cystic, low-grade mucoepidermoid, and acinic-cell carcinomas; it is more common for epidermoid, anaplastic, adenocarcinoma, higher-grade mucoepidermoid carcinomas, and lymphomas. Therapeutic irradiation of the neck is necessary when lymph nodes are involved. Elective irradiation is given only for those tumors that more commonly spread lymphatically (Fig. 8–26). The first echelon of nodes (i.e., the superficial and deep parotid nodes and the submaxillary and upper cervical nodes) are included in the treatment of all patients with parotid carcinoma because of their proximity to the parotid gland.

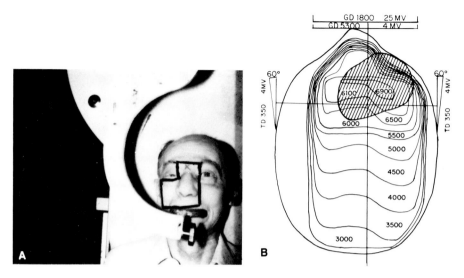

Fig. 8–25. External landmarks *(A)* and dose reconstruction *(B)* for a patient with a large carcinoma involving ethmoids, maxillary antrum, and nasal cavity.

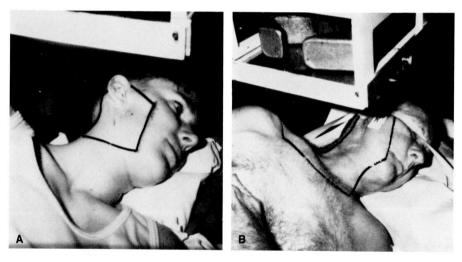

Fig. 8–26. External landmarks for a patient with adenoid cystic carcinoma of the parotid *(A)* and another with adenocarcinoma of the parotid *(B)*.

Field margins for parotid cancer	
Margins	Margins include
Anteriorly	Masseter muscle ⅔ of cheek
Superiorly	Zygoma ⅔ of ear
Posteriorly	Mastoid Posterior cervical nodes
Inferiorly	Hyoid, for low chance of lymph-node involvement Clavicles, for high chance of lymph-node involvement

Rationale for Margins

Margins (see Box) are used with electron-beam treatment that encompass the gland, potential areas of soft-tissue spread, the surgical scar, and adjacent lymph nodes in all patients, and distant lymph nodes in some patients. The tumor depth is calculated at 3 cm to 5 cm depending on the size and extent of the tumor.

Oblique ports with wedges may also be

used to administer a high dose to the parotid area without exceeding spinal-cord and brain-stem tolerance. Care must be taken to avoid having radiation exit through the patient's eyes with the wedge-filter technique.

Temporal Bone

Local Spread

Tumors originating in the external auditory canal may be partly or completely circumferential. They may spread to involve the tympanic membrane and penetrate the anterior wall into the temporomandibular joint. Tumors of the middle ear and mastoid are frequently larger and more advanced than those of the external auditory canal. These may destroy the ossicles in the middle ear, the mastoid air cells, and much of the petrous portion of the temporal bone. They may penetrate superiorly into the dura mater, anteriorly into the pterygomaxillary space, and posteriorly into the posterior cranial fossa.

Lymphatic Spread

Only advanced lesions metastasize to the upper cervical nodes anterior, inferior, and posterior to the sternocleidomastoid muscle.

Field margins for tumors of the temporal bone		
Margins	Margins include	
	Small	Large
Anteriorly	Temporomandibular joint	Pterygomaxillary space
Posteriorly	Mastoid	Posterior fossa
Superiorly	Apex petrous portion of temporal bone	Temporal lobe Middle cranial fossa
Inferiorly	Ear lobe	Neck to clavicles

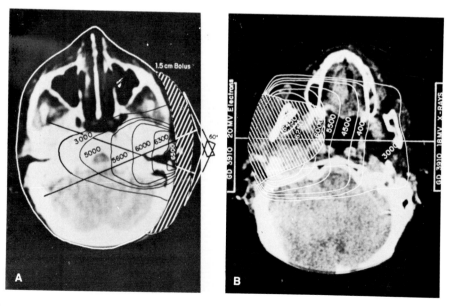

Fig. 8–27. Dose reconstruction superimposed onto a CT scan of a patient with a small squamous cancer of the external auditory canal *(A)* and a patient with a massive carcinoma of the middle ear extending to dura and pterygomaxillary space *(B)*.

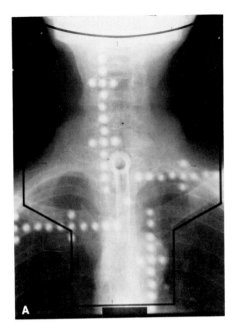
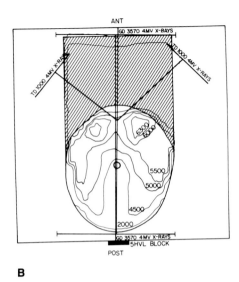

Fig. 8–28. Simulator film *(A)* and dose reconstruction *(B)* for a patient with unresectable anaplastic carcinoma of the thyroid.

Rationale for Margins

Small lesions of the external auditory canal, which seldom spread to lymph nodes, may be treated with small-volume, high-dose techniques. Generally, 5 cm × 7 cm fields are used with 60° wedges 20° to the right and left of vertical (Fig. 8–27A). Because the external auditory canal angles forward, the isocenter is placed just in front of the ear. The canal is filled with vaseline gauze to eliminate the dose perturbation that might result from the air cavity; a wax mold is placed in the concavity of the external ear to raise the surface dose to the outermost portion of the ear canal (Fig. 8–27A).

For large tumors of the middle ear and mastoid, field margins are determined after review of polytomography radiographs and CT scans. These lesions are generally extensive and require a generous field size that includes much of the CNS. An optimized dose distribution can be achieved by irradiating the side of the tumor with electron-beam and the side opposite the

tumor with high-energy x-rays as shown in Figure 8–27B. The neck is routinely irradiated because of the propensity of large temporal-bone tumors to metastasize to lymph nodes.

Thyroid

Local Spread

Thyroid carcinoma can spread locally beyond the thyroid gland to the adjacent trachea, esophagus, muscles of the neck, larynx, and superior mediastinum.

Lymphatic Spread

Regional nodes that may be involved include the Delphian node, the jugular, paratracheal, jugulodigastric, and superior mediastinal nodes.

Field margins for tumors of the thyroid	
Margins	Margins include
Anteriorly	Anterior surface of the neck
Posteriorly	Posterior cervical nodes
Superiorly	Mandible
	Mastoid process
Inferiorly	Clavicle
	Superior mediastinum to carina
	of the trachea

Rationale for Margins

Thyroid carcinomas requiring irradiation are most often anaplastic carcinomas that are frequently large and unresectable. Portals should encompass the thyroid gland, bilateral neck nodes from the mandible to the clavicle, and, usually, the upper mediastinum as well. Care must be taken not to exceed spinal-cord tolerance; AP–PA fields with compensating filters are used. The spinal cord is shielded by a midline posterior-anterior (PA) block and the tumor volume is boosted anteriorly with oblique portals or electron-beam irradiation to achieve a tumoricidal dose within the limits of spinal-cord tolerance (Fig. 8–28).

REFERENCES

1. Gerber, R., Marks, J.E., and Purdy, J.A.: The use of thermal plastics for immobilization of patients during radiotherapy. Int. J. Radiat. Oncol. Biol. Phys. 8:1461, 1982.
2. Haus, A.G., Marks, J.E., and Griem,M.L.: Evaluation of a rapid processable film for imaging during the complete radiotherapeutic exposure. Radiology 107:697, 1973.
3. Marks, J.E. and Haus, A.G.: The effects of immobilization on localization error in the radiotherapy of head and neck cancer. Clin. Radiol. 27185, 1976.
4. Marks, J.E. et al.: The effects of radiation on parotid salivary function. Int. J. Radiat. Oncol. Biol. Phys. 7:1013, 1981.
5. Marks, J.E. et al.: Dose-response analysis for nasopharyngeal cancer: an historical perspective. Cancer 50:1042, 1982.
6. Mikhael, M.A.: Radiation necrosis of the brain: Correlation between computed tomography, pathology, and dose distribution. J. Comput. Assist. Tomogr. 2:71, 1978.
7. Powers, W.E. et al.: A new system of field shaping for external beam radiation therapy. Radiology 108:407, 1973.
8. Prasad, S.C.: Unpublished data. Mallinckrodt Institute of Radiology, June, 1981.
9. Shukovsky, L.J. and Fletcher, G.H.: Retinal and optic nerve complications in a high dose irradiation technique of ethmoid sinus and nasal cavity. Radiology 104:629, 1972.

Chapter 9

RADIATION THERAPY OF CARCINOMA OF THE LUNG AND ESOPHAGUS

Carlos A. Perez

James Purdy

Aly Razek

BRONCHOGENIC CARCINOMA OF THE LUNG

Natural History and Pathologic Features

Knowledge has increased concerning the clinicopathologic behavior of bronchogenic carcinoma. Technologic advances have resulted in improved diagnostic techniques, including mass radiographic screening, fiberoptic bronchoscopy, brush or needle biopsy, and radionuclide scanning; the roles of surgery, radiotherapy, and chemotherapy in the management of the disease have been more clearly defined.[64,84,91,94,95]

It is extremely important to approach lung-cancer patients with a positive attitude and, if there is no clinical evidence of distant metastasis at the time of diagnosis, aggressive radiation therapy or surgical techniques should be used to eradicate the intrathoracic tumor.

As in any other malignant tumor, the basic therapeutic approach should be guided by the natural history and clinicopathologic characteristics of the disease. Bronchogenic carcinoma usually originates in the secondary or tertiary bronchial divisions or, in the case of adenocarcinoma, in the periphery of the lung.

Even before the tumor has reached a clinically detectable size, there is invasion of the regional lymphatics and the blood vessels, resulting in widespread lymphatic and hematogenous dissemination.[21,56] Goldberg et al.[34] reported that mediastinoscopy showed ipsilateral hilar lymph-node involvement in 50% of the patients (Table 9–1). Patients with poorly differentiated or anaplastic tumors have a higher incidence of lymph-node metastasis.[34,56] Figure 9–1 illustrates the lymphatic drainage of the various lobes of the lung. This information is critical to the design of irradiation portals.

As indicated by Hansen and Muggia[42] and Line and Deeley[56] there is a high incidence of visceral distant metastasis, particularly to the brain, liver, bones, and adrenal glands. Abdominal lymph-node involvement has been reported in over 50% of the patients with small-cell undifferentiated carcinoma.[6]

Radionuclide studies may demonstrate subclinical distant metastasis to the bone, liver, or brain. Bone-marrow aspirates have shown tumor invasion in 3.6% of the patients with epidermoid carcinoma, in 12.5% of those with large cell carcinoma, in 18.5% of those with adenocarcinoma,

TABLE 9–1. Lung Carcinoma: Mediastinal Spread.

Pathology	Number of Patients	Mediastinoscopy			
		Positive	Ipsilateral	Contralateral	Bilateral
All cell types	179	86 (48%)	35 (41%)	8 (9%)	43 (50%)
Well-differentiated squamous cell	64	10 (16%)	7 (70%)	2 (20%)	1 (10%)
Large cell Poorly differentiated, undifferentiated, anaplastic	74	47 (68%)	17 (36%)	6 (13%)	24 (51%)
Small cell Undifferentiated, oat cell	23	17 (70%)	5 (30%)	—	12 (70%)
Adenocarcinoma	18	12 (66%)	6 (50%)	—	6 (50%)

(From Goldberg, E.M. et al.: Semin. Oncol. *1*:213, 1974.)

LYMPHATIC DRAINAGE OF THE LUNG

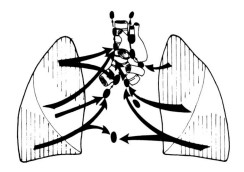

Fig. 9–1. Diagrammatic representation of lymphatic drainage of various lobes of the lung. Almost all lobes drain to the subcarinal nodes and subsequently to the right superior mediastinum.

and in 46.4% of those with small-cell undifferentiated carcinoma.[42] Hansen and Muggia noted that only 16% of the patients with positive bone-marrow biopsy showed roentgenologic evidence of bony metastasis and that 69.2% showed positive bone scans.

Peritoneoscopy and liver biopsies have been performed in an effort to detect clinically inapparent hepatic metastasis, but the yield is low. Hansen and Muggia reported that these procedures showed liver metastases in only 1 patient of 47 with localized disease and 3 of 11 with disseminated tumor.[42]

Many patients with lung cancer, and most of those with advanced disease, have distant metastasis. Matthews et al.,[60] however, studied a group of 131 patients with epidermoid carcinoma of the lung on whom autopsies were performed within 30 days after a curative surgical procedure; 44 patients had persistent disease, but only 22 (50%) had distant metastases. This limited spread becomes a compelling argument for a more aggressive surgical or radiotherapeutic management of patients with clinically localized bronchogenic carcinoma. It is evident that in order to increase cure rates in these patients, we must find an effective systemic adjuvant therapy that can control micrometastases.

Staging Systems

To understand the clinical course of bronchogenic carcinoma and to define target populations that should receive specific therapeutic strategies, all patients must be staged according to the extent of disease. Tables 9–2 and 9–3 show the TNM classification proposed by Mountain et al. and adopted by the American Joint Committee for Cancer Staging with modifications suggested by Rubin.[65,85] It is critical that we distinguish those patients in whom local control by irradiation is possible from those with extremely advanced regional or metastatic disease for whom palliation is the only goal.

The histopathologic characteristics of the tumor are equally important because its behavior and response to therapy is greatly influenced by its pathologic type (Table 9–4).[59,98]

TABLE 9–2.   The Definitions of T, N, and M Categories for Carcinoma of the Lung.*

T Primary Tumors

TO   No evidence of primary tumor

TX   Tumor proven by the presence of malignant cells in bronchopulmonary secretions but not visualized radiographically or bronchoscopically.

T1   A tumor that is 3.0 cm or less in greatest diameter, surrounded by lung or visceral pleura and without evidence of invasion proximal to a lobar bronchus at bronchoscopy.

T2   A tumor more than 3.0 cm in greatest diameter, or a tumor of any size which, with its associated atelectasis or obstructive pneumonitis, extends to the hilar region. At bronchoscopy the proximal extent of demonstrable tumor must be at least 2.0 cm distal to the carina. Any associated atelectasis or obstructive pneumonitis must involve less than an entire lung, and there must be no pleural effusion.

T3   A tumor of any size with direct extension into an adjacent structure such as the chest wall, the diaphragm, or the mediastinum and its contents; or demonstrable bronchoscopically to be less than 2.0 cm distal to the carina; any tumor associated with atelectasis or obstructive pneumonitis of an entire lung or pleural effusion.

N Regional Lymph Nodes

N0   No demonstrable metastasis to regional lymph nodes

N1   Metastasis to lymph nodes in the ipsilateral hilar region (including direct extension).

N2   Metastasis to lymph nodes in the mediastinum.

M Distant Metastasis

MC   No distant metastasis

M1   Distant metastasis, such as in scalene, cervical, or contralateral hilar lymph nodes, brain, bones, lung, liver, etc.

*Each case must be assigned the highest category of T, N, and M that describes the full extent of disease in that case. (From Anderson, W.A.: American Joint Committee for Cancer Staging and End Results Reporting, 1973.)

GENERAL MANAGEMENT OF BRONCHOGENIC CARCINOMA

Non-Oat Cell Type (Epidermoid, Large-Cell Undifferentiated, Adenocarcinoma)

Non-oat cell carcinoma, whenever resectable, should be treated surgically (lobectomy or pneumonectomy—Table 9–5). This implies the absence of mediastinal lymph nodes or distant metastasis (Stages T1, T2-N0,N1). Patients with potentially resectable localized lesions for whom a surgical procedure is precluded due to medical reasons, should be treated with 6000–6500 rad to the primary tumor and 5000 rad to the regional nodes in about 6 to 7 weeks. Several reports have failed to show any improvement in survival with the use of pre- or postoperative radiation[71,82,97] except for patients with apical tumors[71] or in a small group of patients with hilar lymph-node metastasis.[36] Patients with larger, unresectable tumors (T3, any N stage or T1,T2-N2) should receive definitive radiation therapy (minimum 5000 rad to the primary tumor and minimum 4500 rad to the regional lymph nodes in 5 or 6 weeks). Patients with distant metastasis should receive palliative radiation therapy, consisting of 4000 rad tumor dose in 3 or 4 weeks; this can be given with split courses.[1,38,88] Metastatic sites can be treated with doses of 3000 or 4000 rad delivered in 2 or 3 weeks.

Simpson et al.[93] reported on 49 evalua-

TABLE 9–3. **Nodal Categories and Modifications of T Categories Proposed by Radiation Therapy Groups.**

Nodal Categories

N0	No demonstrable spread to lymph nodes
N1	Ispsilateral hilar nodes
N2.1	Subcarinal (ipsilateral) and lower mediastinal (ipsilateral) involvement
N2.2	High mediastinal involvement
N2.3	Contralateral, hilar, and mediastinal nodes
N2.4	Posterior mediastinal nodes and diaphragmatic and pericardial involvement
N3	Supraclavicular nodes and scalene nodes

Modifications of T Categories

T3	(Extrapulmonary, limited and intrathoracic): This group includes primary lesions that invade through the visceral pleura and are adherent to the parietal pleura. Localized bronchogenic cancers within 2 cm of the carina are essentially extrapulmonary. There is no evidence of visceral, vascular, neurologic, osseous, or cardiac (including pericardial) invasion.
T3.1	Primary lesion meeting above criteria and limited to one lobe including associated atelectasis and infiltration.
T3.2	Primary lesion meeting above criteria and limited to two lobes.
T3.3	Primary lesion meeting above criteria and limited to one main bronchus without atelectasis.
T3.4	Primary lesion meeting above criteria with associated pleural effusion with negative cytology, indicating extensive mediastinal adenopathy and venous compression. This type of lesion is modified by virtue of nodal involvement and it is not necessarily an advanced lesion.
	It is important to recognize that thoracic exploration may be required to identify T3 lesions. Such categories as T3.1, T3.2, and T3.3 represent T1, T2, and T3 lesions clinically and radiographically assessed, which are beyond resection due to location or evidence of extrapulmonary invasion uncovered at the time of surgery.
T4	(Extrapulmonary or extrathoracic): This group includes very extensive primary lesions invading the nerves, major vessels, and cardiac and osseous sites. They are beyond the parietal pleura and are in the chest wall, viscera, and deep mediastinal structures.
T4.1	Associated with total collapse of involved lung with any primary lesion
T4.2	Positive pleural effusion cytology with any primary lesion
T4.3	Superior vena caval obstruction with any primary lesion

(Modified from Rubin et al.: *In* Lung Cancer: Natural History, Prognosis and Therapy. Edited by L. Israel and A.P. Chahinian. New York, Academic Press, 1976, p. 160.)

ble patients with advanced non-oat-cell carcinoma of the lung treated with misonidazole (2-nitroimidazole) as a hypoxic-cell sensitizer and radiation. Tumor doses of 600 rad were given twice weekly for 3 weeks for a total of 3600 rad, preceded by 4 to 6 hours with misonidazole in a dose of 2 g/m^2 or 1.75 g/m^2 administered orally. Objective responses were reported in 67% of patients (complete responses in 18%); 70% of the patients have died with a median survival time of 9 months. Of 32 patients eligible for 12-month follow-up, 34% survived more than one year. Grade 2 or 3 peripheral neurotoxicity occurred in 8 of 24 patients (33%) with drug doses

TABLE 9–4. **Comparison of the World Health Organization (WHO), Veterans Administration Lung Cancer Chemotherapy Study Group (VALG), and Working Party for Therapy of Lung Cancer (WP-L) Classifications of Lung Cancer.***

WHO	VALG	WP-L
I. Epidermoid carcinoma	1. Squamous cell carcinoma (10) (a) With abundant keratin (1a) (b) With intercellular bridges: epidermoid (1b) (c) without keratin or bridges: squamoid (1c)	10. Epidermoid carcinoma 11. Well differentiated 12. Moderately differentiated 13. Poorly differentiated
II. Small cell anaplastic carcinoma 1. Fusiform 2. Polygonal 3. Lymphocyte-like 4. Others	2. Small cell undifferentiated carcinoma (20) (a) with oat cell structure (2a) (b) with polygonal cell structure (2b)	20. Small cell anaplastic carcinoma 21. Lymphocyte-like (oat cell) 22. Intermediate cell (fusiform, polygonal, others)
III. Adenocarcinoma 1. Bronchogenic a. Acinar b. Papillary 2. Bronchioloalveolar	3. Adenocarcinoma (30) a. Acinar (3a) b. Papillary (3b) c. Poorly differentiated (3c)	30. Adenocarcinoma 31. Well differentiated 32. Moderately differentiated 33. Poorly differentiated 34. Bronchio-papillary
IV. Large cell carcinoma 1. Solid tumors with mucin 2. Solid tumors without mucin 3. Giant cell 4. Clear cell	4. Large cell undifferentiated carcinoma (40)	40. Large cell carcinoma 41. With stratification 43. With mucin production 42. Giant cell 44. Clear cell

*WHO data [34]; VALG data [67]; WP-L data [42]. (From Matthews, M.J.: Problems in Morphology and Behavior of Bronchopulmonary Malignant Disease. *In* Lung Cancer: Natural History, Prognosis and Therapy. Edited by L.I. Israel and A.P. Chahinian. New York, Academic Press, 1976.)

of 2 g/m², and in 4 of 26 patients (15%) who received 1.75 g/m². Grade 3 or 4 central-nervous-system (CNS) toxicity occurred in 2 patients, both of whom received 2 g/m². Two patients developed serious late radiation complications: 1 was a transverse myelitis that appeared 1 year following delivery of 3600 rad to the spinal cord; a second patient developed a tracheoesophageal fistula and pericarditis 8 months following treatment.

Doses of Radiation

At the present time there is no clear evidence that defines the best dose of radiation to treat non-oat-cell bronchogenic carcinoma. From experience in treatment of the head, neck, and uterine cervix, how-

ever, we know that in order to sterilize the tumor, doses in the range of 6000–7000 rad are necessary.[31] If therapeutic goals are less radical and emphasize the palliation of symptoms and retardation of tumor growth in patients with short expectations of survival, doses in the range of 3000–4000 rad are adequate.

Bromley and Szur[11] reported that localized lung cancer could be eradicated in about 40% of a group of patients given doses of 4700 rad. Bloedorn et al.[8] reported no recognizable tumor cells at the primary site in 54% of a group of 26 patients who received 6000 rad in 6 weeks preoperatively; the mediastinal nodes showed tumor in only 8% of the cases. Hellman et al.[43] reported residual tumor at the pri-

TABLE 9–5.   Non-Oat-Cell Carcinoma of Lung: Recommended Treatment by Stage Grouping.

Stage No.	TNM	Surgery	Target of Radiation Therapy	Chemotherapy
0	T0 N0 M0	Lobectomy	None	None
I	T1 N0 M0	Lobectomy if possible; pneumonectomy if necessary	None	None
I	T1 N1 M0	As above plus hilar node resection	Mediastinal nodes recommended (4500–5000 rads TD)	None
I	T2 N0 M0	As above	Mediastinal nodes optional	None
II	T2 N1 M0	Lobectomy/pneumonectomy plus hilar node resection	Mediastinal nodes recommended (4500–5000 rads TD)	None
III	T3,2 N0 M0	None, but biopsy; resection of diaphragm and chest wall not advised	Definitive radiation therapy; 5000–6000 rad to T, plus mediastinal nodes (4500–5000 rad)	None
III	T1,2 N2 M0	Surgery optional	Definitive radiation therapy 5000–6000 rad to T, mediastinal and supraclavicular nodes (4500–5000 rad)	None
III	T3 N2 M1	None	As above	None
IV	$T_{any}N_{any}M1$	None	Palliative radiation therapy to T—4000 rad/split course, 2000/week-2-3 rest-2000/week	None
IV	$T_{any}N_{any}M1$	None	Palliative to T, palliative to isolated metastases simultaneously	
	M to brain		Palliative 3000 rad/2 weeks	
	M to bone		Palliative 3000 rad/2 weeks (whole bone)	None
	M to liver		Palliative 3000 rad/2 weeks (small field)	None
Special problems				
Superior vena cava obstruction		None	Rapidly daily dose 400 × 3 = 1200 rad; then additional XRT to 4000–5000 rad	None
Pleural effusion			Radiocolloid ^{32}P—rarely	Intrapleural alkylating agent

Patients with small cell undifferentiated carcinoma will receive multidrug chemotherapy. (Modifed from Rubin et al. *In Lung Cancer: Natural History, Prognosis and Therapy.* Edited by L. Israel and A.P. Chahinian. New York, Academic Press, 1976, p. 160.)

mary site in 17 of 24 patients with lung cancer treated with 5500–6000 rad in 5 to 6 weeks approximately 4 to 6 weeks prior to surgery. In 15 of the patients with preoperative radiographic evidence of hilar or mediastinal adenopathy, only 3 had residual tumor in the pathological specimens of the lymph nodes. Rissanen et al.[79] reported no carcinoma in the tumor volume in 18 of 60 patients (30%) treated with doses of 4500–6250 rad over 5 to 10 weeks. In contrast, viable tumor was found more frequently in patients treated with doses below 4000 rad; 7 patients whose therapy was interrupted after doses of 2000 or 3000 rad all showed evidence of malignancy at autopsy.

One of the problems in determining the optimal dose of irradiation for this disease is the high incidence of distant metastasis, which results in an unrelenting poor prognosis, according to some, without regard to the status of the intrathoracic tumor. Roswit et al.[81] reported a slightly increased 1-year-survival rate (22%) in a group of patients treated with 4000–5000 rad in 4 to 5 weeks, in contrast to 16% 1-year-survival rate in a control group given a placebo. In general, the survival rate was the same whether the patients were treated with 4000, 5000, or 6000 rad. Deeley[20] reported a 6% survival rate at 2 years in 51 patients treated with 3000 rad in 20 sessions over 4 weeks and no survivors in 51 patients receiving 4000 rad in 20 fractions over 4 weeks. This suggests that neither dose is adequate to control the tumor. On the other hand, Guttman,[39] Rubin,[85] Salazar et al.,[87] and others have shown improved survival rates in patients receiving higher doses of radiation. This may be due to selection, because the more favorable cases may be treated more radically. Eisert et al.[25] reported local tumor control in 14 of 51 patients (27%) receiving less than 1450 rets in contrast to 75 of 146 patients (51%) treated with higher doses. Better survival was correlated with control of the primary tumor in the lung.

Fractionation

The potential value of split-course radiotherapy has been based on biological concepts, namely reoxygenation of initially hypoxic tumor cells because of reduction in tumor size and improved vascularization between the two or more courses of therapy, which may result in greater tumor sterilization.[88] Some physicians have advocated this type of therapy for economic and convenience reasons.

Deeley,[21] Levitt et al.,[55] and Lee[53] have used different doses of radiation, ranging from 2000–5000 rad in split courses, comparing them with analogous doses delivered with continuous schedules. The survival rates have been similar in the two treated groups in the various series. In contrast, Holsti and Vuorinen[45] reported a slightly higher survival rate (70% at 6 months, 35% at 1 year, and 10% at 2 years) for patients treated with 5000–6000 rad in a split course with a 2- to 3-week interruption between the two courses of therapy in comparison with a group of patients treated to similar doses in continuous course for 6 weeks, 6 fractions per week (54% at 6 months, 32% at 1 year, and 4% at 2 years).

Abramson and Cavanaugh,[1] in their initial report, described a higher survival rate (43% at 1 year) in a group of patients receiving 4000 rad with a split course, compared with a nonrandomized control group treated with 6000 rad for 6 weeks, 5 weekly fractions (14% survival at 1 year). Subsequent analysis of the data, however,[2] shows appreciably lower long-term survival rates in the study group (13% at 2 years and 6.7% at 3 and 4 years).

Results of Recent Radiation Therapy Oncology Group Clinical Trials

In June of 1973, the Radiation Therapy Oncology Group initiated a randomized study to determine the most effective and best tolerated irradiation dose and fractionation schedule in patients with inoperable or unresectable stage III (T1N2, T2N2, T3N0, T3N1, T3N2) non-oat-cell carcinoma of the lung (epidermoid, adenocarcinoma, or large-cell undifferentiated carcinoma).

Randomization was carried out in the following manner: 4000-rad split course (delivering 2000 rad in 1 week, 5 fractions, 2 weeks rest, and an additional 2000-rad dose in 5 weekly fractions); or 4000-, 5000-, or 6000-rad tumor dose in continuous courses delivered in 5 weekly fractions with daily doses of 200 rad ± 10%.

The treatment portals were designed to include all areas of parenchymal involvement and the hilar and mediastinal lymph nodes with at least a 2-cm margin. A 2-cm wide, 5 half-value layer (HVL) spinal-cord block was used for a portion of the treatment to limit the dose to the spinal cord to 4000–4500 rad with the continuous schedule and to 2500 rad with the split-course schedule. Higher maximum doses frequently were delivered to the anterior portal (unequal loading) to reach a mediastinal dose of 4000 rad in those tumor dose groups and 5000 rad in the 5000–6000 rad groups.

A total of 375 cases were analyzed. Approximately two-thirds of the patients had squamous-cell carcinoma and the other third was equally divided between adenocarcinoma and large-cell undifferentiated carcinoma.[77]

Only 8 of 100 patients (8%) in the 4000-rad split-course group showed complete regression of the tumor, in contrast to 18% to 21% in those treated with continuous schedules. The overall complete and partial regression rate was 46% in the patients who received the 4000-rad split course, 51% with the 4000-rad continuous course, 65% in those who were treated with 5000 rad and 61% in the 6000-rad group (Fig. 9–2). The split-course group had a significantly lower complete response rate than the other regimens (p = 0.02). When the 4000-rad patients are compared with the patients receiving 5000 rad or 6000 rad,

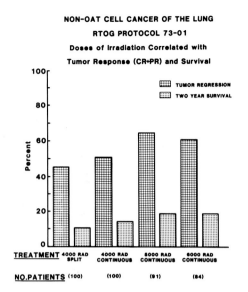

Fig. 9–2. Survival of patients with unresectable non-oat cell carcinoma of the lung in RTOG Protocol No. 73-01, according to treatment regimen. Differences are not statistically significant. (From Perez et al.: Int. J. Radiat. Oncol. Biol. Phys. 6:987, 1980.)

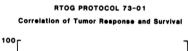
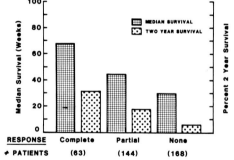

Fig. 9–3. Correlation of survival with degree of local tumor response (RTOG Protocol No. 73-01). (From Perez: Sem. Resp. Med. 4:17, 1982)

the response rates are significantly different (49% vs. 63%, p = 0.005 chi-square test).

The 1-year-survival rate for all groups was about 40%; at 2 years it was 14% to 18% for the patients who were treated with continuous regimens in contrast to only 10% for the split-course group (Fig. 9–3). The differences are not statistically significant. At the present time these survival data should be considered preliminary because 15% of the patients are still known to be alive and some have been followed for only 1 year after therapy.

Patients who showed a complete response had a median survival of 68.8 weeks (63 patients), those with partial response 44.4 weeks (144 patients), and those exhibiting no tumor regression after irradiation 30.6 weeks (168 patients—see Fig. 9–3). Survival for the complete responders is significantly greater than survival for the partial responders ($p = 0.005$, logrank test) and survival for partial responders is significantly greater than survival for the nonresponders ($p = 0.002$, logrank test). There is no apparent difference between the treatments with respect to survival ($p = 0.56$, logrank test). There is also no significant difference in survival among all the patients treated with 4000 rad versus those treated with 5000 or 6000 rad ($p = 0.10$).

Tumor response and survival are correlated with the histology and the stage of the tumor regardless of the dose of irradiation given (Table 9–6). The response-rate difference between the squamous and the adenocarcinoma plus large-cell groups is also signifcant (50% vs. 69%, $p = 0.001$, chi-square test). Stage of disease also has an effect upon response rate ($p = 0.003$, chi-square test). These prognostic factors must be taken into consideration in the analysis of results of definitive radiotherapy in non-oat-cell carcinoma of the lung.

Patients with squamous-cell carcinoma had a complete and partial response rate of 50%; those with adenocarcinoma had a response rate of 65%, and those with large-cell adenocarcinoma had a response rate of 75%. The median survival was about 40 weeks for the squamous-cell-carcinoma and adenocarcinoma patients and 51.9 weeks for those with large-cell undifferentiated carcinoma.

Patients with T1 and T2 tumors had complete and partial response rates of 82% and 67%, respectively, with corresponding median survival of 57.1 and 43.8 weeks. Patients with T3 tumors showed complete and partial reponse rates varying from 46% to 56%; the median survival was 57 weeks for those without radiographic evidence of lymphadenopathy (stage T3N0), in contrast to 37.3 and 34.7 weeks for those with N1 and N2 lymph nodes.

Between 12% and 19% of the patients in the various groups died during the first year after irradiation with persistent regressing intrathoracic tumor and without clinical evidence of tumor regrowth or distant metastasis. The majority of these patients died at home and an autopsy was not performed. The results reported should

TABLE 9–6. **RTOG Protocol No. 73-01. Response Rates and Median Survival by Patient Characteristics.**

Characteristic	Level	Response Rate	Median Survival (weeks)	Two-Year Survival Rate	Number of Deaths/Patients
Histology	Squamous	50%	40.9	13%	229/261
	Adenocarcinoma	65%	39.2	15%	48/57
	Large cell	75%	51.9	26%	38/51
	Other	33%	25.5	0%	5/6
Stage	T1N2	82%	57.1	30%	11/17
	T2N2	67%	43.8	11%	84/95
	T3N0	56%	57.0	32%	46/63
	T3N1	46%	37.7	9%	56/63
	T3N2	47%	34.7	11%	123/137

be considered preliminary because there are many patients on study who may develop a recurrence as follow-up continues.

Of the patients who were treated with a 4000-rad split or continuous course, 36% and 45% respectively showed radiographic evidence of initial intrathoracic recurrence only. In contrast, 28% of the patients who were treated with 5000 rad and 24% of those who received 6000 rad showed such radiographic evidence. Between 14% and 19% of the patients in all groups were reported as showing a combination of local or regional recurrence and distant metastasis. The overall rate of intrathoracic failures was 38% in the patients treated with 6000 rad, 45% in those treated with 5000 rad, 51% for those treated with a 4000-rad split course, and 64% for those treated with a 4000-rad continuous course. The incidence of distant metastases as detected by clinical or radiographic examination is 35% to 50% in all groups.[76]

Analysis of anatomic location of the first failure according to the method of treatment and degree of tumor response indicates that, in the patients treated with 4000 rad, the rate of intrathoracic failure is 42% to 58% as opposed to 33% to 45% in those treated with 5000 or 6000 rad (Fig. 9–4).

Strict quality assurance criteria are necessary in radiotherapy to achieve optimal treatment results. A careful program to evaluate techniques of irradiation and protocol compliance should be maintained to enhance the validity of clinical trials.

An evaluation of protocol compliance was carried out in 301 patients with available data, irradiated at the primary site according to protocol instructions (none or minor variation). Median survival for patients treated to the ipsilateral or contralateral hilar lymph nodes according to the protocol varied from 46 to 50 weeks in contrast to 20 to 30 weeks for those with major protocol variations in nodal irradiation. Variations in ipsilateral and contralateral nodal irradiation correlated with

significant reductions in tumor control (p = 0.02 and p = 0.009, respectively).[75]

In addition to patient and tumor characteristics, the technical factors of irradiation are critical parameters that affect tumor control and survival in patients with non-oat-cell bronchogenic carcinoma.

Limited Small-Cell Carcinoma of the Lung

Although a great number of uncontrolled and a few randomized studies have been reported over the past 10 years on the role of radiation therapy in the treatment of patients with small-cell carcinoma of the lung, a number of questions remain unsettled. The main issues in the management of these patients include the following.

Control of Disseminated Disease. This is crucial because it ultimately determines overall survival. Bone-marrow and distant visceral metastasis is the most common mechanism of failure after definitive treatment. It is important to mention the distant dissemination to sanctuary areas such as the brain, where chemotherapy agents are not transported in adequate concentrations. In attempting to achieve control of systemic disease, effective chemotherapeutic agents are a must. The role of irradiation, either as hemibody or total-body irradiation, has been superficially explored.[86] The irradiation of sanctuary areas, particularly the brain, has been shown to decrease development of clinical disease at these sites, although it has not affected survival.[92]

Local and Regional Tumor Control. Thoracic irradiation enhances tumor control within the irradiated volume. Local-regional (intrathoracic) recurrences are reported in 30% to 60% of the patients receiving thoracic irradiation, depending on the doses given, whereas 75% to 80% of the patients treated with chemotherapy alone exhibit this type of failure.[63] Optimal doses of irradiation have not been definitely established at the present time, optimal volume to be treated remains

INOPERABLE NON-OAT CELL CANCER OF LUNG
ANATOMICAL LOCATION OF RECURRENCES

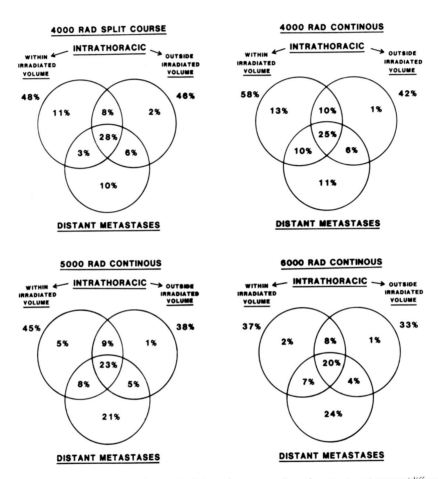

Fig. 9–4. Comparative analysis of anatomical sites of recurrence in various treatment groups (difference in local recurrence between 4000 rad and 6000 rad groups is statistically significant—$p = .04$ using an exact R X C test) (RTOG Protocol No. 73–01). (From Perez et al.: Int. J. Radiat. Oncol. Biol. Phys. 6:987, 1980.)

unknown, and optimal fractionation schedules and the most effective combination with chemotherapeutic agents have not been definitely established.

Careful Analysis of Morbidity of Therapy. This is important because these patients have a poor prognosis. The quality of life after treatment is critically important to the patient because of the low probability of long-term survival.

Role of Radiation Therapy

There is no question that small-cell carcinoma of the lung is sensitive to irradia-

tion. Over 10 years ago, a randomized study by the British Medical Research Council demonstrated 3 survivors in 73 patients treated with moderate doses of irradiation (4000 rad) in contrast to no survivors in 71 patients treated by surgery.[32]

Laing et al.[52] subsequently published a report of 31 patients treated with nitrogen mustard, vincristine, procarbazine, and prednisone (MOPP) compared with 37 patients treated with irradiation (4000 rad). Although the survival at 2 years was the same (below 5%), the median survival for the patients treated with chemotherapy was 4 months as opposed to 12 months for those treated with irradiation.

The Southeastern Cancer Study[51,74] demonstrated in a randomized study involving 53 patients that the concomitant administration of irradiation and chemotherapy yielded a 2-year disease-free survival of 20%, as opposed to less than 10% for the patients treated with radiotherapy alone with delayed chemotherapy upon relapse. The median survival was 27 months for the combined modality group as opposed to 9.9 months for those treated with radiotherapy alone. The intrathoracic failure rate was 40% for patients treated with concurrent combination therapy as opposed to 53% in those treated initially with irradiation alone. This demonstrated that the addition of chemotherapy enhanced the effects of irradiation on the tumor. Of patients who received chemotherapy, 25% had distant metastases compared with those treated with radiation alone, 38% of whom had distant metastases. Since that time, a number of other investigators have reported higher survival rates with more efficacious chemotherapeutic agents combined with thoracic and brain irradiation.[35] Some results are summarized in Table 9–7.

Cox[17] reported on patients treated with chemotherapy and radiotherapy. Local tumor control ranged from 57% to 89%, depending on the type of cytotoxic agents combined with radiotherapy (Table 9–8). When chemotherapy alone was given, the intrathoracic tumor control was only 38%. Similar results have been reported by Mira et al.[63] in a retrospective review of two Southwest Oncology Group (SWOG) protocols (7415 and 7828). In the 7415 protocol the chest received doses of 3000 rad in 2 weeks. The initial relapse in the chest was 24%. Patients treated in protocol 7828 received chemotherapy only and prophylactic brain irradiation without radiotherapy to the chest. The initial relapse in the

chest was 55%, and the overall chest recurrence rate was 73% (Table 9–9).

Of the irradiated patients that had thoracic tumor recurrences, approximately half had tumor relapse in the irradiated volume and half had tumor in other sites within the thorax (e.g., peripheral lung, mediastinum, pleura).

The role of irradiation in the treatment of patients with small-cell carcinoma of the lung is corroborated by a study reported by White et al.[98] on the patients treated in the SWOG protocol 7828. Those patients treated according to the protocol had a 30% 2-year-survival rate, as opposed to only 10% in those treated with major protocol variations (lower doses, inadequate portals, nonstandard dose fractionations). The relapse at the primary tumor site was 55% for those treated according to the protocol and 77% in those treated with protocol variations.

Surgery has not been completely discarded in the treatment of selected patients. Bates[5] reported on 29 patients with tumors initially diagnosed as small-cell undifferentiated carcinoma (6 finally diagnosed as poorly differentiated epidermoid carcinoma), who were treated with preoperative irradiation (1750 rad delivered in 3 days) followed by surgical resection of the tumor. Seven of the 29 patients (24%) survived for 4 years.

Optimal Volume To Be Treated

Current radiation therapy practice is to treat the primary tumor and involved hilar and mediastinal lymph nodes with a 2-cm margin and the contralateral hilum and mediastinum with a 1-cm margin. The supraclavicular lymph nodes are always included in the irradiated volume. Sometimes the volumes treated are large, which gives rise to significant morbidity. The optimal volume that should be treated has not been determined. Hansen et al.[41] reported that patients irradiated only to the thorax had the same survival as patients

TABLE 9–7. Selected Therapy and Survival in Limited-Stage Small-Cell Lung Cancer.

Regimen	Patients (no.)	Median Survival (wk)	One-Year Survival (%)
No specific therapy	31	14	7
Surgery*	270	—	19
Radiotherapy*	235	25	20
Radiotherapy plus			
1 CTX†	27	31	38
2 CTX, VCR†	23	50	50
3 CTX, VCR, ADR†	103	52	50
4 CTX, VCR, ADR, BCG†	19	78	70
5 CTX, VCR, ADR‡	15	76	80
6 CTX, VCR, ADR‡	32	Not reached	75

*Mean values of several studies.
†Radiotherapy given after starting chemotherapy or "sandwiched" between chemotherapy.
‡Radiotherapy given concomitantly with chemotherapy. CTX—cyclophosphamide; VCR—vincristine; ADR—doxorubicin (Adriamycin); BCG—Bacillus Calmette Guerin.
(Modified from: Greco, F.A. et al.: Am. J. Med. 66:626, 1979.)

TABLE 9–8. Small-Cell Carcinoma of Lung—Medical College of Wisconsin: 1974–80.

Study	CR* (%)	Local control of primary tumor	
		Local control (total) (%)	Local control (CR) (%)
I	81	57	65
II	96	81	85
III	72	28	38
IV	67	59	89

*Response of intrathoracic disease.
(From Cox, J.D. et al.: Int J Radiat Oncol Biol Phys 8:191, 1982.)

treated at other sites in addition to the thorax (e.g., the brain, liver and adrenals).

Further investigations in this area are warranted, including the use of whole-body and hemibody irradiation. Salazar et al.[86] in a preliminary report involving 19 patients with disseminated small-cell carcinoma of the lung receiving induction chemotherapy of cyclophosphamide (Cytoxan) and lomustine (CCNU) noted a partial response in 9 of these patients. Upper hemibody irradiation (UHBI) was given (600 rad on day 42 of the program) in addition to localized chest irradiation (2000 rad) to 9 patients. There were 5 overall complete responses of disseminated tumor and 7 complete intrathoracic regressions. The toxicity of this combined treatment was acceptable; only 1 patient developed severe leukopenia (<2000 white blood cells). The first course of maintenance

TABLE 9–9. Chest Relapses After Chemotherapy Response in Two SWOG Studies.

SWOG Study	Area of Chest Irradiated	# of Patients that Relapsed	Initial Relapse in Chest Only**	Overall Chest Relapse
#7415 (Ext. Dis.)	Primary, mediast., supracl*	75	18 (24%)	?
#7828	none	114	63 (55%)	83 (73%)

*3000 rad in 2 weeks
**p = 0.0001
(From Mira, J.G. et al.: Cancer 50:1266, 1982.)

chemotherapy was delayed in only 10% of the patients. The median relapse-free survival was 36 weeks in the patients achieving complete response after UHBI, in contrast to 14 weeks in the 4 who had only a partial response.

Optimal Doses of Irradiation

Johnson et al.[49] and Egan et al.[22] have suggested that doses in the range of 3000 rad delivered in 2 weeks may be adequate to control small-cell undifferentiated carcinoma when combined with intensive multiagent chemotherapy. No autopsy data are available on these patients, however, and intrathoracic recurrences are common.[46]

As reported by Cox et al.[18] and Mira et al.[63] multiple doses and fractionations of irradiation have been used (1500 rad in 1 week, 3000 rad in 2 weeks, 4000–4500 rad in 4–5 weeks, 5000 rad in 5 weeks—Table 9–10). Detailed information on intrathoracic tumor relapses in these patients is not available. In small groups of patients, Choi and Carey[14] reported increased control of primary and regional tumor with higher doses of irradiation (Fig. 9–5).

TABLE 9–10. **Chest Relapse after Chest Irradiation in Lung Small-Cell Carcinoma Treated by Combined Modality Radiotherapy–Chemotherapy.**

Reported by	Disease extent LD/ED*	Chest radiotherapy	Overall chest relapse	Chest relapse in irradiated field
Holoye, P.Y.	LD	6000 rads 20 fractions 8 weeks	—	1/16 (6%)
Abeloff, M.D.	LD	3000 rads 10 fractions 2 weeks	3/6 (50%)	3/6 (50%)
Alexander, M.	LD + ED	3000–5500 rads 15–25 fractions 3–5.5 weeks	8/15 (53%)	5/15 (33%)
Livingston, R.	LD	4500 rads 15 fractions 5 weeks	9/14 (64%)	7/14 (50%)
Levitt, M.	LD	4000 rads 10 fraction 3.5 weeks	8/15 (53%)	5/15 (33%)
Levitt, M.	ED	4000 rads 10 fractions 3.5 weeks	6/15 (40%)	3/15 (20%)
Cox, J.	LD + ED	1200–1800 rets	—	20/66 (30%)
Wittes, R.	LD + ED	3000–5000 rads 10–25 fractions 2–5 weeks	10/19 (53%)	7/23 (30%)
Mira, J.	LD	3000–4500 rads 10–15 fractions 2–6 weeks	7/17 (41%)	2/17 (12%)

*LD: limited disease; ED: extensive disease. (From Mira, J.G. et al.: Cancer 46:2557, 1980.)

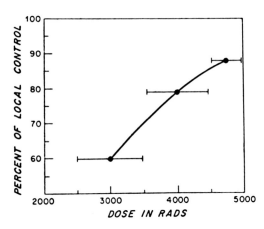

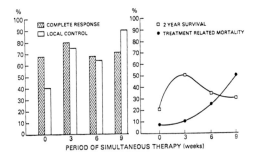

Fig. 9–6. Graph showing tumor control, survival, and treatment-related mortality with administration of irradiation and cytotoxic agents given concurrently or sequentially for the treatment of small cell carcinoma of lung. (From Catane et al.: *Cancer* 49:1936, 1981.)

Fig. 9–5. Control of primary and regional metastases of small cell anaplastic carcinoma over 4 months in relation to radiation dosage. Radiation doses were standardized to a weekly tumor dose of 1000 rad with 200 rad per treatment and 5 treatments weekly. (From Choi, et al: *Cancer* 37:2651, 1976.)

In SWOG protocol 7828, White et al.[98] reported a 30% 2-year disease-free-survival rate in patients receiving 4500 rad as opposed to a 20% 2-year-survival rate in those treated with 3000 rad.

It is apparent that higher doses of irradiation produce better intrathoracic tumor control, although the optimal dose fractionation and the effect on long-term survival are not known.

Cox et al.[16] indicated that doses of irradiation can be modified depending on the chemotherapy regimens used; lower doses of irradiation and chemotherapy show tumor control rates comparable to those for higher doses of radiation alone.

Chronological Administration (Timing) of Irradiation and Chemotherapy

Irradiation and cytotoxic agents have been concurrently or sequentially administered for the treatment of patients with small-cell carcinoma of the lung. A report published by Catane et al.[13] from the National Cancer Institute (NCI) Radiation Oncology Branch, suggests that there is an optimal period of time for simultaneous administration of these therapies. In their experience with small groups of patients

(about 10 per group), this optimal period was 3 weeks. The tumor control in the thorax was improved, and the 2-year survival increased to 40%. With longer, simultaneous administration of these two modalities, however, the morbidity increased greatly and survival declined (Fig. 9–6). One area to be explored in forthcoming protocols is the timing of administration of these modalities.

Value of Elective Brain Irradiation

Several reports indicate that approximately 30% of the patients treated with chemotherapy without prophylactic brain irradiation develop clinical brain metastases. An autopsy series indicated the incidence to be in the range of 45%.[18] Following elective brain irradiation with doses of 3000 rad in 2 weeks to 4000 rad in 3 weeks, the clinical evidence of brain metastasis is decreased to 3% from 5%. No impact on survival has been observed.

The value of elective brain irradiation should be considered within the context of observations reported by Baglan and Marks,[4] who indicate that 70% of the patients who have overt clinical brain metastases have good palliative results with valid doses of cranial irradiation. In elective irradiation, 100 patients would be treated in order to benefit 25% of them, since 5 will recur even if treated electively. With delayed treatment of clinical metastases, 70% of 30 patients (20) would achieve good palliative results. Thus, there is a difference of 5 patients between the two groups that would be benefited by the elective cranial irradiation.

Potential Areas of Future Investigation

The following are areas of potential research in the treatment of limited small-cell carcinoma of the lung:

Chemotherapy
New agents or combinations of drugs
Use of cell kinetics to select optimal drugs, doses, schedules
Adjuncts to improve efficacy of maintenance chemotherapy (reinduction)
Irradiation
Optimal volume to be treated
Optimal dose fractionation
Irradiation of sanctuary sites (local, regional, hemibody, total body)
Use of other techniques (interstitial, high-LET particles, sensitizers)
Combination of Drugs and Irradiation (timing, dose schedules)

Apical Tumors

Apical tumors have been treated with preoperative irradiation (3000–4000 rad in 3–4 weeks) and surgery,[72] a combination of external irradiation and intraoperative implantation of radioactive sources,[44] or external irradiation alone with doses in the range of 6000–6500 rad.[50] Comparable results are observed with these three techniques (25% to 30% survival at 5 years).

CARCINOMA OF THE ESOPHAGUS

Natural History and Pathological Features

Some predisposing conditions that may influence therapeutic decisions have been described (e.g., Plummer-Vinson syndrome, achalasia of the cardia, esophageal peptic ulcer, hiatus hernia, chronic alcoholism, cirrhosis of the liver, and smoking).[23]

Approximately 20% of the primary esophageal carcinomas occur in the cervical esophagus and 80% occur in the thoracic esophagus. Tumors of the thoracic esophagus are more often located in the lower (43%) and the middle (37%) thirds than in the upper third (20%).[83] Squamous-cell carcinoma accounts for 90% of cases, and is usually poorly differentiated, accounting for the high proportion of regional and distant metastases. Adenocarcinoma occurs less frequently and usually appears in the lower third of the thoracic esophagus. Carcinoma of the esophagus commonly exhibits submucosal spread along the muscular layers and frequently extends to lengths of 10 cm or more, forming a scirrhous lesion. Spread by direct contiguity to structures in the neck and mediastinum is common, facilitated by the absence of serosa. Lesions of the cervical esophagus may extend to the carotid arteries, pleura, recurrent laryngeal nerves, and trachea. Lesions of the middle third may invade the mainstem bronchi, the thoracic duct, aortic arch, subclavian artery, intercostal vessels, azygos vein and the right pleura. Tumors of the lower third may extend into the pericardium, left pleura, and descending aorta. These tumors can spread and perforate the mediastinum, causing mediastinitis, or it can spread into the tracheobronchial tree, causing bronchopneumonia. The esophagus has a rich lymphatic supply, and spread of lesion in the upper third of the esophagus leads to involvement of the lymph nodes of the anterior jugular chain and supraclavicular region; tumors of the lower third of the esophagus metastasize mainly to the celiac and perigastric lymph nodes. Hematogenous metastases, noted in 40% of patients with primary carcinoma of the esophagus at presentation are mainly to the liver, lung, bones, and kidneys.[80] The lungs and pleura can become involved by direct extension or hematogenous metastasis. The liver is involved in 52%, the lungs or pleura in 21%, and the bones in 8% of the patients.

Staging Procedures

Dynamic examinations while the patient is drinking barium are very useful in showing a fixed nondistensible esophagus.[23] Esophagoscopy and biopsy definitively establish the diagnosis (endoscopy is accurate in about 96% of the cases). Bronchoscopy is indicated in patients with tumors in the upper and middle thoracic esophagus. Distant metastasis may be detected with chest radiographs, bone scans, liver–spleen scans, and so forth.

The current TNM staging system is shown in Table 9–11.[85] It is to be noted that the cervical lymph nodes are classified because they are easily palpable. The

TABLE 9–11.   Classification* of Carcinoma of the Esophagus.

Regions†
Cervical Esophagus.—(upper third)
Intrathoracic Esophagus.—(middle third)
Distal Part of Esophagus Including Abdominal portion.—(lower third)

Classification

T.—Primary Tumor
  T1.—Tumor confined to one region and not impairing peristalsis or mobility of the organ
  T2.—Tumor confined to one region but impairing peristalsis or mobility of the organ
  T3.—Tumor extending to more than one region
  T4.—Tumor extending to neighboring structures

N.—Regional Lymph Nodes
  a. Cervical esophagus: Regional nodes are the cervical nodes
    N0.—No nodes palpable
    N1.—Movable homolateral nodes
    N2.—Movable contralateral or bilateral nodes
    N3.—Fixed nodes
  b.—Intrathoracic esophagus
  c.—Distal esophagus‡

M.—Distant Metastases
  M0.—No evidence of distant metastases
  M1.—Distant metastases present

*Classification applies only to carcinoma. Extent of disease may be assessed by clinical examination, radiography, and endoscopy.
†Tumor is assigned to the region in which the bulk of it is situated.
‡Since it is impossible to assess the state of intrathoracic and intraabdominal lymph nodes, the symbol NS is used, permitting eventual addition of histological information, thus, NX − or NX +.
(From Rubin, P.: JAMA 226:1545, 1973.)

intrathoracic and abdominal nodes are not classified because they are not clinically accessible. The length of the tumor has a direct relationship to nodal spread. Fifty percent of patients with tumors less than 5 cm in length develop nodal metastases; however, if the length is greater than 5 cm, 90% of the patients develop nodal metastases.

General Management of Esophageal Carcinoma

If no regional or distant metastases are detected, attempted complete resection of the tumor is the basic primary treatment of carcinoma of the esophagus, even though operative mortality for this procedure is high, ranging between 10% and 15%.[12,70] Infiltration of the mediastinum at presentation and a high incidence of nodal or distant metastases markedly limit the indications for surgical resection. In a series done by Ross,[80] only 23% of the patients were treated by radical surgery. Patients with esophageal cancer are more frequently treated with chemotherapy. Several reports have been recently published without significant results.[33,67,89]

Surgery

The tumor is excised with at least a 5-cm margin above the upper limits of any palpable tumor, and below the stomach cardia. The paraesophageal lymph nodes and the paratracheal lymph nodes are excised. Esophagogastrostomy is performed to restore the continuity of the digestive tract.

For tumors at the gastroesophageal junction, a thoracoabdominal exploration is performed. The tumor is excised, as are the whole stomach and the jejunum; the colon is used to restore continuity with the remaining part of the esophagus.[61]

Preoperative Radiotherapy

Preoperative radiotherapy has been used to decrease the size of the lesion and render radical resection more feasible.[3]

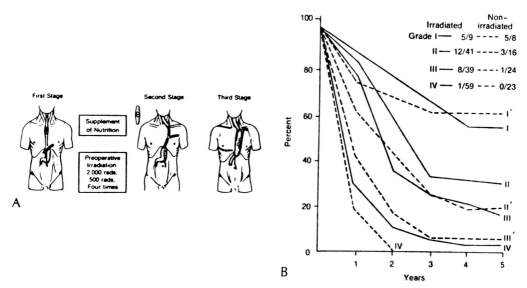

Fig. 9–7. *(A)* Three-stage operation for cancer of the upper and midthoracic esophagus. The first stage consists of celiotomy with removal of lymph nodes and gastrostomy. After 1 to 2 weeks, in the second stage, entire thoracic esophagus is removed. The third stage is esophagogastrostomy performed 6 to 12 months later. *(B)* Relationship between grade of cancer of upper- and mid-thoracic esophagus and effect of preoperative irradiation. (From Nakayama et al.: Cancer 20:778, 1967.)

Nakayama and Kinoshita[66] reported a decrease in the operative mortality from 8.1% in patients treated with one-stage operation to 3.9% in patients treated with three-stage operation (Fig. 9–7A). The latter starts with a celiotomy, removal of the celiac lymph nodes, and gastrostomy. If there is no evidence of tumor spread, this is followed by preoperative irradiation (2000 rad in 3–4 daily fractions); 1 to 2 weeks later the entire thoracic esophagus is removed. In 6 to 12 months, if the patient is tumor-free, an esophagogastrostomy is performed. The 5-year-survival rate with preoperative radiotherapy in the series by Nakayama and Kinoshita was 57.7%, but this is a highly selected population; the survival rate for patients treated by resection only is 19% (Fig. 9–7B). Parker[70] reported 0.6% 2-year-survival rate with surgery alone, 5% with radiotherapy alone, and 9% to 12% with preoperative radiotherapy (4500 rad in 3–4 weeks followed in 6–8 weeks by surgical resection of the tumor). Mortality was reduced from 37%

with surgery alone to 14% with preoperative radiotherapy.

Groves and Rodrigues-Antunez[37] at the Cleveland Clinic described 6 of 24 patients with squamous-cell carcinoma of the esophagus surviving after 2400 rad were delivered in 3 fractions prior to surgery. Four of the 6 surviving patients were followed for more than 2 years postoperatively. Marks[58] reported 3-year-survival rate of 22.8% in 101 patients treated with preoperative radiotherapy (4500 rad in 18 fractions) followed by surgical resection. The 2-year-survival rate was only 5.6% in those not amenable to exploration, and 12.1% in those given high curative radiotherapy. Yamashita et al.[100] described a 35% 5-year-survival rate in patients with carcinoma of the esophagus treated with preoperative irradiation (5000–6000 rad in 4–6 weeks) and surgery, compared to the 14% survival rate for those treated with surgery alone and the 9% survival rate for those treated with radiotherapy alone. Radical resection was feasible in 90% of the irradiated patients in contrast to 30%

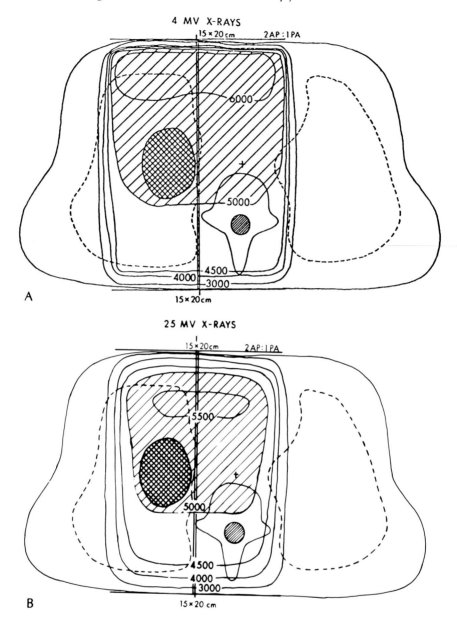

4 MV X-RAYS

15 × 20 cm   2AP:1PA

6000

5000

4500
4000   3000

A   15×20cm

25 MV X-RAYS

15×20cm   2AP:1PA

5500

5000

4500
4000
3000

B   15×20 cm

Fig. 9–8.   *(A)* Isodose distributions for AP–PA portal arrangements using 4 MeV x-rays wih a 2:1 AP–PA loading. *(B)* Dose distribution using 25 MeV x-rays with 2:1 AP–PA loading. The tumor dose (5000 rad) is comparable to 4 MeV x-rays, but the maximum dose is about 15% less because of the improved depth dose with the higher energy beam. (From Perez: Sem. Resp. Med. 4:17, 1982.)

in the nonirradiated. The local recurrence rate was 24% in the patients treated with combined therapy and 50% in those treated with surgery alone.

Definitive Radiotherapy

Pearson[73] reported a 10% survival rate at 5 years for those treated by radical megavoltage irradiation versus 7% survival for those treated by surgery alone in an analysis of 2032 patients with esophageal cancer. The difference was mainly due to operative mortality. He also reports that patients treated radically by irradiation have a better prognosis if the tumor is located high in the esophagus; those treated surgically have a better prognosis the lower the tumor is located. This trend is influenced by the patient's sex and age.

Squamous-cell carcinoma of the esophagus is, on the average, moderately radiosensitive. Tumor infiltration is generally more than 5 cm beyond gross demonstrable margin. As a basic rule the entire esophagus is irradiated, as are the adjacent mediastinum and periesophageal lymph nodes. Anterior–posterior (AP) or oblique portals are used to achieve optimal dose distribution (Figs. 9–8 and 9–9). Casts have frequently been used to aid in the accurate alignment of oblique beams.[73] Rotational techniques are particularly suited for irradiation of the esophagus, although the correction for the varying course of the esophagus in the mediastinum may prove to be extremely difficult (Fig. 9–10).

A three-portal arrangement and dose distribution are illustrated in Figure 9–11.

Pearson[73] recommends delivering 5000

rad in 4 to 5 weeks; he reported a 20% 5-year-survival rate. The dose of radiation necessary to eradicate even a small tumor (i.e., 2–3 cm) is about 6000 rad. A segment of esophagus at least 5 cm above and below the gross lesion should be included in the high-dose volume. Irradiation of more than 1-cm margins beyond demonstrable tumor requires a reduction in tumor dose (maximum of 5500 rad in 6 weeks to long segments of the esophagus). The uninvolved adjacent esophagus and mediastinum should be treated with a tumor dose of about 5000 rad. Doses in the range of 4500 rad provide good palliation in a large proportion of the patients.

The usual fractionation is 180- to 200-rad tumor dose daily with 4 to 5 weekly fractions.

A trial of neutron therapy combined with ^{60}Co gamma rays in carcinoma of the esophagus was reported by Eichhorn et al.[24] The tumor disappeared completely in

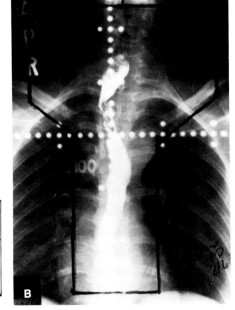

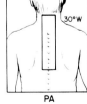

Fig. 9–9. *(A)* Portals used for the treatment of carcinoma of the esophagus with two oblique anterior wedge portals and a posterior open field. *(B)* Simulation film illustrating volume irradiated in patient with carcinoma of the thoracic esophagus. (A. From Radiation Therapy Oncology Group, S. Kramer, Chairman: Standard treatment planning summary: Dosimetry guidelines for cancer of the esophagus, stomach and pancreas, No. 6, p. 34.)

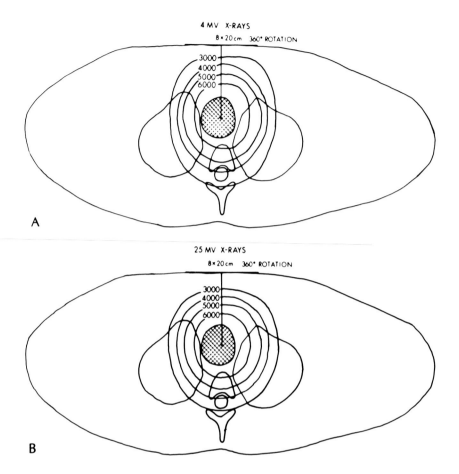

Fig. 9–10. Dose distribution using 360° rotation with 4 MeV *(A)* and 25 MeV *(B)* x-rays. Note the comparable dose distribution obtained with these energies.

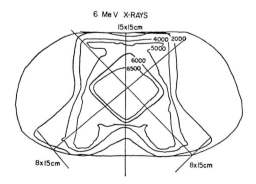

Fig. 9–11. Three portal arrangement using 6 MeV x-rays. Approximately 5000 rad are delivered to the mediastinum with a maximum of 6500 rad to the center of the thorax.

6 of 11 patients treated with combined ^{60}Co gamma rays and a neutron dose proportion of 27%. This appeared superior to ^{60}Co alone, which yielded complete regression of tumor in only 25 of 65 patients treated. The combinations of those beams may be used in the future to obtain better tumor control.

TECHNIQUES OF IRRADIATION

Carcinoma of the Lung: Volume, Portals, and Beam Arrangement

The volume to be treated and the configuration of the irradiation portals should be determined by: (1) the size and location of the primary tumor; (2) the areas of lym-

NON–OAT CELL CA OF LUNG
AP PORTALS

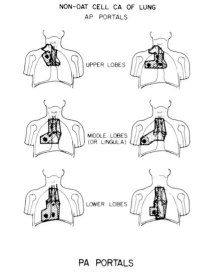

UPPER LOBES

MIDDLE LOBES
(OR LINGULA)

LOWER LOBES

PA PORTALS

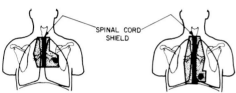

SPINAL CORD
SHIELD

Fig. 9–12. Example of portals used for irradiation of non–oat-cell carcinoma of the lung, depending on the anatomical location of the primary. The tumor and immediate lymph node bearing areas (linear pattern) are treated to higher doses and electively irradiated lymph-node draining sites (dotted pattern) receive a minimum of 4500-rad tumor dose. A shield for the spinal cord could be used on the posterior portals, keeping in mind that if 5 half-value-layer (HVL) blocks are used there is a significant decrease in the dose under the block.

phatic drainage in the hila and mediastinum; (3) the histologic type; and (4) the equipment and beam energy available. It is extremely important to keep in mind the maximum doses tolerated by sensitive intrathoracic structures (e.g., the lung, spinal cord and heart). It is common practice to design the treatment portals with a 2-cm margin around any gross tumor seen on the posterior-anterior (PA) chest radiograph and a minimum 1-cm margin around electively treated regional-lymph-node areas (hilar, upper or lower mediastinal, supraclavicular nodes). To include the appropriate lymph-node draining areas, special attention should be given to the lym-

phatic pathways of each lobe of the right and left lungs.[69] Irregularly shaped fields are preferred, requiring special secondary blocking to spare as much normal tissue as possible (Fig. 9–12). AP and PA fields may suffice with high-energy photon beams (over 20 MeV) or when tumor doses below 4500 rad are delivered with low-energy photons.

In patients with potentially curable lesions to be treated with high doses of irradiation, particularly when only ^{60}Co or 4 MeV x-rays are available, more complicated portal arrangements are necessary, such as the three-field plan shown in Figure 9–11. Oblique or lateral portals are also useful in combination with AP–PA ports, to boost the dose to a particular segment of the lung or the mediastinum. Another technique, widely used in the mediastinum, is 360° or partial-arch rotation. Spinal-cord shielding blocks in the posterior portal must be used judiciously; it is important to recognize the impact of this practice in reducing the mediastinal dose. The spinal-cord block should therefore be used only for a small portion of the treatment; oblique or lateral portals are required to deliver the prescribed tumor dose to the mediastinal and hilar lymph nodes or to centrally located primary tumors, regardless of the photon energy used. Special care should be exercised to restrict the dose to normal lung tissue as much as possible. Large volumes of contralateral, uninvolved lung should not receive doses above 1800 rad.

If the primary tumor is in the upper lobes

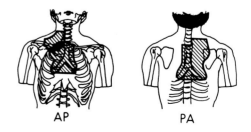

AP   PA

Fig. 9–13. Example of portals used for irradiation of apical tumors.

or if there is evidence of superior mediastinal involvement, the supraclavicular nodes should always be included in the irradiated volume. The portal arrangement varies slightly for apical tumors; the supraclavicular nodes, adjacent vertebral body, and the upper lobe and hilar nodes are included in the fields of irradiation (Fig. 9–13). The same fields can be used for epidermoid carcinoma, large-cell undifferentiated carcinoma, and adenocarcinoma.

Small-cell undifferentiated carcinoma requires more generous portals, which should always include the hilar, mediastinal, and supraclavicular lymph nodes. In the past 5 years, some investigators have advocated elective irradiation of organs with a high incidence of metastatic spread such as the brain; however, this will require further investigation.

Carcinoma of the Esophagus: Volume, Portals, and Beam Arrangement

Special consideration must be given to the location of the primary tumor, the extent of the involvement of the adjacent esophagus, and the location of the mediastinal lymph nodes. Treatment of the supraclavicular lymph nodes (in cervical or proximal thoracic lesions) and the gastroesophageal junction and celiac axis (in distal thoracic esophagus tumors) must also be given special consideration.

In the cervical esophagus, it is preferred to extend the ports from the laryngopharynx to the carina of trachea. The anterior cervical and superior mediastinal lymph nodes should be included in the irradiated volume. For cervical or upper thoracic-esophagus tumors, the portals may be modified to include the supraclavicular lymph nodes. We do not routinely treat the supraclavicular lymph nodes in the middle or distal thoracic esophagus unless they are clinically palpable.

For lesions of the thoracic esophagus, the entire length of the esophagus is included in the irradiated volume. A 5-cm margin beyond the gross tumor is used in the proximal portion; the portals thus include some of the cervical esophagus in the tumors located in the upper thoracic esophagus. In tumors located in the distal third of the thoracic esophagus, we routinely irradiate the gastroesophageal junction and celiac-axis lymph nodes.

To determine the configuration of the portals, a viscous radiopaque substance is given to the patient at the time of the simulation to outline the esophagus. The mediastinum is included with a 1-cm to 2-cm margin. Most portals are 6 cm to 8 cm wide.

In patients treated for palliation, a tumor dose of approximately 4500 rad is given in 4 to 5 weeks using an unequal loading favoring the anterior port (3:2) and holding the spinal-cord dose below 4000 rad. For patients treated with definitive radiotherapy, the same initial approach is used. When a 4500-rad tumor dose is completed, the patients are given 2 weeks rest; upon returning for treatment, anterior or posterior oblique fields with wedges are instituted to raise the dose to a 6500-rad tumor dose (uncorrected for increased lung transmission).

In carcinoma of the esophagus, a posterior spinal-cord block should never be used, for obvious anatomic and dosimetry reasons. A combination of stationary and rotational portals has been used at some institutions to accomplish the same treatment goals.

CONSIDERATIONS IN TREATMENT PLANNING

The choice of appropriate beam energies and loadings, in addition to the volume to be treated, are crucial to the delivery of adequate doses of irradiation to the tumor without producing injury to the adjacent normal tissues. Because of the large diameter of the chest, better dose distributions are achieved with high energy photons (Fig. 9–14A) The use of unequal loading (i.e., 2:1, AP–PA) such as illus-

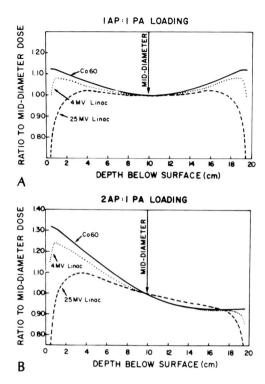

A

B

Fig. 9–14. *(A)* Dose profile with various energies for equal AP–PA loading in irradiation of the thorax. Increasing given (maximum) doses are necessary for 4 MeV x-rays or ^{60}Co in order to achieve the same midplane tumor dose when compared with 25 MeV x-rays. *(B)* Dose profile for same energy beams with a 2:1 AP–PA loading. Even though the doses at the midplane and posteriorly are comparable, there is a 25% greater dose delivered with the ^{60}Co and 15% with a 4 MeV x-rays to the anterior tissues, namely the heart, in comparison with 25 MeV photons.

trated in Figure 9–14B may be used to deliver different doses to the tumor and the normal structures (i.e., the spinal cord) but care must be exercised to avoid undesirably high doses to other sensitive organs (e.g., the heart).

The most significant problems encountered in treatment planning for bronchogenic cancer include: (1) the sloping surface of the chest with decreased diameter at the thoracic inlet; (2) the presence of nonunit density tissues such as the lung; (3) the proximity of sensitive structures (spinal cord, heart, and lung); and (4) the frequent need for irregular-field isodose computations.

The sloping surface of the chest results in varying source–tumor distances over the treatment field and produces a nonuniform dose distribution. One method of compensating for this problem is to use the decreasing-field technique or "poorman's wedge." This achieves an effective isodose distribution by decreasing the field size across the portals axis when a desired tumor dose is achieved at a given point. A disadvantage of this method is that it requires setups for varying field sizes, complicated prescriptions, and multiple calculations at various points.

The sloping-surface effect may be corrected alternatively by the use of compensating filters (Fig. 9–15). Several of these devices have been described in the literature[9,27,40,54,96,99] and some are commercially available. At our Institution, a lucite stepwedge compensating filter is routinely used in the treatment of chest portals. This filter is relatively inexpensive and can be assembled very easily. One must bear in mind, however, that this is a special-purpose filter that compensates only for the midsagittal plane and for surfaces sloping in the cephalocaudad direction only.

A method of compensating for sloping surfaces and tissue heterogeneities over a volume was outlined by Ellis in 1960.[26] He indicated that information on the inhomogeneity of thoracic tissue (obtained by transverse axial tomography at several levels), when used in conjunction with the information derived from standard isodose curves for tumor dose beyond the inhomogeneity, could provide the basis for avoiding errors as large as 30% in dosage to the esophagus. This method, though sound in principle, is difficult in practice without adequate radiographic facilities and a mould-room staff. A more recent report by Ellis and Lescrenier describes a technique that uses film to measure transmitted-beam parameters upon which the construction of individual compensators can be based.[28] The method requires that

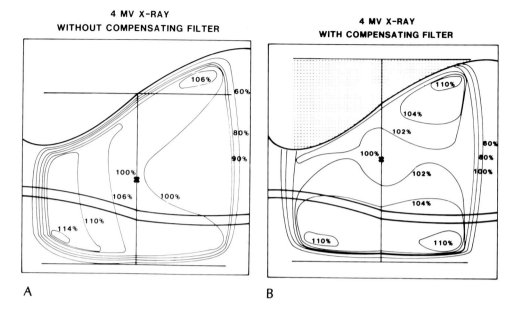

Fig. 9–15. *(A)* Dose distribution in a sagittal plane of the chest showing the increased dose to the spinal cord particularly at the thoracic inlet because of the sloping anterior surface of the chest. *(B)* Effect of compensating filter in normalizing the dose in the chest, thus sparing the spinal cord at the thoracic inlet.

diametrically opposed beams be used. A densitometer is used to monitor the photographic image of the high-energy treatment beam after passage through the patient; this allows one to estimate the amount of matter traversed at each point, whether modified by surface irregularities or tissue inhomogeneities. By compensating for these variations, the entire tissue volume can be covered.

Four inhomogeneities are generally encountered in radiation therapy: air cavities, lung, fat, and bone. Only air cavities and lung are usually considered in treatment planning for lung and esophageal carcinoma. To correct fully for these inhomogeneities, it is necessary to know not only their size, shape, and position, but also their electron density and atomic number; to date, only part of this information has been developed. The usual procedure for accounting for these inhomogeneities is to use a standard water-equivalent-isodose chart and then to calculate correction factors to this data. Several methods have been developed for

this type of correction including: (1) the tissue–air-ratio (TAR) method; (2) the iso-dose-shift method; and (3) the power law TAR method.[47] A modification of the TAR power method has recently been suggested by MacDonald et al.[57] This method appears to be an improvement because it applies separate correction factors to the primary and scatter components of the absorbed dose.

A problem unique to the treatment of tumors in the upper respiratory system with two opposed beams is that a dose inhomogeneity may occur in the transition zone between air and tissue, causing a dose reduction to cells close to the air cavity and possibly accounting for recurrences. Several investigators have measured this effect, indicating an approximate reduction in dose 25%.[29,68,90] The recent advent of computerized tomography has opened new perspectives to assess the effects of inhomogeneities in dose distribution in the thorax (Fig. 9–16).

Another problem in the treatment of lung tumors is encountered when the isocentric

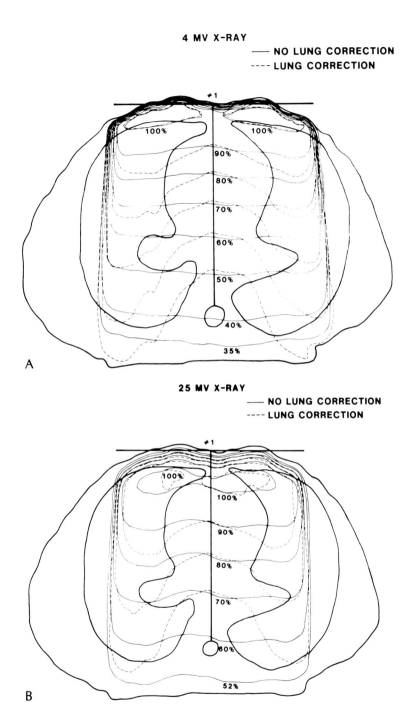

Fig. 9–16. Isodose for single beams of 4 MeV *(A)* and 25 MeV *(B)* x-rays demonstrating the increased transmission in the lung and effect of correction in treatment plan.

technique is used. In this case, the treatment axis is not horizontal when the patient is supine. This problem and its solution are discussed in detail in articles by Besford et al.[7] and Fleming and Orchard.[30] They demonstrated that it is not sufficient to rotate the field direction alone when treating a tilted axis in multiple fixed-field therapy. The authors showed that suitable rotation of the field direction, the couch, and the field-defining diaphragm axis enables the physician to obtain the correct treatment angle with respect to the tilted axis.

It is relatively easy to deliver a 4500-rad tumor dose to the midplane of the mediastinum with AP–PA ports, particularly when high-energy beams are used. Special attention should be paid to the dose delivered to the spinal cord. A common practice to decrease the spinal cord dose has been to insert a 1.5 cm to 2 cm wide shielding block of the posterior port with varying degrees of thickness (1–5 HVL). This technique should be discouraged because it reduces the dose delivered to the midplane of the mediastinum (Fig. 9–17).

When additional doses are required to the hilar or mediastinal lymph node, it is extremely useful to resort to oblique ports that spare the spinal cord. When the treatment plan indicates it, wedges should be used (Figs. 9–18 and 9–19). It is important for the radiation oncologist to become familiar with the anatomy of the chest in oblique-beam arrangements. A useful technique is to identify the volume of interest and outline the appropriate port under fluoroscopic conditions using the simulator on the AP projection. Once this is accomplished, the beam can be rotated with frequent fluoroscopic observation. This permits the physician to observe the progressive distortion of the anatomy with the rotation of the beam. Radiographs and photographs should be obtained to document the setup. The photograph should include the gantry rotation and the specific outline of the port from the patient's skin.

The large, irregularly shaped treatment fields commonly used for carcinoma of the lung necessitate the calculation of dose by an approximation method or by using the scatter-calculations method described by Clarkson.[15] Two commonly used approx-

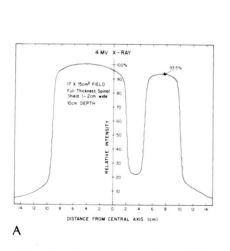

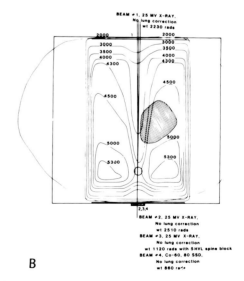

A   B

Fig. 9–17. *(A)* Dose profile with open field or with interposition 2 cm (5 HVL) midline block used for the spinal cord. Note the 20% dose level below the block because of scattered irradiation where a 3% dose level below the block from primary beam transmission only would be expected. *(B)* Treatment plan showing reduced midline dose to mediastinum because of posterior spinal-cord block.

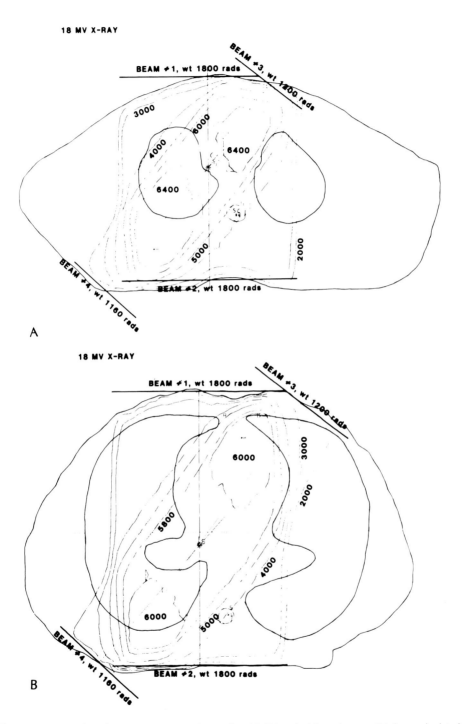

Fig. 9–18. Examples of various treatment plans using AP–PA and oblique beams. *(A)* dose calculated at thoracic inlet, *(B)* dose calculated at central axis, midthorax level.

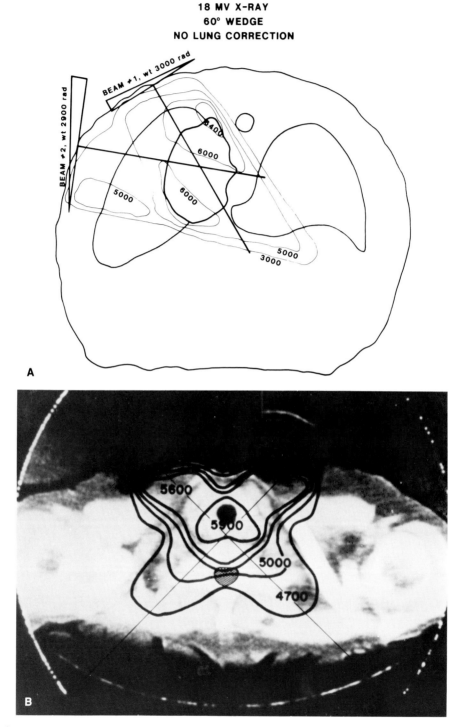

18 MV X-RAY
60° WEDGE
NO LUNG CORRECTION

Fig. 9–19. Examples of oblique beams using wedges for the treatment of tumors in the superior mediastinum.

imation methods involve either a geometric approximation, in which the irregular treatment field is approximated by a rectangular field, or empirically determined correction factors, which give the variation of the treatment setup from a standard phantom setup. The accuracy of these approximations is dependent upon the particular type of radiation unit, field size and shape used for measurement, and the points chosen for calculation.

Clarkson's more general approach using either scatter functions or scatter–air ratios has been explained in detail for manual calculations by Cundiff et al.[19] and Johns and Cunningham.[48] With this approach, the dose to any point within the patient is calculated as a summation of the primary and scattered radiation contributions to that point. If the variation in source–skin distances and the variation of dose rate across the field are taken into consideration, the Clarkson method is reasonably accurate.

RADIATION TOLERANCE OF INTRATHORACIC ORGANS

Meticulous techniques are necessary in order to decrease the dose to a variety of sensitive normal tissues in the thorax, particularly the lungs. In the absence of chemotherapy, the following are accepted tolerated doses for intrathoracic structures:

Ipsilateral normal lung
  a 2000-rad tumor dose is the maximum tolerated, unless required to treat tumor and lymph nodes
Contralateral normal lung
  no irradiation unless absolutely unavoidable, in which case a 2000-rad tumor dose is the maximum tolerated
Entire heart
  a 4500-rad tumor dose in 5 weeks is the maximum. Less than 50% of the heart may receive a 5000-rad maximum in 6 weeks
Spinal cord
  4000-rad tumor dose in 5 weeks is the maximum (2500-rad tumor dose in 1–2 weeks with split-course therapy regimen)
Esophagus
  5500-rad tumor dose/5 weeks is the maximum

Table 9–12 shows the major complications observed in the patients treated on RTOG protocol 73-01 for the various doses of irradiation given.

The addition of chemotherapy has been shown to significantly enhance the effect of irradiation. Phillips and Margolis[78] reported a 50% incidence of radiation pneumonitis in patients treated with radiation alone in doses of about 2650 rad in 20 fractions. When actinomycin D was added,

TABLE 9–12.   RTOG Protocol No. 73-01: Definitive Radiation Therapy in Unresectable Carcinoma of the Lung.

Severe Complications of Treatment							
	4000 Rad Split		4000 Rad Continuous		5000 Rad Continuous		6000 Rad Continuous
Pneumonitis	3	2*	—		2	1*	3 1*
Pulmonary fibrosis	8		1		1		3
Esophagitis	2		1		1		1
Pneumothorax	1		—	1*	—		—
Bronchial obstruction	—		—		—		— 2*
Esophageal stricture	—		1		—		1
Total	14 & 2*		3 & 1*		4 & 1*		8 & 3*

*Life-threatening complications

the incidence of pneumonitis was 50% with doses of 2050 rad in 20 fractions. Patients receiving bleomycin may develop interstitial pulmonary fibrosis, which can accentuate the similar effects of irradiation. Decreased pulmonary function frequently occurs following irradiation, particularly if large volumes of lung are treated to doses over 2000 rad. In the initial phases of radiation therapy, pulmonary capacity may improve because of decreased bronchial obstruction and atelectasis. Brady et al.[10] and Deeley[20] have pointed out that there is a progressive, decreased ventilatory and diffusing capacity as a result of alveolar-cell degeneration and interstitial fibrosis.

Johnson et al.[49] reported several cases of esophageal fibrosis with stenosis following the administration of 3000 rad in 2 weeks combined with intensive triple agent chemotherapy (Doxorubicin Hydrochloride, vincristine sulphate, and cyclophosphamide) given the same day every 3 to 4 weeks. Also, the well-known cardiotoxicity of adriamycin, coupled with the effects of radiation on the heart, makes this combination more toxic. When these two agents are combined, it is recommended that no more than 400-rad tumor dose be given to the entire heart, or that a maximum of 450 mg/m^2 total dose of adriamycin be administered.

The effects of combined irradiation and chemotherapy on the spinal cord have not been properly evaluated, but it is reasonable to believe that there may be an additive or potentiating effect.

REFERENCES

1. Abramson, N., Cavanaugh, P.J.: Short-course radiation therapy in carcinoma of the lung. Radiology 96:627, 1970.
2. Abramson, N., Cavanaugh, P.J.: Short-course radiation therapy in carcinoma of the lung: A second look. Radiology 108:685, 1973.
3. Akakura, I. et al.: Surgery of carcinoma of the esophagus with preoperative radiation. Chest 57:47, 1970.
4. Baglan, R.J., Marks, J.E.: Comparison of symptomatic and prophylactic irradiation in brain metastases from oat cell carcinoma of the lung. Cancer 47:41, 1981.
5. Bates, M., Hurt, R., Levison, V., Sutton, M.: Treatment of oat-cell carcinoma of bronchus by preoperative radiotherapy and surgery. Lancet 1:1134, 1974.
6. Bell, J.W.: Abdominal exploration on one-hundred lung carcinoma suspects prior to thoracotomy. Ann. Surg. 167:199, 1968.
7. Besford, H., Sivyer, A., Brain, E.W.: A planning device for use with beam direction shells. Br. J. Radiol. 37:391, 1964.
8. Bloedorn, F.G. et al.: Preoperative irradiation in bronchogenic carcinoma. AJR 92:77, 1964.
9. Boge, J.R., Edland, R.W., Matthes, D.C.: Tissue compensators for megavoltage radiotherapy fabricated from hollowed styrofoam filled with wax. Radiology 111:193, 1974.
10. Brady, W.L., Germon, P.A., Cander, L.: The effects of radiation therapy on pulmonary function in carcinoma of the lung. Radiology 85:130, 1965.
11. Bromley, L.L., Szur, L.: Combined radiotherapy and resection for carcinoma of the bronchus: Experiences with 66 patients. Lancet 2:937, 1955.
12. Cancer of the oesophagus (editorial). Br. Med. J. 2:135, 1976.
13. Catane, R. et al.: Small cell lung cancer: Analysis of treatment factors contributing to prolonged survival. Cancer 48:1936, 1981.
14. Choi, C.H., Carey, R.W.: Small cell anaplastic carcinoma of lung. Reappraisal of current management. Cancer 37:2651, 1976.
15. Clarkson, J.R.: A note on depth doses in fields of irregular shape. Br. J. Radiol. 14:265, 1941.
16. Cox, J.D. et al.: Dose-time relationships and the local control of small cell carcinoma of the lung. Radiology 128:205, 1978.
17. Cox, J.D. et al.: The role of thoracic and cranial irradiation for small cell carcinoma of the lung. Int. J. Radiat. Oncol. Biol. Phys. 8:191, 1982.
18. Cox, J.D., Kamaki, R., Byhardt, R.W., Kun, L.E.: Results of whole-brain irradiation for metastases from small cell carcinoma of the lung. Cancer. Treat. Rep. 64:957, 1980.
19. Cundiff, J.H. et al.: A method for the calculation of dose in the radiation treatment of Hodgkin's disease. AJR 117:30, 1973.
20. Deeley, T.J.: A clinical trial to compare two different tumor dose levels in the treatment of advanced carcinoma of the bronchus. Clin. Radiol. 17:299, 1966.
21. Deeley, T.J.: In Monographs on Oncology—The Chest. Woburn, MA, Butterworth, 1973, p. 84.
22. Eagan, R.T., Maurer, L.H., Forcier, R.J., Tulloh, M.: Combination chemotherapy and radiation therapy in small cell carcinoma of the lung. Cancer 32:371, 1973.
23. Edwards, D.A.W.: Carcinoma of the oesophagus and fundus. Postgrad. Med. J. 50:223, 1974.
24. Eichhorn, H.J., Lessel, A., Matschke, S.: Comparison between neutron therapy and ^{60}Co gamma ray therapy of bronchial, gastric and

oesophagus carcinomata. Europ. J. Cancer 10:361, 1974.

25. Eisert, D.R., Cox, J.D., Komaki, R.: Irradiation for bronchial carcinoma: Reasons for failure. Cancer 37:2665, 1976.

26. Ellis, F.: Accuracy in compensation for tissue heterogeneity in treatment by x-rays, supervoltage x-rays and electron beams. Br. J. Radiol. 33:404, 1960.

27. Ellis, F., Hall, E.J., Oliver, R.: A compensator for variations in tissue thickness for high energy beams. Br. J. Radiol. 32:421, 1959.

28. Ellis, F., Lescrenier, C.: Combined compensator for contours and heterogeneity. Radiology 106:191, 1973.

29. Epp, E.R., Logyeed, M.N., McKay, J.W.: Ionization buildup in upper respiratory air passage during teletherapy with Co-60 radiation. Br. J. Radiol. 31:361, 1958.

30. Fleming, J.S., Orchard, P.G.: Isocentric radiotherapy treatment planning where the treatment axis is not horizontal. Br. J. Radiol. 47:34, 1974.

31. Fletcher, G.H.: Clinical dose-response curves of human malignant epithelial tumours. Br. J. Radiol. 46:1, 1973.

32. Fox, W., Scadding, J.G.: Medical Research Council comparative trial of surgery and radiotherapy for primary treatment of small-celled or oat-celled carcinoma of bronchus. Lancet 2:63, 1973.

33. Fujimaki, M. et al.: Role of preoperative administration of bleomycin and radiation in the treatment of esophageal cancer. Jap. J. Surg. 5:48, 1975.

34. Goldberg, E.M., Shapiro, C.M., Glicksman, A.S.: Mediastinoscopy for assessing mediastinal spread in clinical staging of lung carcinoma. Semin. Oncol. 1:205, 1974.

35. Greco, F.A. et al.: Small cell lung cancer, complete remission and improved survival. Am. J. Med. 66:626, 1979.

36. Green, N., Kurohara, S.S., George, F.W., Crews, Q.E., Jr.: Postresection irradiation for primary lung cancer. Radiology 116:405, 1975.

37. Groves, L.K., Rodriguez-Antunez, A.: Treatment of carcinoma of the esophagus and gastric cardia with concentrated preoperative irradiation followed by early operation. A progress report. Ann. Thorac. Surg. 15:333, 1973.

38. Guthrie, R.T., Ptacek, J.J., Hass, A.C.: Comparative analysis of two regimens of split course radiation in carcinoma of the lung. AJR 117:604, 1973.

39. Guttman, R.: Radical supervoltage therapy in inoperable carcinoma of the lung. *In* Modern Radiotherapy: Carcinoma of the Bronchus. Edited by T.J. Deeley. New York, Appleton, 1971, pp. 181–195.

40. Hall, E.J., Oliver, R.: The use of standard isodose distributions with high energy radiation beams: The accuracy of a compensator technique in correcting for body contours. Br. J. Radiol. 34:43, 1961.

41. Hansen, H.H. et al.: Prophylactic irradiation in bronchogenic small cell anaplastic carcinoma. A comparative trial of localized versus extensive radiotherapy including prophylactic brain irradiation in patients receiving combination chemotherapy. Cancer 46:279, 1980.

42. Hansen, H.H., Muggia, F.M.: Staging of inoperable patients with bronchogenic carcinoma with special reference to bone marrow examination and peritoneoscopy. Cancer 30:1395, 1972.

43. Hellman, S., Kligerman, M.M., Von Essen, C.F., Scibetta, M.P.: Sequelae of radical radiotherapy of carcinoma of the lung. Radiology 82:1055, 1964.

44. Hilaris, B.S., Luomanen, R.K., Beattie, E.J., Jr.: Integrated irradiation and surgery in the treatment of apical lung cancer. Cancer 27:1369, 1971.

45. Holsti, L., Vuorinen, P.: Radiation reaction in the lung after continuous and split-course megavoltage radiotherapy of bronchial carcinoma. Br. J. Radiol. 40:280, 1967.

46. Hornback, N.B. et al.: Oat cell carcinoma of the lung: Early treatment results of combination radiation therapy and chemotherapy. Cancer 37:2658, 1976.

47. International Commission on Radiation Units and Measurements: Determination of absorbed dose in a patient irradiated by beams of x or gamma rays in radiotherapy procedures. ICRU 24, Washington, D.C., 1976.

48. Johns, H.E., Cunningham, J.R.: The Physics of Radiology, 3rd ed. Springfield, Ill., Charles C Thomas, 1971.

49. Johnson, R.E., Brereton, H.D., Kent, C.H.: Small-cell carcinoma of the lung: Attempt to remedy causes of past therapeutic failure. Lancet 2:289, 1976.

50. Komaki, R., Roh, J., Cox, J., Lopes da Conceicao, S.: Superior sulcus tumors: Results of irradiation of 36 patients. Cancer 48:1563, 1981.

51. Krauss, S. et al.: Combined modality treatment of localized small-cell lung carcinoma: A randomized prospective study of the Southeastern Cancer Study Group. Cancer Clin. Trials 3:297, 1980.

52. Laing, A.H., Berry, R.J., Newman, C.R., Smith, P.: Treatment of small-cell carcinoma of bronchus. Lancet 1:129, 1975.

53. Lee, R.E.: Radiotherapy of bronchogenic carcinoma. Semin. Oncol. 1:245, 1974.

54. Leung, R.M.K., Van Dyk, J., Robins, J.: A method of large irregular field compensation. Br. J. Radiol. 47:805, 1974.

55. Levitt, S.H., Bogardus, C.R., Ladd, G.: Split-dose radiation therapy in the treatment of advanced lung cancer. Radiology 88:1159, 1967.

56. Line, D.H., Deeley, T.J.: The necropsy findings in carcinoma of the bronchus. Br. J. Dis. Chest 64:238, 1971.

57. MacDonald, S.C., Keller, B.E., Rubin, P.: Method for calculating dose when lung tissue lies in the treatment field. Med. Phys. 3:210, 1976.

58. Marks, R.D., Scruggs, H.J., Wallace, K.M.: Pre-

operative radiation therapy for carcinoma of the esophagus. Cancer 38:84, 1976.

59. Matthews, M.J.: Morphology of lung cancer. Semin. Oncol. 1:175, 1974.

60. Matthews, M.J., Kanhousa, W., Pickren, J., Robinette, D.: Frequency of residual and metastatic tumor in patients undergoing curative surgical resection for lung cancer. Cancer Treat. Rep. 4:63, 1973.

61. Miller, C.: Carcinoma of the thoracic oesophagus and cardia: A series of 405 cases. Br. J. Surg. 49:507, 1962.

62. Mira, J.G., Livingston, R.B.: Evaluation and radiotherapy implications of chest relapse patterns in small cell lung carcinoma treated with radiotherapy-chemotherapy: Study of 34 cases and review of the literature. Cancer 46:2557, 1980.

63. Mira, J.G., et al.: Influence of chest radiotherapy in frequency and patterns of chest relapse in disseminated small cell lung carcinoma. A Southwest Oncology Group Study. Cancer 50:1266, 1982.

64. Mountain, C.F.: Surgical therapy in lung cancer: Biologic, physiologic and technical determinants. Semin. Oncol. 1:253, 1974.

65. Mountain, C.F., Carr, D.T., Anderson, W.A.D.: A system for the clinical staging of lung carcinoma. AJR 120:130, 1974.

66. Nakayama, K., Kinoshita, Y.: Surgical treatment combined with preoperative concentrated irradiation. JAMA 227:178, 1974.

67. Nelson, C.S.: Chemotherapy as the definitive form of therapy in esophageal carcinoma. J. Thorac. Cardiovasc. Surg. 63:817, 1972.

68. Nilsson, B., Schell, P.O.: Build-up effects of air cavities measured with thin thermoluminescent dosimeters. Acta Radiol. (Ther) (Stockh) 15:427, 1976.

69. Nohl, H.C.: An investigation into the lymphatic and vascular spread of carcinoma of the bronchus. Thorax 11:172, 1956.

70. Parker, E.F., Gregorie, H.B.: Carcinoma of the esophagus. Long term results. JAMA 235:1018, 1976.

71. Paterson, R., Russell, M.H.: Clinical trials in malignant disease. IV. Lung cancer. Value of post-operative radiotherapy. Clin. Radiol. 13:141, 1962.

72. Paulson, D.L. et al.: Combined preoperative irradiation and resection for bronchogenic carcinoma. J. Thorac. Cardiovas. Surg. 44:281,1962.

73. Pearson, J.G.: The present status and future potential of radiotherapy in the management of esophageal cancer. Cancer 39:882, 1977.

74. Perez, C.A. et al. and the Southeastern Cancer Study Group: Thoracic and elective brain irradiation with concomitant or delayed multiagent chemotherapy in the treatment of localized small cell carcinoma of the lung: A randomized prospective study by the Southeastern Cancer Study Group. Cancer 47:2407, 1981.

75. Perez, C.A. et al.: Impact of irradiation technique and tumor extent in tumor control and survival of patients with unresectable non-oat cell carcinoma of the lung: Report by the Radiation Therapy Oncology Group. Cancer 50:1091, 1982.

76. Perez, C.A. et al. and the Radiation Therapy Oncology Group: Patterns of tumor recurrence after definitive irradiation for inoperable non-oat cell carcinoma of the lung. Int. J. Radiat. Oncol. Bio. Phys. 6:987, 1980.

77. Perez, C.A. et al.: A prospective randomized study of various irradiation doses and fractionation schedules in the treatment of inoperable non-oat carcinoma of the lung: Preliminary report by the Radiation Therapy Oncology Group. Cancer 45:2744, 1980.

78. Phillips, T., Margolis, L.: Radiation pathology and the clinical response of lung and esophagus. In Frontiers of Radiation Therapy and Oncology, Vol 6. Edited by J.M. Vaeth. Baltimore, University Park Press, 1972, pp. 254–273.

79. Rissanen, P.M., Tikka, U., Holsti, L.R.: Autopsy findings in lung cancer treated with megavoltage radiotherapy. Acta Radiol. (Ther) (Stockh) 7:433, 1968.

80. Ross, W.M.: Radiotherapy of carcinoma of the oesophagus. Proc. R. Soc. Med. 67:19, 1974.

81. Roswit, B., Higgins, G.A., Shields, W., Keehn, R.J.: Preoperative radiation therapy for carcinoma of the lung: Report of a national VA controlled study. In Frontiers of Radiation Therapy and Oncology, Vol. 5. Edited by J.M. Vaeth. Baltimore University Park Press, 1970, pp. 163–176.

82. Rubin, P., Ciccio, S., Setisarn, B.: The controversial status of radiation therapy in lung cancer. In Proceedings of the 6th National Cancer Conference. Philadelphia, Lippincott, 1970, pp. 855–865.

83. Rubin, P.: Cancer of the gastrointestinal tract. II. Esophagus: Treatment—Localized and Advanced. JAMA 227:175, 1974.

84. Rubin, P., Perez, C., Keller, B.: The logical basis of radiation treatment policies in the multidisciplinary approach to lung cancer. In Lung Cancer: Natural History, Prognosis and Therapy. Edited by L. Israel and A.P. Chahinian. New York, Academic Press, 1976, p. 160.

85. Rubin, P.: Cancer of the gastrointestinal tract. I. Esophagus: Detection and Diagnosis. JAMA 226:1544, 1973.

86. Salazar, O.M. et al.: Half-body and local chest irradiation as consolidation following response to standard induction chemotherapy: An Eastern Cooperative Oncology Group pilot report. Int. J. Radiat. Oncol. Biol. Phys. 6:1093, 1980.

87. Salazar, O.M. et al.: The assessment of tumor response to irradiation of lung cancer: Continuous versus split-course regimes. Int. J. Radiat. Oncol. Biol. Phys. 1:1107, 1976.

88. Sambrook, D.K.: Split-course radiation therapy in malignant tumors. AJR 91:37, 1964.

89. Sandeman, T.F.: The roles of radiotherapy and cytotoxic drugs in the management of carcinoma of the oesophagus. Aust. NZ. J. Surg. 42:373, 1973.

90. Scrimger, J.W.: Effect of air gap on absorbed dose in tissue. Radiology *102*:171, 1972.

91. Seydel, H.G., Chait, A., Gmelich, J.T.: Cancer of the Lung. New York, John Wiley & Sons, 1975.

92. Seydel, H.G., Creech, R.H., Mietlowski, W.L., Perez, C.A.: Preliminary report of cooperative randomized study for the treatment of localized small cell lung carcinoma. Int. J. Radiat. Oncol. Biol. Phys. 5:1445, 1979.

93. Simpson, J.R. et al.: Large fraction radiotherapy plus misonidazole for treatment of advanced lung cancer: Report of a Phase I/II trial. Int. J. Radiat. Oncol. Biol. Physics. 8:303, 1982.

94. Smart, J.J.: Can lung cancer be cured by irradiation alone? JAMA 159:1034, 1966.

95. Straus, M.J.: The growth characteristics of lung cancer and its application to treatment design. Semin. Oncol. *1*:167, 1974.

96. van de Geijn, J.: The construction of individual intensity modifying filters in cobalt 60 teletherapy. Br. J. Radiol. *38*:685, 1964.

97. Warram, J.: Preoperative irradiation of cancer of the lung: Final report of a therapeutic trial— a collaborative study. Cancer 36:914, 1975.

98. White, J.E. et al.: The influence of radiation therapy quality control on survival, response and sites of relapse in oat cell carcinoma of the lung: Preliminary report of a Southwest Oncology Group Study (unpublished data).

99. Wilks, R., Casebow, M.P.: Tissue compensation with lead for ^{60}Co therapy. Br. J. Radiol. 42:452, 1969.

100. Yamashita, H., Okura, J., Yoshioka, F.T., Tanaka, Y.: Preoperative irradiation in treatment of carcinoma of the oesophagus. Aust. Radiol. 16:250, 1972.

Chapter 10

BRAIN TUMOR LOCALIZATION: DETERMINATION OF EXTENT AND VOLUME FOR RADIATION TREATMENT

Chu H. Chang

Sadek K. Hilal

Preoperative localization of brain tumors is a precise and difficult task in which the neurosurgeon and neuroradiologist map the operative approach. Postoperative brain-tumor localization is by no means a less demanding job; the radiation oncologist, neurosurgeon, and neuroradiologist plan for treatment of the residual or inoperable tumors. In most cases, a postoperative computerized tomographic (CT) scan or arteriogram is desirable in order to assess the amount of tumor removed and to visualize the shift or redistribution of the postoperative "avascular silent space." A competent and prudent radiation oncologist should acquire a full knowledge of the extent and volume of a brain tumor before proceeding with treatment planning and radiotherapy.

A working knowledge of the brain-tumor types and the incidence of various types of brain tumors are essential in day-to-day management of patients with brain tumors. A Brain Tumor Classification, published by the American College of Pathology, with partial modification by Walker,[5] is shown in Table 10–1. The incidence of various brain tumors, obtained by the combination of several large reported series, is shown in Table 10–2.

ANATOMY AND TOPOGRAPHY OF THE BRAIN

For accurate localization of brain tumors, it is necessary to have a precise topographic knowledge of the brain structures, especially the anatomic and physiologic delineation of the cerebral lobes, cortical functioning areas, and deep structures.

The brain is conventionally divided into the following five major divisions: telencephalon (endbrain); diencephalon (interbrain); mesencephalon (midbrain); metencephalon (afterbrain, contains pons and cerebellum); and myelencephalon (medulla oblongata).

The cerebrum comprises the telencephalon, diencephalon, and upper midbrain. The brain stem is a collective term for the diencephalon, mesencephalon, metencephalon, and myelencephalon, exclusive of the cerebellum. The brain stem is subdivided by its topographic relation to the tentorium into the supratentorial divisions (diencephalon) and the infratentorial division (midbrain, pons, and medulla oblongata).

Each cerebral hemisphere is conventionally divided into six lobes (Fig. 10–1):

TABLE 10–1.   Brain Tumor Classification (Neuroectodermal Tumors).

Benign	Malignant
GLIOMAS	
Pilocytic astrocytoma (I)	Anaplastic astrocytoma (III)
Astrocytoma (II)	
Protoplasmic astrocytoma	Glioblastoma multiforme (IV)
Fibrillary astrocytoma	Giant cell glioblastoma
Gemistocytic astrocytoma	Mixed glioblastoma-sarcoma
Oligodendroglioma (I)	Anaplastic oligodendroglioma (II–III)
Ependymoma (I)	Anaplastic ependymoma (II–III)
Gangliocytoma	Anaplastic gangliocytoma
Pineocytoma	Pineoblastoma
	Medulloblastoma
OTHER	
Neurofibroma	Anaplastic neurofibroma
Meningioma	Anaplastic meningioma
Neurilemoma	Anaplastic neurilemoma
Pituitary adenoma	
Chromophobe adenoma	Meningeal sarcoma
Basophilic adenoma	
Acidophilic adenoma	Hemangioblastoma
	Neoplasm metastatic

(From Walker, M.D.: Brain and peripheral nervous system tumors. *In* Cancer Medicine. Edited by J.F. Holland and E. Frei III. Philadelphia, Lea & Febiger, 1982.)

frontal, parietal, occipital, temporal, central (insula or island of Reil), and limbic. The boundaries of the frontal, parietal, temporal, and occipital lobes on the lateral surface of the cerebral hemisphere are cerebral sulci. The most prominent lateral cerebral sulcus (sylvian fissure) separates the temporal lobe from all other lobes of the hemisphere. The prominent vertical sulcus (central sulcus) separates the frontal lobe from the parietal lobe and the parieto-occipital sulcus separates the parietal lobe from the occipital lobe.

The medial surface of the cerebral hemisphere can be subdivided into the limbic lobe and portions of the frontal, parietal, and occipital lobes (Fig. 10–2).

The limbic lobe is the ring of cortex around the ventricular system of the cerebrum. The limbic cortex is of interest because it is phylogenetically older than the neocortex. The neocortex constitutes the bulk of the cerebral cortex in man, exclusive of the limbic lobe, and is the phylogenetically new cortex of the mammals.

The two cerebral hemispheres are connected by the corpus callosum. Beneath the corpus callosum are the midline structures (e.g., third ventricle, pineal body, and midbrain) and the deep paramedian structures (e.g., lateral ventricles, caudate and lentiform nuclei, thalamus, and hypothalamus).

The functional cortical localization of three speech areas of the dominant hemisphere is important because most neurosurgeons are reluctant to operate on tumors that are located in or near the motor or major speech areas (Fig. 10–3). The *Broca's speech area* is in the anterior speech cortex, which is a part of the inferior frontal gyrus (Brodmann's areas 44

TABLE 10–2.   Incidence of Different Brain Tumor Types.

	% of Brain Tumors
Gliomas	43
Glioblastoma multiforme	23
Astrocytoma	13
Ependymoma	1.8
Oligodendroglioma	1.7
Mixed and other	1.9
Medulloblastoma	1.6
Meningioma	16.0
Pituitary adenoma	8.2
Nerve sheath tumor	5.7
Craniopharyngioma	2.8
Sarcoma	2.5
Hemangioblastoma	2.7
Pineal tumor	1.1
Metastatic	13.0
Other	5.0

Number of brain tumors studied = 17,580. (From Walker, M.D.: Brain and peripheral nervous system tumors. *In* Cancer Medicine. Edited by J.F. Holland and E. Frei III. Philadelphia, Lea & Febiger, 1982.)

and 45). This is known as Broca's motor aphasia of the expressive speech center. The *Wernicke's speech area* is in the posterior speech cortex, which is the auditory association area on the lateral surface of the posterior portion of the superior temporal gyrus (Brodmann's area 22). This is known as Wernicke's receptive aphasia area. The *inferior parietal speech* area is in the angular and supramarginal gyri (Brodmann's areas 39 and 40), which is at times associated with Gerstmann's syndrome of dysgraphia, left-right confusion, and finger agnosia.

DIAGNOSTIC STUDIES AND LOCALIZATION OF BRAIN TUMORS

Plain Radiograph of the Skull

The plain radiograph of the skull is the initial diagnostic step. It provides gross anatomic and angiographic landmarks of various cerebral lobes (Fig. 10–4), location of calcified normal structures (such as pineal body and choroid plexuses), calcified tumors (such as suprasellar craniopharyngioma, meningioma, and some cerebral gliomas), evidence of increase of intra-cranial pressure (separation of cranial sutures), and measurable size of the sella turcica, optic foramen, and internal auditory canal (diagnostic for certain specific tumors).

Cerebral Angiography

It is previously widely held among neuroradiologists that cerebral angiography should be performed in the vast majority of cases prior to pneumoencephalography (PEG). It should be performed as the first special procedure in almost all patients suspected of having a supratentorial tumor. The angiographic sylvian triangle serves as a useful guide for localizing deep, paramedian tumors arising from the adjacent areas between the posterior parietal, frontotemporal, and parietotemporal regions (Fig. 10–5). The angiography may show single displacement of vessels from their normal position without tumor vascularity. It may depict the blood supply to the tumors, tumor stain or tumor blush, and change in arterial and venous flow, which may permit prediction of malignancy of the tumor (such as an early filling vein). It may define the size of the ventricles, and the posterior fossa structures. It may show the displacement or herniation of vital structures. It frequently provides valuable vascular landmarks for neurosurgeons and assists in determining operability. Angiography does, however, carry some risk.

Air Studies

The ventriculogram and the PEG are very useful for demonstration of ventricular size and for delineation of tumor arising within the ventricles and within adjacent structures outside the ventricle or cisterns. PEG almost always results in a more definitive examination than ventriculography.

Radionuclide Imaging

Radionuclide imaging may depict small and deep lesions slightly greater than 2.5

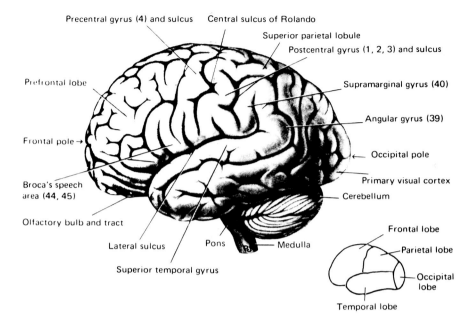

Fig. 10–1. Lateral surface of the left cerebral hemisphere. Several major sulci divide the cerebral cortex into 4 major lobes: frontal, parietal, occipital, and temporal. (From Noback, C.R. and Demarest, R.J.: The Human Nervous System, 2nd ed. New York, McGraw–Hill, 1975.)

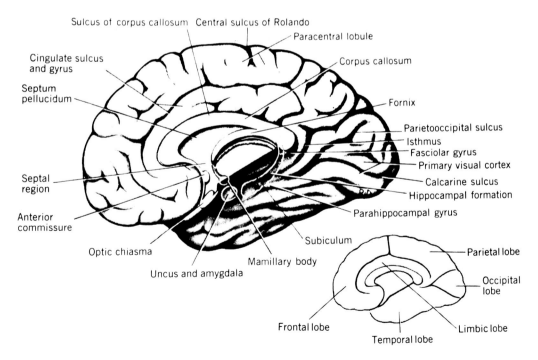

Fig. 10–2. Medial surface of the cerebral hemisphere. This medial surface is subdivided into the limbic lobe and portions of the frontal, parietal, and occipital lobes. (From Noback, C.R. and Demarest, R.J.: The Human Nervous System, 2nd ed. New York, McGraw–Hill, 1975.)

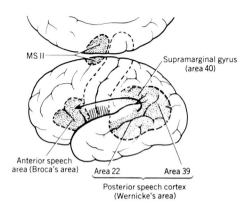

MS II

Supramarginal gyrus (area 40)

Anterior speech area (Broca's area)

Area 22

Area 39

Posterior speech cortex (Wernicke's area)

Fig. 10–3. Location of some of the major functional speech association areas of the cerebral cortex. Numbers refer to Brodmann's areas. (From Noback, C.R. and Demarest, R.J.: The Human Nervous System. New York, McGraw–Hill, 1975.)

cm in diameter in 85% of patients. Such lesions are usually missed by angiography. Angiography detects some slowly growing avascular or cystic tumors not seen by the imaging camera.

Computerized Tomography

The CT scan is a revolutionary contribution not only to the detection of but also to the accurate localization of intracranial lesions by a method almost devoid of risk. Its accuracy rate in detection of brain tumors may equal or surpass that of radionuclide scanning and angiography. It is now widely used in the screening of brain tumors prior to angiography. Because of its ability to define the extent of tumor, to obtain, quantitatively, the "absorption density" of the anatomic structures in the sections and to develop isodose curves with inhomogeneity correction, the potential for its use in tumor localization and radiation treatment planning[4] is unsurpassed.

Nuclear Magnetic Resonance

With the advent of nuclear magnetic resonance (NMR) imaging in medicine, three dimensional views of a brain tumor are readily obtained. However, further improvement of spatial resolution of proton NMR imaging for supratentorial brain tumors is needed. NMR offers the great potential of describing both morphology and function. Recent advances have permitted the separate imaging of each compound of phosphorous, which is key to the study of regional metabolism. The potential of NMR in providing an index of malignancy appears quite encouraging. Radiation therapy dose scheme can be designed, in the near future, according to both the volume and grade of the malignancy in the involved tissues as shown in the NMR brain tumor imaging.

DEFINITIONS AND GUIDELINES IN TREATMENT PLANNING FOR TUMORS OF THE CENTRAL NERVOUS SYSTEM

It is generally agreed by members of Radiation Therapy Oncology Group (RTOG)[2] and among many other radiotherapists and physicists that a set of working definitions and guidelines in treatment planning for tumor of the central nervous system (CNS) are needed for conducting clinical trials in order to achieve uniformity of treatment and good quality control. Several commonly used terms and treatment policies are defined as follows:

1. Tumor Volume—A three-dimensional reconstruction of the volume of a tumor as determined by tumor localization with CT scan and other diagnostic procedures.

2. Target Volume—Extended tumor volume to encompass local or regional extension or spread of tumor (e.g., direct tumor infiltration, tumor-cell seedings, or multicentric tumors; in this sense and in practice, the target volume is the irradiation volume. Within the target volume, dose inhomogeneity of more than 15% should not be permitted. For low grade astrocytoma, oligodendroglioma, and pituitary adenoma,

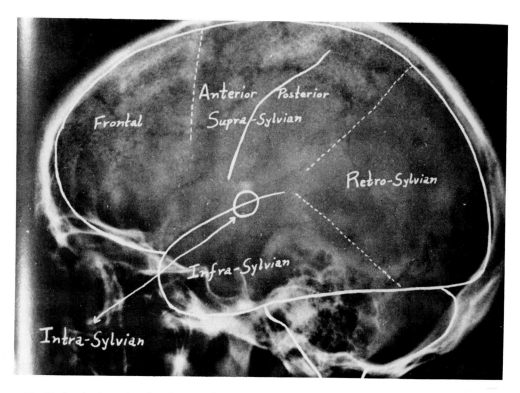

Fig. 10–4. Angiographic classification of brain-tumor location. The subdivision of these tumor locations corresponds well to those used in the localization of intracranial masses when diagnosed by pneumography. (From Taveras, J.M. and Wood, E.H.: Diagnostic Neuroradiology. Baltimore, Williams & Wilkins, 1964.)

the target volume is the extended tumor volume, about 1 cm to 2 cm beyond the margin of tumor. For malignant glioma, lymphoma, leukemia, metastatic brain tumor, and malignant pineal tumor, the entire brain is the target volume. For medulloblastoma, meningeal carcinomatosis, and a certain number of ependymoma and pinealoma, the entire CNS is the target volume.

3. Booster-Target Volume—A reduced target volume encompassing the initial tumor volume with about 1 cm additional margin. This is commonly used for boosting the dose to the initial tumor site of malignant glioma, cerebellar medulloblastoma, ependymoma, pinealoma, and other tumors following initial target volume irradiation.

The radiotherapist is responsible for determining the tumor volume, translating the tumor volume into target volume, and drawing the outline (blue line) of the target volume on radiographic film or on the appropriate treatment planning sheet. The radiotherapist should also evaluate the portal arrangement with the treatment-planning team. The guidelines for prescribing target volume and booster-target volume are based on clinical information, tissue and cytology diagnosis, institutional treatment policy, and the group-protocol requirement.

Tolerance of Critical Organs to Irradiation

A tissue-tolerance dosage guideline[3] pertinent to treatment planning for brain tumor has been compiled and is presented in Table 10–3. These reflect only our present knowledge of this subject; the table

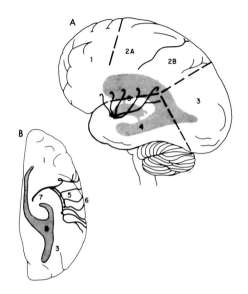

Fig. 10–5. Angiographic sylvian triangle, which serves as a basis for classification of supratentorial tumors. *(A)* Lateral view of sylvian triangle. The base of the triangle is formed by the 4 or 5 loops of the primary branches of middle cerebral artery under the frontal or parietal opercula. Tumors may be found anterior to, above, behind, or beneath this triangular configuration. *(B)* Coronal view of sylvian triangle. Tumor may be found lateral or medial to the triangle, or in the sylvian fissure. **1,** frontal; **2A,** anterior suprasylvian; **2B,** posterior suprasylvian; **3,** retrosylvian; **4,** infrasylvian; **5,** intrasylvian; **6,** laterosylvian; **7,** centrosylvian; **8,** intraventricular. (From Wood, E.H., Taveras, J.M., and Tenner, M.S.: The Brain & the Eye: An Atlas of Tumor Radiology. Chicago, Year Book Medical Publishers, 1975.)

will be modified as new findings and additional data become available.

Case Illustrations

Sellar and Parasellar Tumors

Pituitary Adenoma. The pituitary adenoma is usually confined to the sella turcica, causing varying degrees of sellar enlargement and extrasellar extension.

Tumor Localization. The dense sella is an excellent landmark for tumor localization under fluoroscopy provided by a modern simulator. For a large pituitary tumor, it is pertinent to determine the presence or absence of suprasellar, parasellar, or retrosellar extension by PEG, CT, or arteriography.

Case Illustration. A 30-year-old woman who 2 years previously had undergone a craniotomy with partial removal of a pituitary chromophobe adenoma and who had received a postoperative course of radiotherapy (4000 rad in 4 weeks), was suffering from a decrease of vision, headaches, lethargy, and general weakness. The diagnostic workup included a PEG, which demonstrated a high suprasellar extension of an intrasellar mass with tumor impinging the floor of the third ventricle (Fig. 10–6). A CT scan showed a large suprasellar enhancing mass (Fig. 10–7).

Portal Arrangement. A pituitary tumor centrally located in the base of the skull is an ideal tumor for a full 360° rotational or 220° arc technique. Two parallel-opposed temporal ports or a third midfrontal port are acceptable when a rotational facility is not available. The port size is usually 4 cm × 4 cm or 5 cm × 5 cm for an average-size tumor with minimal extrasellar extension. For a large tumor that extends into the third ventricle, a larger port size is needed to encompass the entire tumor. For this illustrated case, a 5 cm × 7.5 cm port was needed to encompass the pituitary-suprasellar mass with a 1 cm free margin. A 360° rotational technique was used for the second course for 4500 rad in 6 weeks (Fig. 10–8).

Precaution. It is important to avoid overdose to the optic nerves and chiasm. In our experience, an initial tumor dose of 5000 rad in 5½ to 6 weeks in daily fractionation with a fraction size of 180 to 200 rad is safe. Daily fractions greater than 200 rad should be avoided. No radiation optic neuritis, vasculitis, or blindness was recorded at this fractionation. The risk of a second course of radiotherapy is undoubtedly increased but was dictated by clinical need in this case.

Craniopharyngioma. Craniopharyngioma grows slowly and produces its effect by pressure on surrounding organs (e.g., chiasm, hypothalamus, and pituitary gland). Surgery is the initial treatment of choice but the recurrence rate is high.

TABLE 10–3.   Tolerance of Critical Organs—A Dosage Guideline for Brain Tumor Treatment Planning.

Organ	Radiation Injury	*TTD$_{5/5}$ (rad)	**TTD$_{50/5}$ (rad)	Volume Irradiated (Whole or Partial)
Brain	necrosis	6000	7000	Whole
		7,000	8000	Partial (25% of whole)
Spinal cord	necrosis	4500	5500	10 cm in length
Peripheral nerve	neuritis	6000	10000	10 cm in length
Lens	cataract	500	1200	Whole or partial
Retina	loss of vision	5500	7000	Whole
Optic nerve	loss of vision	6000	8000	Whole or partial

(Modified from Rubin, P., Cooper, R., and Phillips T.L. (eds): Radiation Biology and Radiation Pathology Syllabus [Set R.T.1: Radiation Oncology.] Chicago, Am. College of Radiology, 1975.)
*TTD$_{5/5}$ is defined as that tissue tolerance dose associated with a 5% rate of complications occurring within 5 years of radiation treatment.
**TTD$_{50/5}$ is defined as that tissue tolerance dose associated with a 50% rate of complications occurring within 5 years of radiation treatment.

Radiotherapy in high dosage is recommended postoperatively.

Tumor Localization. Craniopharyngioma is a highly calcified tumor in the juxtasellar region that provides good landmarks for localization; however, the tumor often contains a cystic component and the solid part of the tumor usually extends beyond the calcified part of the tumor. CT scan and PEG are sometimes both necessary for accurate localization. Not infrequently, the tumor extends into the third ventricle and obstructs the foramen of Monro, producing hydrocephalus.

Case Illustration. A 25-year-old woman had a history of headaches, visual loss, and bitemporal visual field defect. A CT scan showed a lucent lesion in the suprasellar region with partial enhancement by contrast medium (Fig. 10–9). It was interpreted to be a solid tumor containing a large cystic component. A subtotal resection was performed and a tissue diagnosis of craniopharyngioma was made. A post-operative course of radiotherapy was recommended.

Portal Arrangement. A 360° rotational or 220° arc technique is most commonly used for a relatively small, centrally located tumor. A three-portal technique, using 2 lateral-wedged ports and a superior open port is recommended for a large tumor. The port size in this case was 6 cm × 6 cm (tumor dose: 5000 rad/6 weeks).

Precaution. It is important to avoid overdose to the optic nerve, chiasm, and hypothalamus. A daily dose should not exceed 200 rad.

Optic-Nerve Glioma. Optic-nerve gliomas represent 1% to 4% of all intracranial tumors in children. In about 30% of patients, it involves the optic nerve alone; in about 65% of patients it involves the optic nerve and chiasm. In less than 5% of patients it involves the chiasm alone. The majority of optic-nerve gliomas are low-grade astrocytomas, but some chiasmal gliomas are higher grade and require more aggressive treatment.

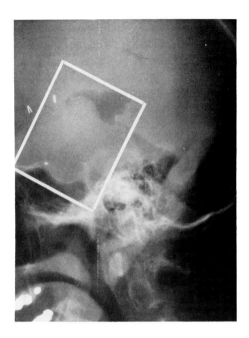

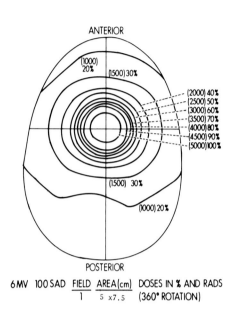

Fig. 10–6. Pituitary adenoma. Lateral view of pneumoencephalograph showed a large suprasellar extension of an intrasellar tumor causing a smooth crescent-like indentation on the floor of the third ventricle and providing a good landmark for upper tumor extent. A 5 cm × 7.5 cm port encompassed the tumor and provided a 1 cm margin for target volume irradiation.

Fig. 10–8. Isodose distribution with a 6 MeV accelerator, 5 cm × 7.5 cm portal area in full 360° rotation (same patient as in Fig. 10–6). (From Keller, et al.: Standard Treatment Planning Atlas. Philadelphia, Radiation Therapy Oncology Group, 1976.)

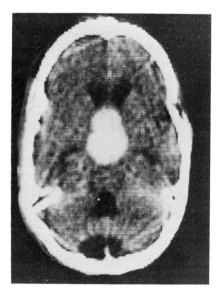

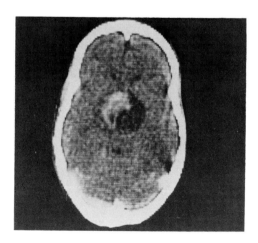

Fig. 10–7. CT scan showed a dense enhancing suprasellar mass, overshadowing the third ventricle and producing no dilatation of lateral ventricles. The tumor is longer in AP than in bilateral projection.

Fig. 10–9. Recurrent craniopharyngioma. CT scan showed a round, lucent suprasellar mass lesion with partial intratumoral enhancement, most likely representing a recurrent solid tumor with cystic degeneration.

Tumor Localization. PEG and CT scan are indispensable for tumor localization. It is essential to determine whether the intraorbital portion, intracranial portion, chiasm, or third ventricle is involved.

Case Illustration. A 2-year-old girl had a 3-month history of progressive failing of vision with mild proptosis of the left eye. A PEG showed a J-shaped sella and a chiasmal mass without ventricular dilatation. A CT scan showed a large fusiform tumor in the intraorbital portion of the left optic nerve with chiasmal contrast enhancement. There was no ventricular dilatation (Fig. 10–10). Because the chiasm was also involved, surgery was contraindicated and radiotherapy was recommended.

Portal Arrangement. If the intraorbital portion of the optic nerve is involved, the port has to be extended to include the posterior globe. If the chiasm and hypotha-

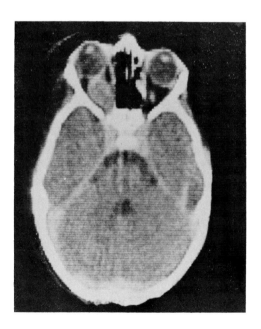

Fig. 10–10. CT scan showed a large fusiform tumor in right posterior orbit conforming with the intraorbital portion of the optic nerve and enlargement of the right optic canal. A contrast enhancement of the suprasellar tissue indicates involvement of the chiasm. There was no dilatation of the ventricles. The tumor was localized as involving the intraorbital portion, intracranial portion of the left optic nerve and the chiasm.

lamic region are involved, the port should be extended to encompass the third ventricle. Usually bilateral parallel-opposed ports with 15° obliquing are used to spare the uninvolved eye. The port size is determined by the extent of tumor. In this case, two lateral parallel-opposed ports with 15° obliquing were used, and the port size was 5 cm × 4 cm (Fig. 10–11).

Precaution. To avoid overdose to the chiasm and the uninvolved eye on the opposite side, the daily dose should not exceed 180 rad. A tumor dose of 4000 to 5000 rad delivered over 5 to 6 weeks is used, depending on the age of the child.

Meningioma. The majority of meningiomas are benign and relatively radioresistant. They can be adequately treated by radical surgery. Routine postoperative radiotherapy is not indicated. A few meningiomas, however, are vascular, consisting of angioblastic or sarcomatous types of tumor cells or of a small group of tumors that involve the cavernous sinus, visual pathway, and other strategic locations that prevent it from being removed surgically. It is with these groups of meningioma that postoperative irradiation should be considered.

Tumor Localization. Cerebral arteriogram and CT scan appear to be the most useful tools in the localization of the volume and blood supply of this tumor.

Case Illustration. A 52-year-old woman had a 2-year history of progressive headaches and decrease of vision in her right eye. A CT scan showed a large and densely enhanced mass in the right parasellar and right posterior sphenoid wing (Fig. 10–12). A cerebral arteriogram demonstrated the external carotid blood supply and confirmed the diagnosis of sphenoid-wing meningioma. A right temporal craniotomy was done and the tumor was found to have invaded the cavernous sinus; a subtotal resection of the tumor was therefore made. The tissue diagnosis was meningioma of the angioblastic type.

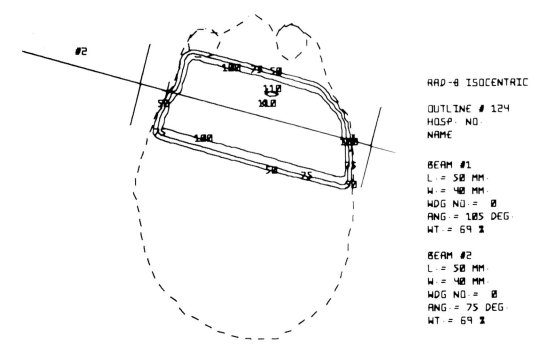

RAD-8 ISOCENTRIC

OUTLINE # 124
HOSP. NO.
NAME

BEAM #1
L = 50 MM
W = 40 MM
WDG NO. = 0
ANG = 105 DEG
WT = 69 %

BEAM #2
L = 50 MM
W = 40 MM
WDG NO. = 0
ANG = 75 DEG
WT = 69 %

Fig. 10–11. The portal arrangements. Two oblique–opposed lateral ports that encompass the whole length of left optic nerve from the posterior globe to the optic chiasm. The right eye is spared. The port size was 5 cm × 4 cm.

A postoperative course of radiotherapy was recommended.

Portal Arrangement The portal arrangement should encompass a limited target volume using a three-portal technique with the aid of wedge filters (Fig. 10–13).

Precaution. It is important to avoid overdose to the optic nerve, chiasm, and lens. 5000 rad/6 weeks is a safe dose.

Supratentorial Tumors

Frontal Tumors (Astrocytoma). The incidence of astrocytoma (low grade) is about 25% to 35% of all brain tumors. Although a cerebellar astrocytoma usually presents no further therapeutic consideration after complete removal of a cystic tumor containing a solid mural nodule, a cerebral astrocytoma frequently shows local infiltration or low-grade malignancy. Our treatment policy is to give a postoperative course of radiotherapy if an astrocytoma is incompletely removed.

Tumor Localization. A CT scan and arteriogram are the most useful tools for localization of frontal tumors.

Case Illustration. An 8-year-old girl had a 2-month history of lethargy and intermittent vomiting and a 1-week history of frontal headaches and diplopia. On admission she was dehydrated and inattentive; she had bilateral marked papilledema, left sixth-cranial-nerve palsy, and right hemiparesis. A CT scan showed a large well-marginated lucent mass 7.5 cm in diameter in the left frontoparietal region containing a peripheral enhancing nodule about 3 cm in diameter (Fig. 10–14). A cerebral arteriorgram showed a large left frontal vascular mass with a nodular stain. There was a 9-mm left-to-right midline shift. A left frontoparietal craniotomy was done with gross total removal of a 45-cm³ (3 × 5 × 3 cm) nodular tumor from a cystic capsule; about 250 ml cystic fluid was evacuated from the cystic capsule.

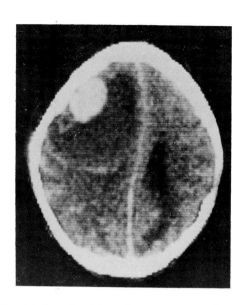

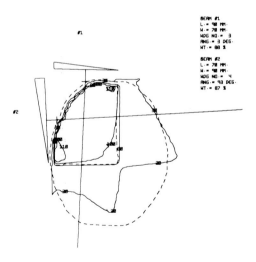

Fig. 10–12. Sphenoid wing meningioma. CT scan showed a large and densely enhancing mass in the right parasellar and right sphenoid wing with peritumoral edema extending posteriorly to the right parietal lobe and compressing the right lateral ventricle. There was a 12-mm midline shift from right to the left.

Fig. 10–14. Frontal cystic astrocytoma. CT scan showed a large well-marginated lucent mass lesion 7.5 cm in diameter containing a 3-cm enhancing mural nodule. There was considerable left to right midline shift.

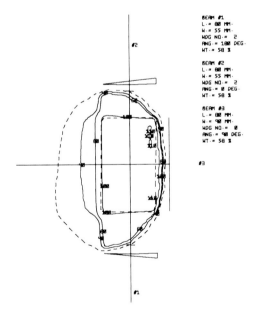

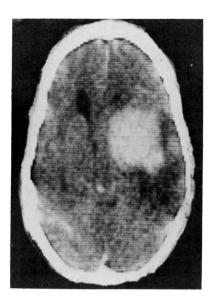

Fig. 10–13. Portal arrangement from Fig. 10–12. The tumor volume (including peritumoral edema) was determined to be 4 cm × 6.5 cm and the target volume to be 5.5 cm × 8 cm × 9 cm. A three portal technique with two AP–PA opposed and wedged ports and one right lateral open port was plotted as shown.

Fig. 10–15. Portal arrangement and isodose distribution: a left lateral port and a left frontal right-angled port with wedge filters. The port's size was 7 cm × 9 cm encompassing the target volume (same patient as in Fig. 10–14).

The final tissue diagnosis was astrocytoma with areas of astroblastomatous features. Postoperative radiotherapy was advised.

Portal Arrangement. Our treatment technique for cerebral astrocytoma is to irradiate the tumor bed with a limited target volume. Left-lateral and left-anterior ports at right angles to wedge filters were used. The port size was 7 cm × 9 cm each, determined by direct measurement of tumor size plus a 2-cm extended margin from CT scan (Fig. 10–15).

Precaution. A tumor dose of 5000 rad delivered in 5½ weeks to a limited target volume in the frontal region should present no problem. In this young age group, however, high-dose irradiation to the hypothalamic region may cause late hypothalamic-pituitary hormonal deficiency.

Retrosylvian Tumors (Parietal and Parieto-Occipital). The retrosylvian region is the common site for harboring glioblastoma multiforme and other gliomas. Glioblastomas grow rapidly by direct and extensive infiltration. They may occasionally reach the ventricle or grow to the brain surface, thereafter metastasizing to other parts of the CNS through the cerebrospinal fluid (CSF) pathway.

Tumor Localization. In this location, cerebral arteriograms usually permit precise tumor localization by depicting tumor vascularity and vascular displacement. CT scan may provide even better tumor localization with a contrast-enhancement technique. The usually densely enhanced tumor with peripheral edema and secondary-mass effect permits direct measurement of the extent of the tumor after appropriate modification by a CT magnification factor.

Case Illustration. A 62-year-old woman presented with a 2-month history of progressive left hemiparesis, 1-month history of mental slowing, visual-field defect, and agitation. A cerebral arteriogram showed a right-parietal mass lesion. A CT scan showed a large, right-parietal mass with ring enhancement and central, irregular

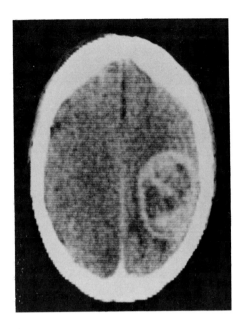

Fig. 10–16. Glioblastoma, right parietal lobe. CT scan showed a large elongated mass lesion with ring enhancement and central irregular lucency suggestive of necrosis. There was minimal peripheral edema and no midline shift.

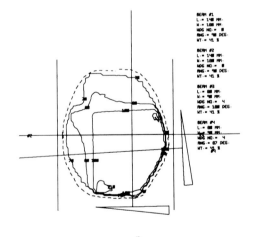

Fig. 10–17. Portal arrangement and isodose distribution. Whole brain was the target volume (requirement of RTOG malignant-glioma protocol). Two parallel-opposed lateral ports were used. The port size was extended 2 cm beyond the normal contour of the calvarium. A booster target volume was encompassed by two posterior and lateral right-angled and wedged ports.

lucency suggestive of tumor necrosis. There was minimal peritumoral edema (Fig. 10–16). There was a small enhancing mass in the left-parietal region suggestive of a multicentric glioblastoma (not shown in Fig. 10–16).

A right-parietal craniotomy was done with subtotal removal of a grossly infiltrative malignant glioma. The tissue diagnosis was glioblastoma multiforme (Astrocytoma Grade IV).

Portal Arrangement. The policy for malignant glioma in adult patients is that the whole brain is the target volume for the initial treatment (RTOG Protocol requirement). The simplest portal arrangement to fulfill this requirement is two large parallel-opposed lateral ports. The port size should be extended about 2 cm beyond the patient's calvarial contour in order to achieve more homogeneous dose gradients within the calvaria. The booster-target volume may be irradiated with two right-angled fields with the aid of wedge filters after whole-brain irradiation with 6000 rad delivered in 6 to 7 weeks (Fig. 10–17).

Precaution. Shielding of the retina and lens of both eyes with a beam-blocking technique must be an important consideration in treatment planning.

Infrasylvian Tumors (Temporal). The temporal lobe is probably the most common site of gliomas. Owing to their rapid involvement of the speech areas, neurosurgical resection is often rejected. On the other hand, the temporal lobe is often the site of some long-standing gliomas that may be effectively treated by resection.

Tumor Localization. There is a practical need for precise localization of an infrasylvian temporal-mass lesion because surgical resectability is limited to the more anterior portion of the temporal lobe. In this regard, cerebral and vertebral angiography appears to be indispensable. As the tumor extends deeply toward the thalamus, diagnosis is aided by delineation of the posterior circulation, particularly the

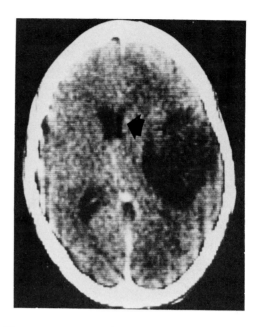

Fig. 10–18. CT scan showed an approximately 6 cm × 7 cm, elongated, lucent mass in the right temporal lobe with little enhancement following contrast injection. There is pressure deformity and partial collapse of right lateral ventricle with some midline shift *(arrow).*

demonstration of changes in the posterior choroidal vessels. CT scan has proved very helpful in localizing the extent of the tumor in all directions and especially in demonstrating any cystic component of the tumor.

Case Illustration. A 26-year-old man presented with a 4-year history of intermittent grand mal seizures. The subsequent diagnostic workup showed bilateral papilledema. There was no localizing sign. A radionuclide brain scan was negative. A CT scan showed a large, lucent, right-middle cranial-fossa mass with cystic component and with some midline shift (Fig. 10–18). A right-internal-carotid arteriogram showed elevation and medial displacement of the right-middle cerebral artery by an avascular mass (Figs. 10–19 and 10–20). He underwent a right temporal craniotomy with subtotal removal of a right temporal tumor with cystic component. The tissue diagnosis was astrocytoma with malignant change (Grade

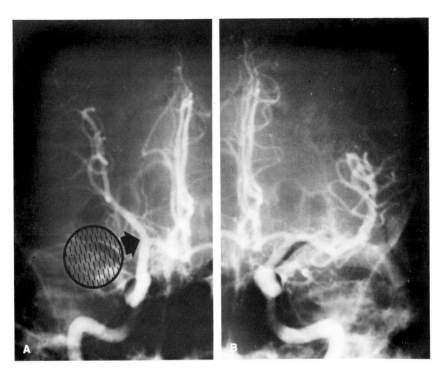

Fig. 10–19. *(A)* Anteroposterior view of right cerebral arteriogram showed marked medial displacement and elevation of right middle cerebral artery above the internal carotid siphon *(arrows* and *shaded circle).* The anterior cerebral artery is shifted to the left. There are no tumor stains. *(B)* Anteroposterior view of left cerebral arteriogram of the same patient shown for comparison.

II–III). A postoperative course of radiotherapy was recommended.

Portal Arrangement. The present policy for all adult malignant gliomas is to use whole-brain irradiation with two parallel-opposed lateral ports for 5000 rad in 5 weeks, to be followed by booster-volume irradiation to the temporal tumor for an additional 1000 rad in 1 week (Fig. 10–21).

Precaution. It is important to avoid overdose to the brain stem and ears, and to take special care of the ear for otitis in irradiation of a temporal-lobe tumor.

Centrosylvian Tumors (Thalamic and Corpus Callosal). Tumors in the centrosylvian region are usually deep gliomas of the thalamus and corpus callosum. Owing to their deep location, they are usually inoperable, although biopsy and decompression are occasionally attemped with great

risk. Most of these tumors are irradiated without tissue diagnosis.

Tumor Localization. Cerebral arteriogram and CT scan are most useful for localization of tumors in this deep location.

Case Illustration. A 4-year-old girl had a 2-month history of some right facial weakness and progressive weakness of the right leg and later of the right arm. She also had some behavioral change.

A cerebral arteriogram demonstrated a large left suprasylvian-staining mass involving corpus callosum and uncinate gyrus. A CT scan showed two large, enhancing oval conglomerate masses of about 4 cm to 5 cm in diameter, situated in the left-parietal region with extension to the corpus callosum beyond the midline (Fig. 10–22). A bifrontal craniotomy was done for biopsy. The tissue diagnosis was malignant glioma in the corpus callosum.

Portal Arrangement. The present policy

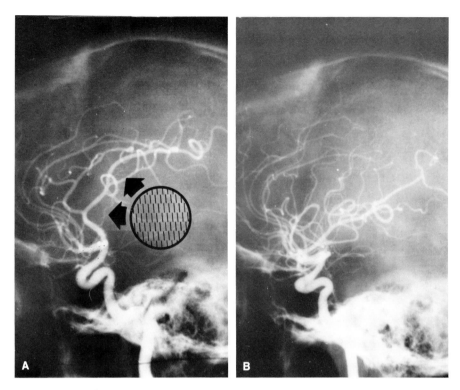

Fig. 10–20. *(A)* Lateral view of right cerebral arteriogram showed marked elevation and displacement of right middle cerebral artery *(arrows* and *shaded circle).* The opercular branches were stretched. The anterior choroidal artery was prominent. *(B)* Left lateral cerebral arteriogram of the same patient shown for comparison.

for malignant glioma in children is whole-brain irradiation for 4000 to 4500 rad in 4 to 5 weeks to be followed by booster-target-volume irradiation for an additional 1000 rad using two parallel-opposed lateral ports (similar to Fig. 10–21).

Precaution. It is important to avoid overdose to the thalamic midbrain region. Brain necrosis and hormonal deficiency may result, especially in children.

Intraventricular and Posterior Third-Ventricle Tumors. Posterior third ventricular and ectopic pinealoma (including suprasellar germinomas) form a special group of uncommon tumors in children that appears to respond well to radiotherapy with a high long-term-survival rate.

Tumor Localization. This group of tumors is best localized by PEG and CT scan with a contrast-enhancement technique.

Case Illustration. A 15-year-old girl with midline pineal tumor who received 4000 rad to the tumor volume was found to have recurrent tumor at the primary site 2 years later. She received an additional 4500 rad in 5 weeks to the whole brain and 3500 rad in 4½ weeks to the spinal axis. She is alive and well 5 years after the second course of radiotherapy without evidence of recurrence.

Portal Arrangement. Our present policy is to use two parallel-opposed lateral ports to encompass the whole brain (target volume) for the delivery of 4000 rad in 4 to 5 weeks and two parallel-opposed lateral small ports to encompass the booster-target volume for the delivery of an additional 1000 rad in one week (Fig. 10–23). If the CSF contains tumor cells, the spinal axis is irradiated with 4000 to 4500 rad in 5 to 6 weeks.

Precaution. It is important to immobi-

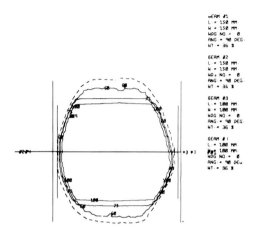

lize the child carefully and to tattoo the lower margin of the cranial port for possible future irradiation to the spinal axis for spinal seeding. Avoid overdose to the brain stem, hypothalamus, and chiasm.

Infratentorial Tumors

Brain-Stem Glioma. Tumor growing in the brain stem and midbrain are nearly always gliomas of various degrees of malignancy. About 30% of brain-stem gliomas are glioblastomas. Because of their location, gliomas of the brain stem, if untreated, may quickly expand and cause irreparable damage to the CNS, which is quickly followed by death. Most neurosurgeons consider surgical intervention to be extremely hazardous and useless.

Fig. 10–21. Same patient. The portal arrangement and isodose distribution for the medium grade malignant glioma. The whole brain is the target volume and the temporal tumor site is the booster target volume. There are two large parallel-opposed lateral ports for whole brain irradiation and two smaller parallel-opposed lateral ports for the booster dose.

Tumor Localization. PEG is the key to diagnosis and localization of the tumor; however, CT scan can provide useful and necessary anatomic information for delineation of the tumor extent. Some neurologists believe that CT scan can confirm the clinical diagnosis and should replace the more hazardous procedure of PEG.

Case Illustration. A 16-year-old boy had a 6-week history of dizziness, nausea and vomiting, diplopia, and slurring of speech. He had an unsteady gait that veered to the left, and mild difficulty in drinking liquid.

A PEG showed that the fourth ventricle was well-filled with air. Its floor was displaced posteriorly by a large midbrain, pontine mass (Fig. 10–24). A CT scan showed lucency in the region of the brain stem, which seemed to be enlarged. The fourth ventricle seemed to be elevated. An angiogram showed widening of the brain stem consistent with a brain-stem glioma.

Neurological examination showed a bilateral decrease of spontaneous facial expression, of right corneal reflex, and of gag reflex. There was trunkal ataxia. The clinical diagnosis was a brain-stem glioma.

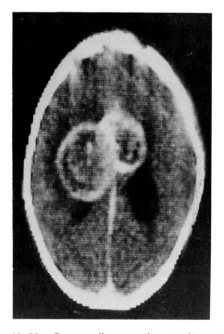

Fig. 10–22. Corpus callosum malignant glioma. CT scan showed two oval conglomerate enhancing masses of about 4–5 cm in diameter, each in the left medial parietal and corpus callosum. The irregular central lucency and zone of peritumoral edema indicate tumor necrosis and malignancy.

Portal Arrangement. Our present policy

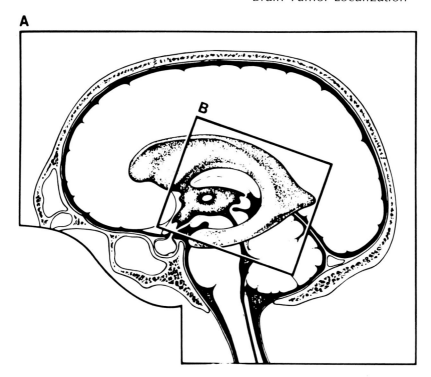

Fig. 10–23. Portal arrangement for pinealoma or metastatic brain tumor requiring whole brain irradiation and subsequent booster tumor volume treatment. Familiar two parallel-opposed lateral ports were used.

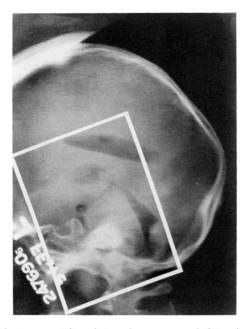

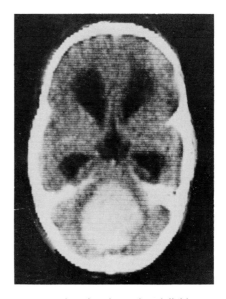

Fig. 10–24. A lateral view of pneumoencephalography showed that the floor of fourth ventricle and aqueduct of Sylvius were displaced posteriorly, presumably by a large midbrain and pontine glioma. Two 11 cm × 14 cm parallel-opposed lateral ports, as outlined on left lateral view, encompassing the mid-brain down to the C1 vertebral level were used for radiotherapy.

Fig. 10–25. A densely enhanced medulloblastoma, almost fills the entire fourth ventricle. The third and both lateral ventricles appear markedly dilated due to tumor obstruction in the aqueduct of Sylvius. There was no evidence of enhancement of the ventricular wall of the third or lateral ventricles that would suggest tumor seeding.

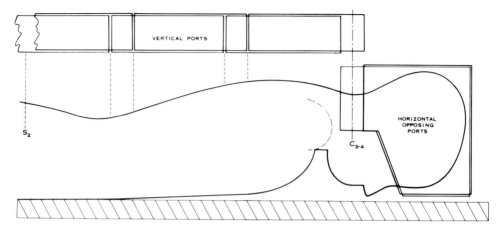

Fig. 10–26. Portal arrangement for medulloblastoma. Two horizontal parallel-opposed lateral cranial ports in relationship to three vertical spinal ports with moving gaps were depicted. The junction between the cranial port and spinal port was as shown. The cerebellum region was boosted with an additional dose.

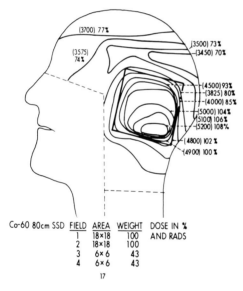

Co-60 80cm SSD	FIELD	AREA	WEIGHT	DOSE IN %
	1	18×18	100	AND RADS
	2	18×18	100	
	3	6×6	43	
	4	6×6	43	

17

Fig. 10–27. Isodose distribution for medulloblastoma with portal arrangement as shown in Fig. 10–26. The boostered primary cerebellar tumor site obtained a 100% dose versus 70–75% dose in the remaining whole brain. (From Keller, et al.: Standard Treatment Planning Atlas. Philadelphia, Radiation Therapy Oncology Group, 1976.)

× 14 cm, with beam-shaping technique. A few authors recently recommended whole-brain irradiation to be followed by an additional dose to the booster-target volume.

Precaution. Brain-stem necrosis following injudicious irradiation is a well known phenomenon. A tumor dose of 5000 to 5500 rad in 6½ to 7 weeks for brain-stem glioma is well tolerated. This may be delivered with 180 rad per fraction and 5 fractions per week.

Fourth-Ventricular Tumors (Medulloblastoma, Ependymoma). Medulloblastoma is the most common primary intracranial tumor in children and is recognized as the most sensitive to radiation. More than 80% of patients with medulloblastoma have subarachnoid spread of tumor with spinal seeding. The 5-year-survival rate greatly improved after the introduction of the whole-neuraxis-irradiation concept and technique.

Tumor Localization. The vast majority of medulloblastomas originate from the midline vermis of the cerebellum with a rapid extension to the fourth ventricle and the cerebellar hemisphere. A staging system based on the size of the primary medulloblastoma and the presence or absence of seedings has been developed.[1] With the

is to irradiate the entire brain stem and midbrain using two parallel-opposed lateral ports to encompass the midbrain and the brain stem, including the cerebellum and the fourth ventricle. The port size for this patient was determined to be 10 cm

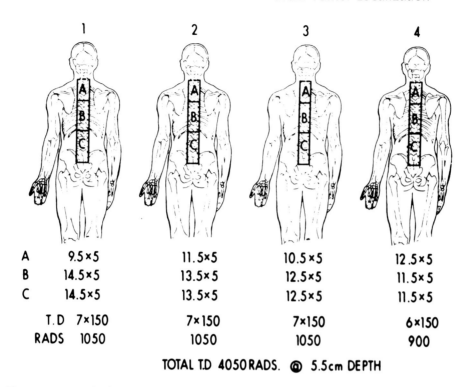

	1	2	3	4
A	9.5×5	11.5×5	10.5×5	12.5×5
B	14.5×5	13.5×5	12.5×5	11.5×5
C	14.5×5	13.5×5	12.5×5	11.5×5
T.D	7×150	7×150	7×150	6×150
RADS	1050	1050	1050	900

TOTAL T.D 4050 RADS. ⊚ 5.5cm DEPTH

Fig. 10–28. Spinal column ports in tandem with several gaps. The spinal ports were "gapped" at several places as shown to avoid large dose gradients due to beam unflatness. (From Keller, et al.: Standard Treatment Planning Atlas. Philadelphia, Radiation Therapy Oncology Group, 1976.)

advent of CT scan, the location and extent of the primary tumor and ventricular seeding can be visualized following contrast enhancement.

Case Illustration. An 11-month-old girl who had a normal perinatal period was well until 1 month prior to admission, when she developed a rapid progression of nausea, vomiting, and other signs of an increase of intracranial pressure. An arteriogram showed a midline posterior fossa mass. A CT scan demonstrated a large midline enhancing mass that almost filled the entire fourth ventricle associated with marked enlargement of the third and lateral ventricles (Fig. 10–25). The patient underwent a suboccipital craniectomy with subtotal removal of a vascular tumor. The tissue diagnosis was medulloblastoma.

Portal Arrangement The entire neuraxis is the target volume for irradiation.

Our portal arrangement consists of two horizontal parallel-opposed lateral ports encompassing the whole brain and the vertical spinal ports with moving gaps between the ports (Figs. 10–26, 10–27, 10–28). The posterior-fossa target is boosted with an additional dose in order to reduce the incidence of local recurrence of the primary tumor.

Precaution. Immobilization during the extended neuroaxial treatment is the most important part of the technique. A special couch with an adjustable head holder to help keep the patient comfortable in the prone position should be available. Avoiding overdose to the brain stem, spinal cord, and ocular lens is critically important. Some other techniques may deliver excessive doses to the lens, thyroid, and thymus. Because the entire spinal column is irradiated, frequent blood counts should be done in order to avoid severe bone-marrow depression.

Metastatic Brain Tumors

Metastatic brain tumors are usually multiple and require whole-brain irradiation for palliation. Localization of an individual tumor is therefore less important unless a booster dose is planned for a large residual tumor. Our portal arrangement is that of two parallel-opposed lateral ports encompassing the whole brain with an additional margin of 2 cm beyond the contour of the calvarium in order to achieve more homogeneous dose gradients across the brain (Fig. 10–22).

REFERENCES

1. Chang, C.H., Housepian, E.M., Herbert, C.: An operative staging system and a megavoltage radiotherapeutic technique for cerebellar medulloblastomas. Radiology 93:1351, 1969.
2. Keller, B.E., Grant, W., Suntharalingam, N.: Standard Treatment Planning Atlas. Philadelphia, Radiation Therapy Oncology Group, 1976.
3. Rubin, P., Cooper, R., and Phillips, T.L. (Eds): Radiation Biology and Radiation Pathology Syllabus (Set R.T. 1: Radiation Oncology). Chicago, Am. College Radiology. 1975.
4. Timmerman, R.A., Bilaniuk, L.T., Grundy, G., Littman, P.: Computed tomographic localization for radiotherapy of cerebral tumors. Radiology 119:230, 1976.
5. Walker, M.D.: Brain and peripheral nervous system tumors. *In* Cancer Medicine. 2nd Ed. Edited by J.F. Holland and E. Frei III. Philadelphia, Lea & Febiger, 1982.

Chapter 11

GYNECOLOGIC CANCERS: PELVIC EXAMINATION AND TREATMENT PLANNING

Luis Delclos

DIAGNOSTIC STUDIES AND DETERMINATIONS OF TUMOR EXTENT AND VOLUME

Diagnostic Examinations

At the M. D. Anderson Hospital and Tumor Institute, patients with gynecologic malignancies are first seen in the gynecology clinic, where the initial evaluation is done. Initial evaluation consists of a regular history, a physical examination, laboratory studies (complete blood count, blood chemistry, and urinalysis), electrocardiogram, and x-ray studies (chest radiograph in orthogonal projections and intravenous pyelogram). The general condition of the patient (e.g., the presence of additional illness, and the patient's mental attitude) are important, because the patient will be treated by irradiation for an extended period of time and will require several hospital admissions for intracavitary irradiation or additional surgery. Interruption of the treatment jeopardizes the chances of success. The patient is given a cystoscopy to eliminate or confirm bladder involvement; a complete pelvic examination is done in the established way,[2,16,21,29] which includes visual inspection, speculum examination, bimanual abdominovaginal and bidigital rectovaginal palpations, and biopsies from the uterine cervix (four quadrants, endocervix, and endometrium).

A lower-extremity lymphangiogram is recommended for all patients with disease involving more than one quadrant of the uterine cervix. The external iliac nodes, including the obturator node, located in the medial group of the external iliac chain, and the common iliac and para-aortic nodes can be consistently visualized on a lymphangiogram; however, the hypogastric and presacral nodes cannot be identified by lymphangiography because they are not in the same lymphatic pathway. The lymphangiogram is of great value only when positive; a node that is not traversed by lymphatic channels and a crescent defect in a node always indicate a metastatic disease.[36]

Cancer of the uterine cervix spreads in a very predictable manner. In patients with relatively early disease, in whom tumor volume is small and involvement of the paracervical, vaginal, and paracolpium areas is minimal, the common iliac and para-aortic nodes are very rarely involved; in this situation, there is less need for the lower-extremity lymphangiogram because the external-beam irradiation fields cover the lymph nodes most likely to be involved (external iliac, hypogastric, presacral, and distal common iliac) up to the level of the upper surface of L5. A positive lower-extremity lymphangiogram is, however, of extreme value in patients with larger tumors where the common iliac and para-aortic nodes may be involved; in these instances, the external-beam irradiation portals have to be progressively extended to cover the involved areas and an adequate margin.

Proctoscopy and barium enemas are recommended only in patients with posterior tumor extension or massive fixation to the left pelvic wall when the tumor could be wrapped around, or could involve, the rectum or sigmoid colon. Metastatic bone surveys and liver scans are not routinely recommended. Renal scans are necessary

only if the patient is allergic to the contrast dye, ruling out an intravenous pyelogram.

After the initial diagnostic workup, the patient is seen by the gynecologist and the radiotherapist at the gynecology-radiotherapy disposition clinic. A therapeutic recommendation is made, assigning the patient to treatment with one of the high-energy units (18–25 MV photons).

Preirradiation Evaluation of the Patient

The steps described here are those usually followed for patients who have carcinoma of the uterine cervix; they can be extrapolated for use with other gynecologic tumors.

The patient record is carefully scrutinized by the radiotherapist, not only to verify the extent of the cancer, but also to assure that additional illnesses are treated adequately. Special attention is paid to any

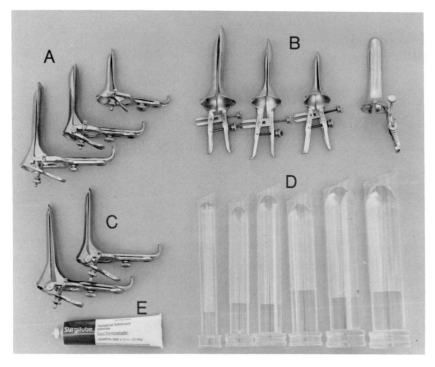

Fig. 11–1. A variety of vaginal speculums of different length, diameter, and shape should be available to meet any anatomical situation. *(A)* Graves anteroposterior blade aperture. *(B)* Devilbiss lateral blade aperture for visual inspection of the anterior and posterior vaginal walls. *(C)* Pederson narrow-blade (see also Fig. 11–2). *(D)* Cylindrical speculums, particularly useful for patients with cystocele or rectocele. *(E)* Sterile surgical lubricant and Xylocaine lubricant should be available.

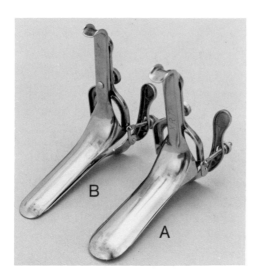

Fig. 11–2. Comparison of Graves *(A)* and Pederson *(B)* vaginal speculums. Note that Pederson blades are narrower.

previous curative process, such as abdominal surgery or pelvic infections, that could have promoted adhesions. This is very important, because a bowel entrapped by adhesions becomes less tolerant to both external and intracavitary irradiation, and adjustments in field size, dose rate, and total dose have to be made initially and during the treatment.

The patient is first examined in the supine position. Both supraclavicular and inguinal areas are checked for enlarged nodes. The abdomen is checked for an enlarged liver, large omental, para-aortic, or lower abdominal masses, and for ascites.

The patient's pelvis is then examined with the patient in the lithotomy position. There are many excellent books that describe the proper way to perform a thorough pelvic examination.[2,16,21] Some aspects of the pelvic examination are paramount and should be emphasized for their role in determining tumor extension and tumor volume, and in selecting and sequencing treatment modalities (e.g., ex-

ternal irradiation first versus intracavitary irradiation first) and techniques to be employed (e.g., parallel opposed fields, extended or reduced fields, four field "box" technique).

The pelvic examination begins with visual inspection of the external genitalia; then, a gloved finger is inserted into the vagina to determine the size and shape of the speculum to use. Inspection of the uterine cervix and all vaginal walls is very important in determining the shape of the cervix, the clinical variety of the cervical component of the tumor, and the amount of vaginal extension of the tumor; for this inspection a variety of speculums is necessary (Figs. 11–1 and 11–2). Figure 11–3 shows other instruments necessary for a good pelvic examination.[4] The size and shape of the vagina are noted, because they affect the sequence of treatment and the type and size of colpostat to be used. They also affect the positioning of the lower edge of the treatment field and the amount of external irradiation to be given.

After the uterine cervix and vagina have been inspected, the uterine cavity is probed with a calibrated malleable hysterometer. This sounding is of extreme importance, not only for determining the length, width, and position (e.g., retroflexed, anteverted, fixed to one side) of the uterus, but also for detecting and draining a possible pyometra. Probing is repeated at the weekly examinations throughout the treatment. Bimanual abdominovaginal examination follows the speculum examination. Although it is of some merit to examine the pelvis bimanually before the speculum examination, in patients with tumors of the uterus this manipulation may cause vaginal hemorrhage, hampering completion of the examination.

Bimanual abdominovaginal examination should be done with both hands (Figs. 11–4, 11–5, and 11–6) because the left hand can reach deeper into the left pelvis and the right hand can reach deeper into the right pelvis; it also allows a better com-

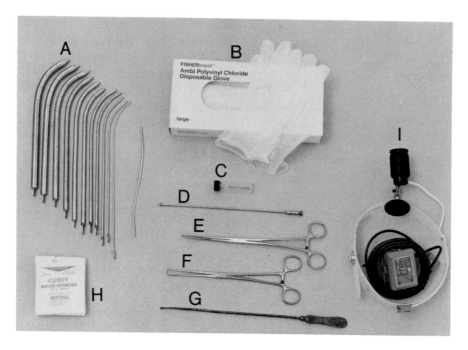

Fig. 11–3. *(A)* Calibrated uterine dilators[6] and regular Hegar or Hanks' dilators; *(B)* disposable gloves; *(C)* silver seeds; *(D)* seed implanter; *(E)* Bozeman uterine packing forceps; *(F)* Braun or Barrett uterine forceps; *(G)* malleable hysterometer; *(H)* Sponges; *(I)* Direct-focusing headlight with simple focusing sleeve.

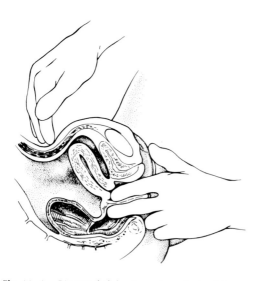

Fig. 11–4. Bimanual abdominorectovaginal pelvic examination. (From Greenhill, J.P.: Office Gynecology, 9th ed. Chicago, Year Book Medical Publishers, 1971, p. 28.)

parison of the findings in either side, which is not easy when only one hand is used because of the necessary rotation of the hand to feel the opposite side.

After the bimanual abdominovaginal examination, the physician proceeds to a bidigital vaginorectal examination. The index finger is introduced in the vagina and the middle finger of the same hand in the rectum (see Figs. 11–4 and 11–6). This allows a more accurate outlining of the pelvic organs and structures than the use of the index finger alone for the rectal examination. The middle finger is longer than the index finger (1–2 cm) and can reach higher. The bidigital examination produces firmer pressure against the perineal body; moreover, the rectal finger establishes very clearly the extent of disease in the uterosacral areas, broad ligament, and cardinal ligament. Determining tumor extension posteriorly as well as anteriorly along the pubocervical fascia is very important to the selection of field arrange-

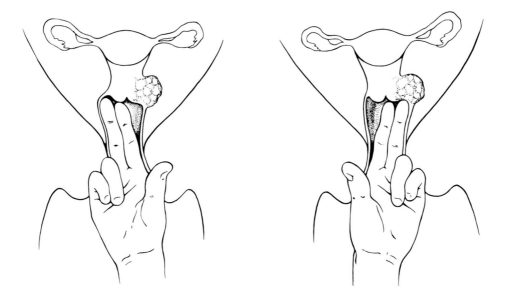

Fig. 11–5. Bidigital vaginal examination. (From del Regato, J.A. and Spjut, H.J.: Female Genital Organs/ Cervix. *In* Cancer, 5th ed. Edited by Ackerman and del Regato. St. Louis, C.V. Mosby, 1977, p. 733.)

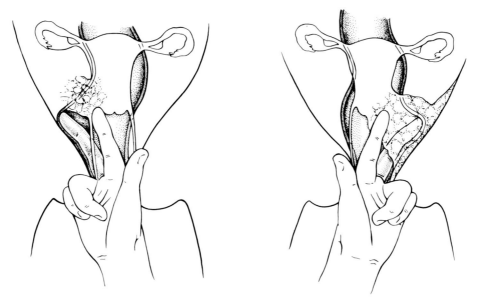

Fig. 11–6. Bidigital rectovaginal examination.

ment. When the tumor includes these areas, the physician cannot use the four-field "box" technique; he is limited to the use of parallel-opposed-fields arrangement in order to cover adequately the areas of tumor extension.

Determining the tumor volume is very important regardless of tumor extension. Large bulky tumors are always treated with external-beam irradiation first, for two reasons: the need to reduce tumor volume, reducing the number of tumor cells and improving tumor oxygenation, and the need to improve conditions in the pelvis so that the colpostats and intrauterine tandem can be placed in the best position for effective intracavitary irradiation.

LOCALIZING GYNECOLOGIC MALIGNANCIES FOR TREATMENT PLANNING

Megavoltage radiation therapy with 18- to 25-MV photons allows high doses of radiation to be delivered to the pelvis with simple field arrangements providing satisfactory dose distribution. The shape of the pelvic portals depends on whether treatment is to be given to the parametria and pelvic lymph nodes, as a supplement to intracavitary irradiation, or to the whole pelvis, including the primary tumor and the adjacent pelvic and lymphatic areas. The number of portals depends on the tumor volume and extensions of the tumor

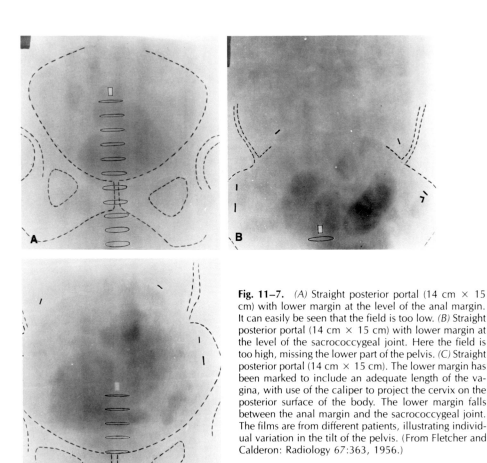

Fig. 11–7. *(A)* Straight posterior portal (14 cm × 15 cm) with lower margin at the level of the anal margin. It can easily be seen that the field is too low. *(B)* Straight posterior portal (14 cm × 15 cm) with lower margin at the level of the sacrococcygeal joint. Here the field is too high, missing the lower part of the pelvis. *(C)* Straight posterior portal (14 cm × 15 cm). The lower margin has been marked to include an adequate length of the vagina, with use of the caliper to project the cervix on the posterior surface of the body. The lower margin falls between the anal margin and the sacrococcygeal joint. The films are from different patients, illustrating individual variation in the tilt of the pelvis. (From Fletcher and Calderon: Radiology 67:363, 1956.)

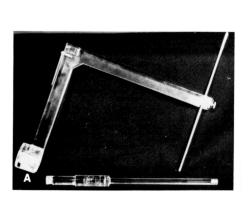
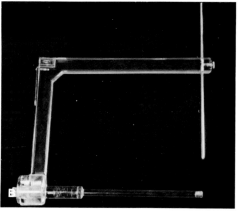

Fig. 11–8. Simplified Fletcher cervical localizer: *(A)* The removable vaginal arm with the lead tip at the distal end is shown disconnected from the L-shaped arm with the sliding rod. *(B)* Both arms are connected showing the alignment of the lower tip of the sliding rod with the leaded tip on the removable arm. Note that there is an inserted level on the proximal end of the horizontal branch of the L-shaped arm and on the proximal end of the removable arms.

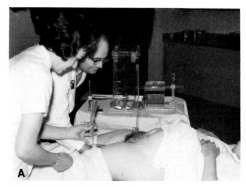
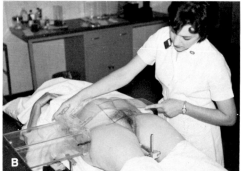
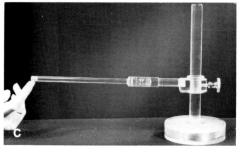

Fig. 11–9. The removable arm of the cervical localizer is introduced into the vagina and guided by the examining finger until it is in contact with the uterine cervix or with the vaginal extension of the tumor. This point is then transferred to the skin with the sliding rod at the tip of the L-shaped arm *(A)*. The level in the L-shaped arm assures that the horizontal branch of the arm is truly horizontal. The L-shaped arm is then detached from the removable arm, and the removable arm is left in the vagina and mounted on a stand *(B)*. C shows details of the vaginal arm and stand. In B we can see the nurse-technician setting the lateral fields while the vaginal arm is in the vagina. *(A.B.* From Fletcher, G.H. and Hamberger, A.D.: *In* Textbook of Radiotherapy, 3rd ed. Edited by G.H. Fletcher. Philadelphia, Lea & Febiger, 1980, p. 761.)

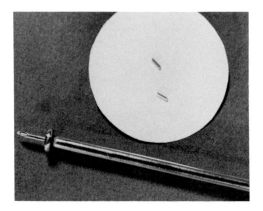

Fig. 11–10. Details of the cervical marker and silver seeds. The seeds are small pieces of silver wire or inactive gold grains. The implanter is a 10-inch rigid radon implanter to which a small flange has been soldered so that the silver or gold grain is always introduced to the same depth. (From Delclos: Radiology 93:695, 1969.)

(i.e., laterally along the broad and cardinal ligaments, posteriorly along the uterosacral ligaments, or anteriorly along the pubocervical fascia).

Treatment of the primary lesions with intracavitary radium and moderate supplementary radiation to the lateral parametria and pelvic wall nodes has achieved excellent results and a low incidence of complications in patients with small tumor volumes and suitable anatomy. Management of some clinical varieties of stage I tumors, and of all stages II, III, and IV lesions is more complex. In these more extensive tumors, external irradiation plays a greater role, intracavitary irradiation is more individualized, and in some instances irradiation is combined with surgery.

The practice of taking localization radiographs with the therapy unit,[10,13] and more recently with both the simulator and the therapy unit,[12] has shown that there are too many anatomic variables to rely on the surface and bony landmarks in all patients. For example, the pubic symphysis anteriorly, or the tip of the coccyx posteriorly, cannot be used routinely as landmarks for the lower margin of the portal (Fig. 11–7).[13]

Anatomic Relationships

The anatomic structures of the pelvis relevant to the planning of external-beam

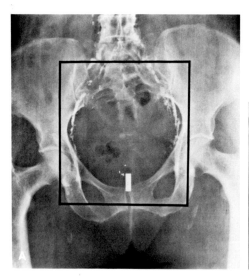
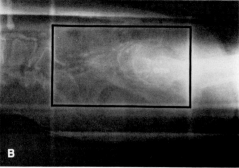

Fig. 11–11. Anteroposterior *(A)* and lateral simulator *(B)* x-ray films showing the leaded tip of the vaginal arm of the simplified Fletcher cervical localizer against the uterine cervix and four silver seeds implanted into the cervix (two seeds, one in the anterior and one in the posterior cervical lip are enough). Seeds are also implanted in the lowest vaginal extension of the tumor. (From Fletcher, G.H. and Hamberger, A.D.: In Textbook of Radiotherapy, 3rd ed. Edited by G.H. Fletcher. Philadelphia, Lea & Febiger, 1980, p. 761.)

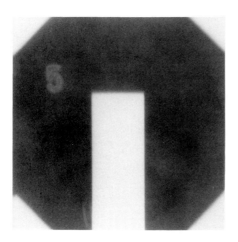

Fig. 11–12. Inverted "U" field. This is a pelvic portal (AP and PA) for parametrial irradiation. The midline is partially blocked by a lead shield mounted on the tray or by the compression cone. This block diminishes the dose to the bladder and rectum at the area of higher dose at the junction of tandem and ovoids. (From Fletcher, G.H. and Rutledge, F.N.: Carcinoma of the uterine cervix. *In* Modern Radiotherapy. Edited by T.J. Deeley. London, Butterworths, 1971.)

therapy were divided into two groups by Fletcher and Calderon in the early 1950s.[13] The first group included the vagina, uterine cervix, paracervical and paracolpal areas, the body of the uterus, and the medial aspect of the broad and uterosacral ligaments. The second group included the lateral aspects of the broad and uterosacral ligaments and the so-called pelvic wall lymph nodes. This distinction is very important because the structures in the second group have a fairly consistent fixed relationship to the bony pelvis, whereas for those in the first group the relationship varies considerably, depending on the age of the patient, the amount of disease, previous surgery, and so forth. Due to the tilt of the pelvis in the prone and supine positions, the relationship between the bony pelvis and the surface landmarks is inconsistent.

The length of vagina to be treated is determined by the extent of the disease in the vagina. In planning for external-beam therapy, therefore, the structures to be covered (e.g., the cervix and the lower extent

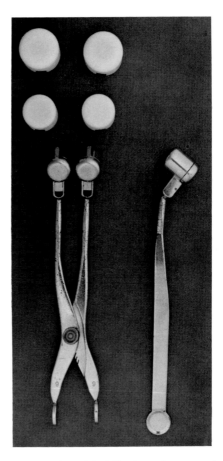

Fig. 11–13. The original Fletcher colpostat, preloadable, with three cylinder sizes (smallest, 2 cm in diameter; medium, 2.5 cm in diameter, and largest, 3 cm in diameter) obtained by adding Teflon jackets to the small metal cylinder. The colpostat has interlocking handles. Although the diameter of the colpostats is the same as in the Manchester ovoids,[11,14,34] they are cylindrical and, therefore, the surface of the colpostat does not follow an isodose curve. This and the additional shielding (Fig. 11–8) reduces the dose to the poles of the ovoids. On the left of the picture, there is a single ovoid designed to be used alone against the uterine cervix in patients with very narrow vaginas.

of the vaginal tumor infiltration) must be projected to the anterior and posterior surfaces, and to the lateral surface when lateral portals are employed.

The location of the pelvic nodes has been well established in the past[18,35] and confirmed more recently by lymphangiograms.[8,9] The so-called obturator node belongs to the medial group of the external iliac chain and lies against the pelvic wall,

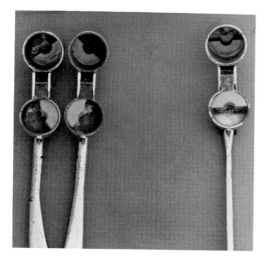

Fig. 11–14. Original preloadable Fletcher colpostats (double and single cylinder)[6] opened to show the position of the tungsten shielding in the upper and lower poles of the cylinders.

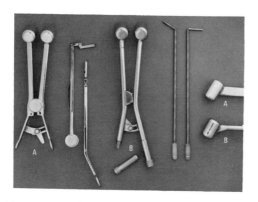

Fig. 11–15. Fletcher afterloading colpostats: *(A)* Fletcher–Suit rectangular-handle model; *(B)* current round-handle, lighter model. Both models are acceptable. The round-handle model, however, is less bulky and the sources insertion (radium holder) is simpler. (From Delclos, et al.: Cancer *41:972, 1978.*)

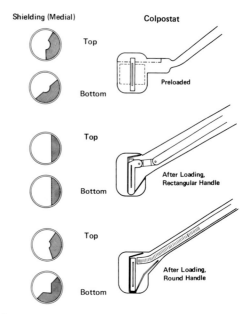

Fig. 11–16. Drawing of *(from top to bottom)* the original Fletcher preloadable colpostat, Fletcher-Suit rectangular-handle afterloading colpostat, and round-handle afterloading colpostat (current model). The tungsten shielding, present in all three models, is rotated in the Fletcher-Suit rectangular-handle model; it has been returned to the original position in the current round-handle model. (From Delclos et al.: Cancer *41:974, 1978.*)

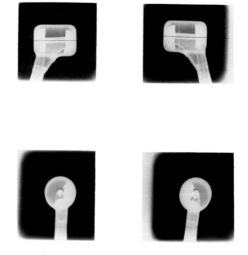

Fig. 11–17. Roentgenogram of the round-handle afterloading colpostat, current model. As in all Fletcher models, the radioactive source is on the central axis of the colpostat and tungsten shielding is in the upper and lower poles.

slightly higher than the center of the acetabulum. The hypogastric or internal iliac group is located in the vicinity of the bifurcation of the common iliac into the external iliac and hypogastric arteries, and is about 4 cm to 5 cm posterior to the obturator node. The remaining external iliac nodes spread along the pelvic inlet, and the sacral nodes lie anterior to the second or third sacral segments. The common iliac nodes extend from the junction of the

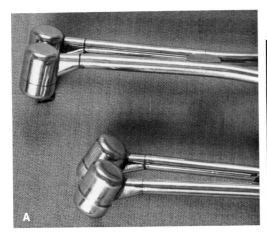
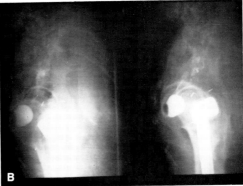

Fig. 11–18. The round-handle afterloadable colpostat is available in two models with different angles between handle and colpostat *(A)*. *(B)* On the right, the colpostat with greater angle fits poorly against the cervix (outlined with silver grains in the anterior and posterior cervical lip). On the left, the colpostat with the more obtuse angle fits properly against the cervix. (From Delclos et al.: Int. J. Radiat. Oncol. Biol. Phys. 6:1197, 1980.)

external and hypogastric chains in front of the sacral wing, and go as high as the top of L5.[8,13]

The projection of the uterine cervix or vaginal tumor extension to the anterior, posterior, and lateral surfaces of the pelvis can be determined either by using a cervical localizer[13] or by implanting pieces of silver wire or inactive gold grains with a cervical marker[3] into the uterine cervix "portio vaginalis" and vaginal extension of the tumor.

Cervical Localizer

The cervical localizer is a caliper constructed with one removable arm (Fig. 11–8). The removable arm of the caliper is a plastic cylinder with a lead tip. The other arm is L-shaped and attaches to the base of the removable arm. At the tip is a sliding rod in line with the lead tip of the plastic cylinder.

With the patient in the supine position, the removable arm is introduced into the vagina, guided by the examining finger until it is in contact with the cervix or with the vaginal extension of the tumor (Fig. 11–9A). This point is then transferred to the skin with the sliding rod. The same

procedure is done with the patient in the prone position. When the radiographs are taken, the L-shaped arm is detached from the vaginal arm with the lead tip, and the vaginal arm is held on a stand (Fig. 11–9B and C). The position of the tip of the rod is checked with the L-shaped arm. The vaginal arm is maintained horizontal (there is a level inserted into the arm), and films are taken with either the treatment unit or the simulator, or both. This cervical localizer is particularly useful when taking treatment-unit films because the piece of lead at the tip is large enough for film definition.

Cervical Marker

Bits of silver wire or gold seeds are implanted by means of the uterine cervix marker (Fig. 11–10).[3] They are useful not only in placing the external portals, but also, at the time the intrauterine tandem and colpostats are inserted, in checking the positions of the uterine cervix, vaginal tumor, intrauterine tandem, and colpostats relative to one another. Several radiographic techniques have been described for megavoltage-therapy radiographs.[17,26] Figure 11–11 shows antero-

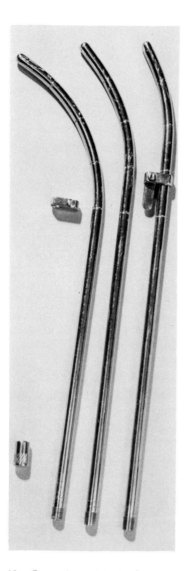

posterior and lateral simulator films, indicating the relationships between the uterine cervix, as marked with seeds, the cervical localizer, and the treatment portals.

Positioning the Pelvic Portals

The lower margin of the pelvic fields should be set 2 cm or 3 cm below the projection of the cervix or the vaginal tumor involvement. This margin is necessary to allow for daily variations in the setup, the field-edge falloff, and potential submucosal tumor extension along the vagina. When tumor extension requires low fields, the anterior field is tilted 10° toward the feet to minimize irradiation of the vulva.

Lateral portals with 18- to 25-MV photons can be used effectively to cover the areas of tumor involvement. When the uterosacral ligaments, are being irradiated, the portals are slightly enlarged posteriorly to include these areas and the presacral lymph nodes. The selection of pelvic portals and extended fields is described in detail by Fletcher.[12]

When irradiation is given to complement intracavitary radium, the lateral aspects of the parametria, uterosacral ligaments, and pelvic wall nodes are irradiated with minimal doses to the midline. This is accomplished by placing a 3-cm or 4-cm wide lead block to cover the midline of the anterior and posterior fields, thus blocking the area of the higher dose at the junction of the intrauterine tandem and vaginal ovoids (Fig. 11–12).

AFTERLOADABLE INTRACAVITARY APPLICATORS

The Fletcher Colpostats

The Fletcher preloadable colpostats (Fig. 11–13)[11,14] were designed in the early 1950s to provide a colpostat for standard radium tubes that would insert easily and would remain in position in the lateral fornices. The colpostats increase irradiation to the paracervical and parametrial

Fig. 11–19. Current intrauterine tandems are available in three curvatures to fit most uteri. The greatest curvature is for the longest uterine cavities, measured in the axis of the uterus. The smallest curvature is for the smallest cavities. Sometimes this rule does not apply, but because localization x-ray films are taken in the operating room, the tandem can be replaced immediately. At the distal end, the tandem is flat at the top to allow for checking the position of the tandem in the uterus throughout the packing procedure. (From Delclos et al.: Int. J. Radiat. Oncol. Biol. Phys. 6:1197, 1980.)

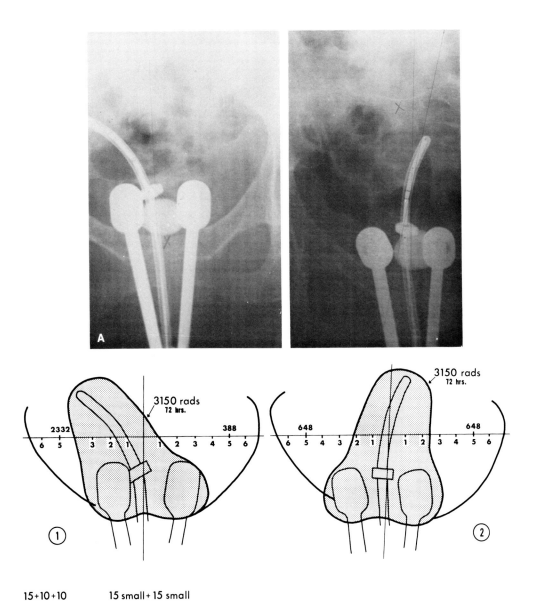

Fig. 11–20. *(A)* Radiographs and *(B)* drawings showing the intrauterine tandem**(1)** tilted to one side and **(2)** at the midline. If the intrauterine tandem is left in the midline on the axis of the pelvis, the dose contribution to the lateral pelvic walls is approximately the same. (From Delclos et al.: Int. J. Radiat. Oncol. Biol. Phys. 6:1198, 1980.)

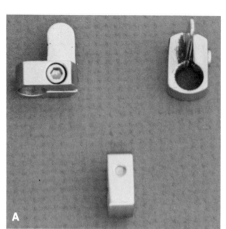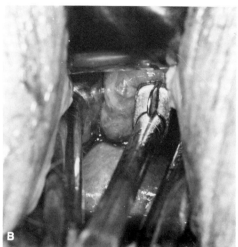

Fig. 11–21. *(A)* Flange with keel and without keel. The keeled flange is placed on the intrauterine tandems when the tandem is used in combination with Fletcher colpostats. *(B)* Tight packing around the keel minimizes rotation of the tandem. The flange without keel is used on tandems in combination with vaginal cylinders (see also Fig. 11–24). (From Delclos et al.: Int. J. Radiat. Oncol. Biol. Phys. 6:1199, 1980.)

tissues by more effectively placing the radium sources then earlier applicators.[34] Bladder and rectal shielding are provided (Fig. 11–14). In the late 1950s, Suit et al.[33] developed the first afterloadable Fletcher colpostat for standard radium tubes (Fig. 11–15A). The design restrictions were basically the same as those in the original Fletcher colpostats, although the shielding was rotated medially because of some mechanical difficulties. This displacement was not considered significant in the overall effectiveness of the applicator.

In the mid 1960s, Green et al.[15] redesigned the afterloading colpostats to precisely match the original colpostat designed by Fletcher. In the late 1960s, at M. D. Anderson Hospital, the Fletcher-Suit rectangular-handle colpostats were converted to a lighter model with round handles (Fig. 11–15B) and the bladder and rectal shielding, as in Green's model, were returned to the original position. Figure 11–16 shows the position of the shielding in the three models. Figure 11–17 is a roentgenograph of the current round-handle model showing the central position of the radium tube along the axis of the colpostat and the medial position of the shielding. In a recent paper,[6] the design restrictions and some problems encountered with poorly manufactured colpostats are discussed in detail. Two angles between colpostat and handle are available (Fig. 11–18A) for a better fitting of the ovoids in the lateral fornices or against the cervical "portio vaginalis" (Fig. 11–18B).

Intrauterine Tandems

The intrauterine tandems are available in three curvatures (Fig. 11–19) that fit the majority of uterine cavities. As a rule, the greatest curvature is used when the uterine cavity measures more than 6 cm. The lesser curvature is used for small uterine cavities.

Because the intrauterine tandem is independent from the colpostats, it can be kept in the axis of the pelvis, equidistant from the pubis, sacral promontorium, and lateral pelvic walls (Fig. 11–20). A tandem curvature is occasionally changed to fit a special situation.

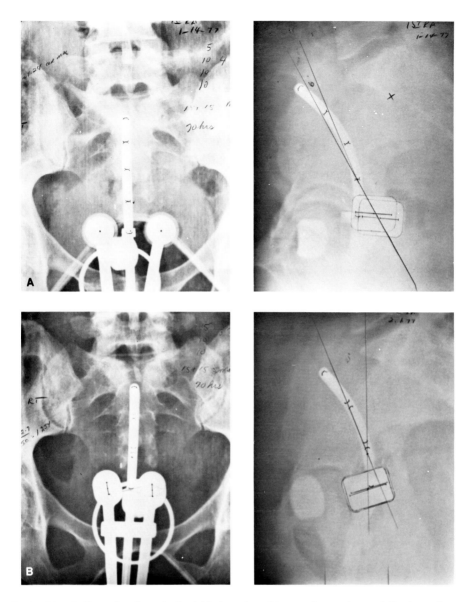

Fig. 11–22. Radiographs of an afterloadable insertion of intrauterine tandem and Fletcher colpostats showing in *(A)* the posterior displacement of the colpostats into the posterior cul-de-sac. This frequently occurs in patients when the anterior fornix is flush and there is a large posterior fornix. In *(B)* the colpostats have been maintained in the proper position by holding the tandem and the ovoids together with the yoke (see also Fig. 11–17). (From Delclos, et al.: Int. J. Radiat. Oncol. Biol. Phys. 6:1199, 1980.)

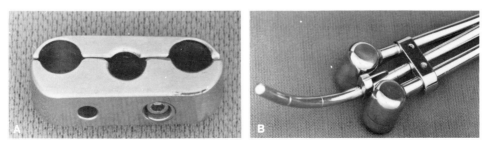

Fig. 11–23. The yoke *(A)* to hold tandem and colpostats together *(B)* in a selected situation. (From Delclos et al.: Int. J. Radiat. Oncol. Biol. Phys. 6:1199, 1980.)

207

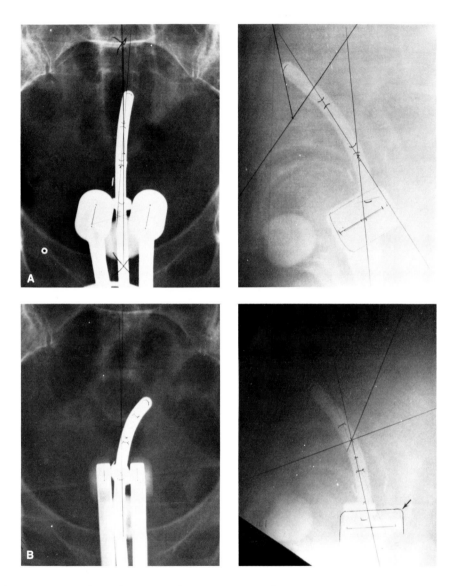

Fig. 11–24. *(A)* Radiographs of an afterloadable insertion of an intrauterine tandem and small Fletcher colpostats in a patient with a narrow vagina. The colpostats are too low and anterior because the upper vagina did not accommodate the small colpostats. This can be solved by using separate tandem and colpostat insertions as recommended by Fletcher,[3] which requires two hospital admissions. The mini-colpostats (8 mm radius) were designed to give the intracavitary treatment in one single insertion (one hospital admission). In *(B)* we see the minicolpostats against the uterine cervix. (From Delclos et al.: Int. J. Radiat. Oncol. Biol. Phys. 6:1200, 1980.)

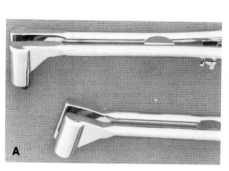
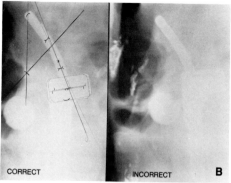

Fig. 11–25. *(A)* The minicolpostats *(B)* are available in two angles to fit adequately against the lateral fornix or uterine cervix. The original afterloading minicolpostats have no shielding at the poles. With the radioactive source equidistance from the poles, the dose at the poles is reduced to 30% to 35% of the lateral surface dose. The surface dose in each minicolpostat (8 mm radius) with 10 mg radium is similar to the surface dose with small Fletcher colpostats (1 cm radius) loaded with 15 mg radium. (From Delclos et al.: Int. J. Radiat. Oncol. Biol. Phys. 6:1201, 1980.)

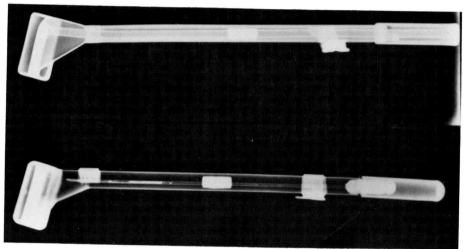

Fig. 11–26. Roentgenogram of two current models of minicolpostats for standard radium sources. There is no shielding on these two models, but shielding is available in a recently developed colpostat for smaller cesium sources. (From Delclos, et al.: Int. J. Radiat. Oncol. Biol. Phys. 6:1201, 1980.)

Flange with Keel

The purpose of the flange (Fig. 11–21) is to keep the intrauterine tandem in the selected position. The keeled flange was designed by Suit in the early 1960s. It is attached to the intrauterine tandem at the precise height of the uterine cavity, as measured with the hysterometer. It should be flush against the external os, or if this has been destroyed by tumor, against the lowest cervical surface. The packing around the keel minimizes displacement or rotation of the intrauterine tandem.

Yoke

Fletcher[12] emphasizes the use of separate intrauterine tandems and vaginal colpostats in order to deliver a higher dose to the largest cervical tumor area. When the anterior fornix is flush with the uterine cervix and the posterior fornix is voluminous, however, it is difficult to keep the colpostats against the laternal fornices or the uterine cervix "portio vaginalis" because the colpostats tend to fall into the posterior fornix (Fig. 11–22A) The yoke was designed to maintain the proper align-

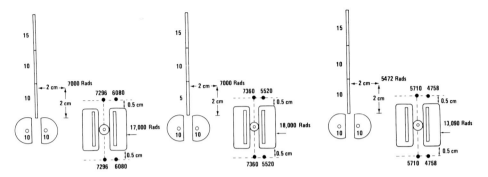

Fig. 11–27. The minocolpostats were designed for narrow vaginas, to be used in combination with intrauterine tandems. Because of the patient's anatomy, the intrauterine and vaginal sources are very close and adjustment has to be made to reduce the dose to the bladder and rectum either by reducing the loading or by reducing the time of the insertion. Note, from left to right, that the planned dose of 7000 rad at point A may be prohibitive for the bladder and rectum. An unsuccessful effort was made to reduce this dose by loading the intrauterine tandem with 15-10-5 mg radium instead of 15-10-10 mg radium. In order to keep the bladder and rectal doses low, it was necessary to reduce the dose to point A to 5500 rad (5472 rad in the drawing). (From Delclos et al.: Int. J. Radiat. Oncol. Biol. Phys. 6:1201, 1980.)

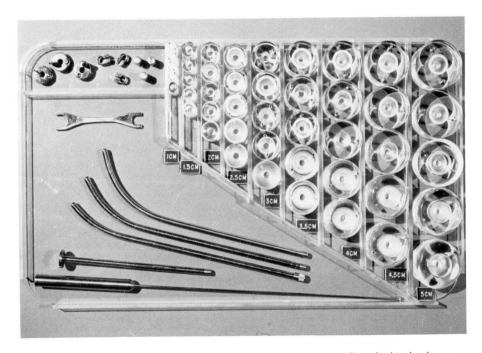

Fig. 11–28. Tray with afterloadable tandems and cylindrical colpostats. The cylindrical colpostats are 2.5 cm in height each, and are available from 1 cm to 5 cm in diameter to fit any vaginal width. As many cylinders as needed are mounted on the vaginal component of an intrauterine tube (see Fig. 11–24). To enable identification of the cylinder and their relationship to the uterine cervix or to the extension of the tumor along the vagina, each cyclinder has two lead markers inserted at the top and at the bottom (see also Fig. 11–25). (From Delclos et al.: Int. J. Radiat. Oncol. Biol. Phys. 6:1202, 1980.)

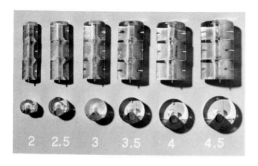

Fig. 11–29. Selection of cylinders with segments of incorporated lead to partially shield the vagina, the rectum or the urinary bladder and urethra. (From Delclos et al.: Int. J. Radiat. Oncol. Biol. Phys. 6:1202, 1980.)

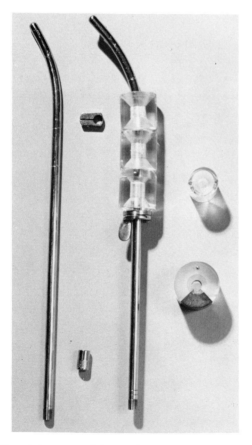

Fig. 11–30. From left to right: intrauterine tandem, flange without keel, sample of three vaginal cylinders mounted on the vaginal component of the intrauterine afterloading tandem, keeled flange (see also Fig. 11–26), and top view of two cylinders, one with and one without lead shielding. (From Delclos: Radiology 96:666, 1970.)

ment of the colpostats and tandem (Figs. 11–22B and 11–23). Several yokes can be manufactured for different colpostat separations and intrauterine tandem lengths.

Minicolpostats

Although it is always desirable to use the largest pair of colpostats to take advantage of the inverse square law, when the vagina is narrow or distorted and there is no visible or palpable tumor involving the vagina, it is less important to irradiate the vagina with margins beyond the tumor. One can use either separate insertions of tandems and colpostats or one insertion with minicolpostats (Fig. 11–24). The minocolpostats are designed with a radius of 8 mm and a flat inner surface (Fig. 11–25), and are used in conjunction with the intrauterine tandem. When loaded with 10-mg radium (radium tubes, active length = 1.5 cm, 1-mm platinum filtration) they deliver about the same surface dose at the lateral surface as do the small Fletcher colpostats (radius 10 mm) with 15 mg radium.

The minicolpostats are no substitute for the Fletcher colpostats. In the original design they do not have shielding (Fig. 11–26) because of lack of space for the radium tubes (2.2 cm total length); shielding, however, is desirable and is available in some minicolpostats constructed for smaller cesium sources. The dose at the top and bottom of one minicolpostat is about one-third of the dose at the lateral-surface. Because the overall diameter of the colpostats and tandem between them is small, there is an increase in dose to the top and bottom areas (midline) when adding the dose contribution from both mini-colpostats and the intrauterine tandem. A preselected dose to point A of 7000 rad would result in an overdose to small areas of bladder and rectum (Fig. 11–27). The dose, therefore, should be adjusted to bladder and rectal tolerance doses by manipulating time and loading.

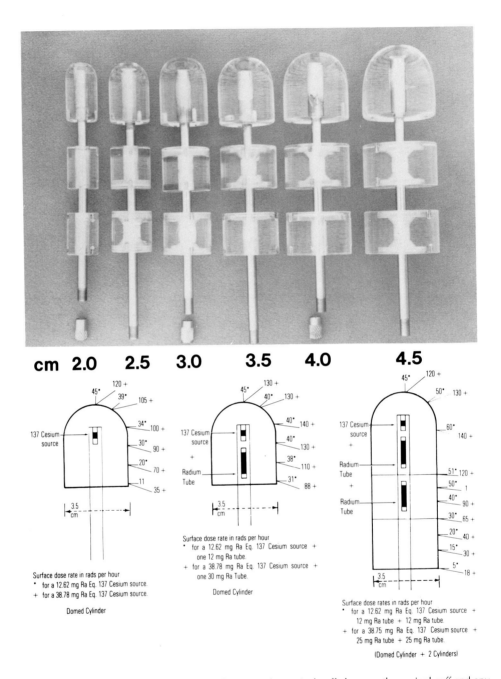

Fig. 11–31.   The dome colpostats were made to treat the vaginal cuff alone, or the vaginal cuff and any selected vaginal length on a patient who has had a hysterectomy. The curvature of each dome cylinder follows an isodose of a ^{137}Cs minisource placed at an adequate distance from the dome in the afterloading stem. The previously described vaginal cylinders can be added to the dome cylinders as shown here. Any length of vaginal surface can be treated by combining a ^{137}Cs minisource with radium tubes or cesium sources. Some examples of loading are shown. (From Delclos, L., Wharton, J.T., and Rutledge, F.N.: Tumors of the vagina and female urethra. *In* Textbook of Radiotherapy, 3rd ed. Edited by G.H. Fletcher. Philadelphia, Lea & Febiger, 1980.)

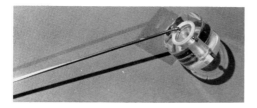

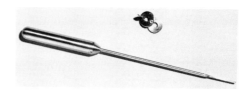

Fig. 11–32. Detail of vaginal cylinder and the hook used to remove it from the vagina. Note the inside groove to facilitate the individual removal of cylinders. This is important when the cylinders are too tight. Note also the lead pellets for identification on the localization film. (From Delclos et al.: Int. J. Radiat. Oncol. Biol. Phys. 6:1202, 1980.)

Fig. 11–33. The fixation round flange with keel, and the long-handle Allen range. The keeled round flange, fixed by tightening the Allen screw, is packed. The labia are then sutured. This minimizes rotation of the intra-uterine tandem. (From Delclos et al.: Int. J. Radiat. Oncol. Biol. Phys. 6:1203, 1980.)

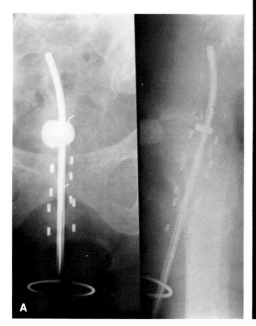

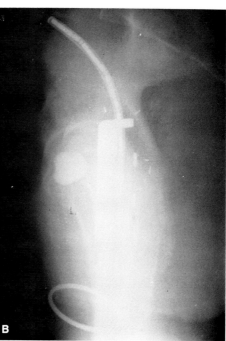

Fig. 11–34. *(A)* Radiogram of an intrauterine tandem with three vaginal cylinders along the vaginal component of the tandem. Note the two silver seeds in the anterior cervical lip, one in the posterior lip and two in the posterior vaginal wall, marking the lower extent of the vaginal tumor extension. The position of the cylinders and dummy sources in relation to the tumor can be identified easily, allowing the proper placement of the radioactive sources. *(B)* Same system with a leaded set of cylinders that reduces the dose to the bladder and urethra. (From Delclos et al.: Int. J. Radiat. Oncol. Biol. Phys. 6:1203, 1980.)

Vaginal Cylinders

The afterloadable vaginal cylinders were designed in the mid 1960s[7] to irradiate the vagina when disease extends from the uterine cervix along the vaginal walls. They are also used to hold a vaginal source when the vaginal anatomy is compromised (too narrow for ovoids), and to irradiate some vaginal tumors.

Cylinders are available in various diameters (1–5 cm) to fit any vaginal width (Fig. 11–28). They can be used in the same diameter, or combined in different diameters to fit conical vaginas. Cylinders are provided with added lead shielding to

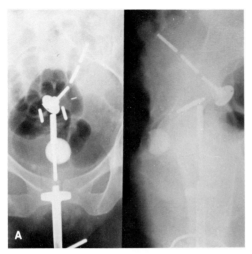

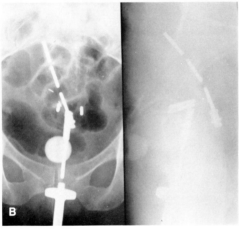

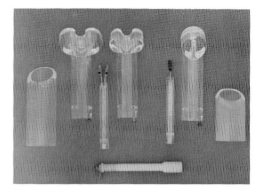

Fig. 11–36. Afterloadable Bloedorn colpostats with double and single ovoids. The diameter of the cylinder is increased by adding plastic sleeves. The inserters that hold the radioactive sources (radium tubes or cesium rods) are shown outside the colpostats. (From Delclos et al.: Int. J. Radiat. Oncol. Biol. Phys. 6:1204, 1980.)

Fig. 11–35. Two examples of disalignment of a pre-loaded, separate intrauterine tandem and Bloedorn colpostat. In both cases, the ovoids of the Bloedorn colpostat are in front of the uterine cervix. This can be avoided by using an afterloadable intrauterine tandem with vaginal cylinders as shown in Figure 11–34. (From Delclos et al.: Int. J. Radiat. Oncol. Biol. Phys. 6:1204, 1980.)

protect selected vaginal areas, the bladder, or the rectum (Fig. 11–29). The cylinders are mounted in the vaginal component of the intrauterine tandem (Fig. 11–30), or along the afterloadable stem of vaginal dome cylinders (Fig. 11–31). The cylinders are fitted into the vaginal component of the intrauterine tandem after the tandem has been inserted into the uterus.

The cylinders have an inside groove on the distal side (Fig. 11–32). With the proper hook, the cylinders can be removed one by one if the system is tight at the time of removal, minimizing the possibility of vaginal tears.

Surface-dose tables for standard radium tubes are available from the Radium Chemical Company (161 East 42nd St., New York, NY 10017), and elsewhere for selected cesium sources.[31]

To minimize the rotation of the intra-uterine tandem when the cylinders are used in combination with a tandem, a flat, round flange with keel (Fig. 11–33) is placed below the last cylinder and is kept in position with some packing. The labia are sutured to prevent the system from slipping out and causing a severe vulvar reaction. Figures 11–34 and 11–35 show examples and advantages of the use of the intrauterine tandem and vaginal cylinders.

Dome Cylinders

Dome cylinders (see Fig. 11–31) were designed to irradiate the vaginal cuff alone, or added areas of the vagina, or the whole vaginal surface, in patients who have had a hysterectomy. To obtain a uniform isodose around the dome, a minicesium source must be used at the top rather than radium sources, which are too long.

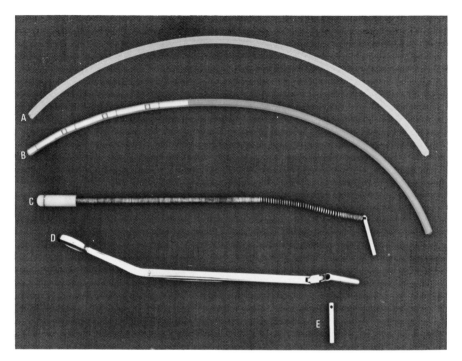

Fig. 11–37. *(A)* Empty Teflon tube narrowed at one end; *(B)* three radium or cesium dummies with spacers in the Teflon tube carrier; *(C)* dummy source attached at the end of a spring for afterloading of the round-handle ovoids; *(D)* source carrier for the Fletcher–Suit rectangular-handle ovoid; *(E)* dummy radium source with eyelet. (From Roosenbeek et al.: The Radioactive Patient: Care, Precautions, Procedures in Diagnosis and Therapy. Flushing, New York, Medical Examination Publishing, 1975, p. 59.)

The cesium source can be used alone or in combination with radium or other cesium sources. As many cylinders as necessary can be added to treat all or part of the vagina.

Bloedorn Colpostat

The original preloadable Bloedorn colpostats have been described briefly in several papers and textbook chapters.[1,30] The Bloedorn colpostat is a combination of vault colpostats and vaginal cylinders designed to irradiate the vagina in a single insertion. This is simpler than the two applications considered necessary when separate vault colpostats and cylinder insertions are used to treat the whole vagina. This colpostat has been used mainly to prevent vaginal recurrences in patients with adenocarcinoma of the endometrium. Since the early 1960s, when it was shown that vaginal recurrences are rare and occur usually in the apex of the vagina,[5] Fletcher colpostats have been used at M. D. Anderson Hospital. When it is desired to treat the whole vagina, the dome cylinder is used. To reduce the dose to the bladder and rectum, the Bloedorn colpostat is used. It is available in different diameters and lengths, with one or two vault colpostats of different sizes. It was adapted for afterloading in the late 1960s (Fig. 11–36).

Tandem Inserter

Radium, or cesium tubes are afterloaded into the applicators in the patient's room. The sources have been previously mounted in the radium laboratory in a Teflon tube of a smaller diameter than the stainless steel tandem (Fig. 11–37A and B). The Teflon tubing is narrowed at one end by pulling a copper wire around the Teflon and heating it with an air heat gun.

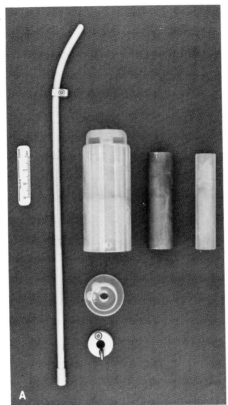

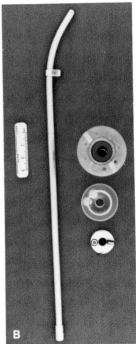

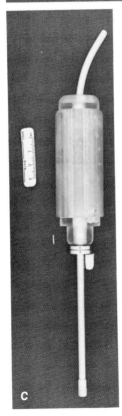

Fig. 11–38. *(A & B)* A dismantled, short-distance, surface-cylinder, afterloading colpostat. Note the holes in the cylinder periphery that accommodate the radioactive sources (radium, cesium needles, or iridium wires) and the central lead core that shields the opposite side. *(C)* The cylinder mounted on the vaginal component of an intrauterine tandem.

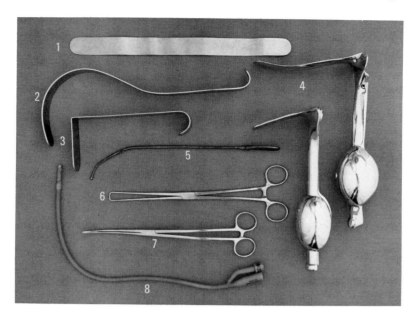

Fig. 11–39. Instruments for inserting afterloadable intrauterine tandems and colpostats. *(1)* Flexsteel ribbon retractor. It should be available in 1-, 1½-, and 2-inch widths; *(2)* Deaver retractor available in 1-, 1½-, and 2-inch widths (two of each); *(3)* Heaney or Kristeller retractors, available in 1-, 1½-, and 2-inch widths (two of each); *(4)* Auvard weighted retractors, 3, 4, and 5 inches in length (one of each); *(5)* malleable hysterometer (one); *(6)* Braun or Duplay uterine tenaculum (two). *(7)* Boseman or De Lee uterine packing forceps (two). *(8)* #16–18 Foley catheter with a 5-ml balloon.

The radium tubes are maintained in position inside the Teflon tube by a plastic-coated wire of adequate size.

Colpostat Inserter

On a round-handle colpostat (present model), the radioactive source is mounted permanently at the end of a wire or spring (Fig. 11–37C). The source is introduced into the colpostat along the handles. For the rectangular-handle model (original Suit model),[33] the radioactive sources are dropped inside a hollow carrier mounted on the handle insert with two hinges to maneuver the carrier around the angle between the handle and ovoid (Fig. 11–37D).

The Fletcher colpostats can be purchased from several firms, either in the preloadable original model or the afterloadable model, both for radium and cesium sources.*

Special Vaginal Surface Applicators

There are situations where it is necessary to treat selected areas of the vagina while minimizing irradiation to the opposite side (i.e., when the patient has had previous irradiation). Customized cylinders are manufactured that keep the radioactive sources at a short treating distance from the selected surface, and add shielding to protect the opposite side (Fig. 11–38). This customized cylinder can be mounted along the vaginal component of an intrauterine tandem if the uterus is present, or along the stem of the dome cylinder if there is no uterus.

A tray should be arranged, as shown in Figure 11–39, with the instruments for the insertion of intrauterine tandems, colpostats, capsules, dilators, and inserters.

Any applicator, even when purchased from a reliable manufacturer, must be checked before use. Figure 11–40 shows several applicators, misnamed Fletcher or Fletcher-Suit colpostats, manufactured by

---

*Radium Chemical Company, 161 East 42nd Street, New York, NY 10017; 3M Company, Product Technical Service, Nuclear Medical Laboratory, New Health Care Enterprises Department, Saint Paul, Minnesota 55101; Nuclear Associates, Inc., 100 Voice Road, Carle Place, New York 11514.

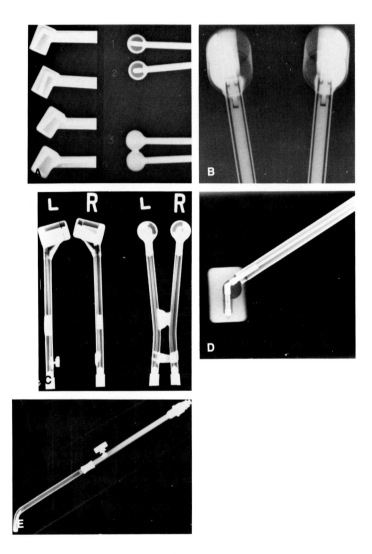

Fig. 11–40. Roentgenograms of some afterloadable applicators manufactured without proper supervision or ignoring the basic features described in several papers.[6,11,14,33] *(A)* The source carrier is not in the axis of any of the ovoids. No tungsten shielding is in the poles. The walls of the ovoids are made with different thicknesses of stainless steel.[6] *(B)* The tungsten shielding is in the wrong side of the ovoids.[6] *(C)* The tungsten shielding is also in the wrong side of the ovoid. The source carrier on the right ovoid is not in the axis of the ovoid. *(D)* There is no tungsten shielding. The source is too close to the lower pole (rectal side), resulting in an increase in rectal dose. *(E)* The pellet sources in this remote-controlled colpostat are too close to the upper pole (the ovoid case is made of plastic and, therefore, is not seen here). This results in a high dose to the urinary bladder.

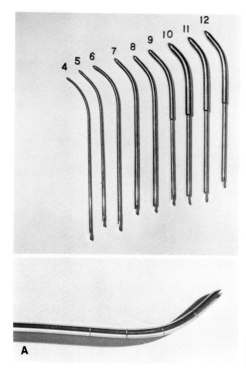

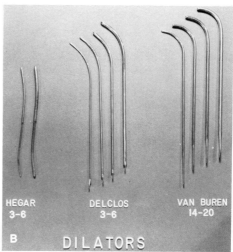

Fig. 11–41. *(A)* Uterine cervix dilators of intermediate curvature. They are calibrated along their long axis in centimeters or inches to check the depth of the uterine cavity during dilatation, thereby minimizing the incidence of uterine perforation. *(B)* The dilator features are compared with those of the Hegar and Van Buren dilators. They are available from 2 mm to 12 mm in diameter. The dilator number, as in the Hegar, represents the diameter of the dilator. (From Delclos: Radiology 93:1201, 1969.)

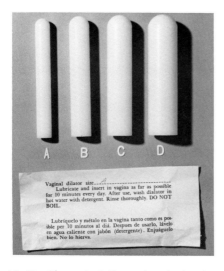

Fig. 11–42. The vaginal dilators described in the text.

different firms that do not adhere to the rules established in the early 1950s[11,14] and maintained through the afterloadable models.[6,15,33]

The Uterine Cervix Dilators

The uterine cervix dilators were designed in the mid 1960s (Fig. 11–41A).[4] They have a longer handle than the Hanks and Hegar uterine dilators. The diameter, like the Hegar's, is calibrated in millimeters (e.g., #4 is 4 mm in diameter). They are longitudinally calibrated either in inches or centimeters, allowing precise checking of the uterine cavity length during dilatation and minimizing the incidence of uterine perforations. The curvature is intermediate between the uterine cervix dilator (Hanks and Hegar) and the male Van Buren's urethra dilator (Fig.

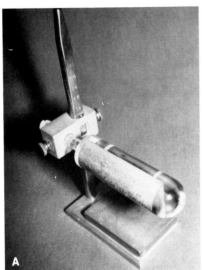

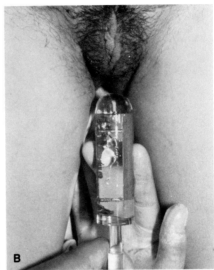

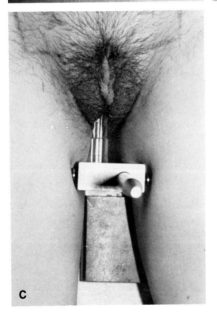

Fig. 11–43. A leaded vaginal cylinder shields a selected area of the vagina during external irradiation. *(A)* The leaded cylinder mounted into the holding stand. *(B)* Before placement in the vagina. *(C)* Placed in the vagina and mounted on the holding stand. (From Fletcher, G.H., Delclos, L., Wharton, J.T., and Rutledge, F.N.: Tumors of the vagina and female urethra. *In* Textbook of Radiotherapy, 3rd Ed. Edited by G.H. Fletcher. Philadelphia, Lea & Febiger, 1980.)

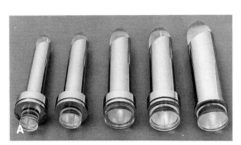

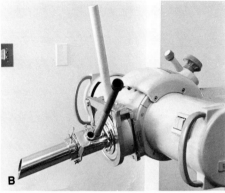

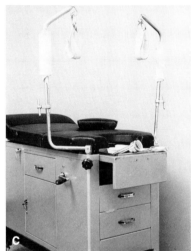

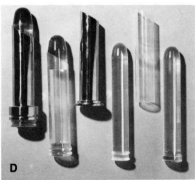

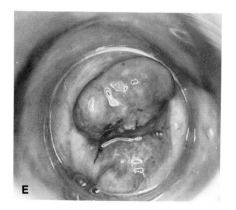

Fig. 11–44.   Equipment for transvaginal irradiation with an orthovoltage apparatus: *(A)* transvaginal treatment cones of different diameters; *(B)* a transvaginal cone mounted on the periscope attached to the kilovoltage therapy unit; *(C)* the gynecologic table for transvaginal therapy; *(D)* plastic transvaginal cones for examination purposes and metal treatment cones. *(E)* tumor around the cervical external os seen through a plastic examination cone.

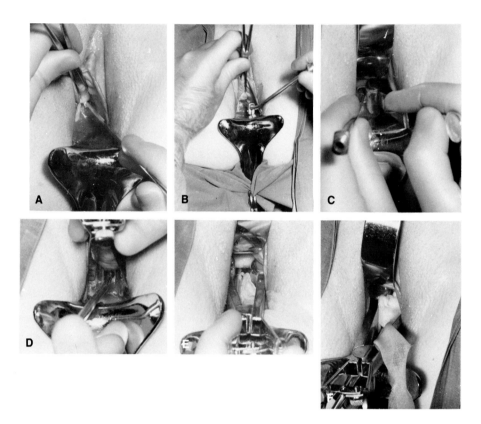

Fig. 11–45.   Sequence of insertion of afterloadable intrauterine tandem and colpostats. *(A)* Seeds, silver or gold, are implanted in the anterior and posterior cervical lip (or at the lower edge of the vaginal extent of the disease). *(B)* The intrauterine tandem, with the keeled flange set at the selected tandem length, is introduced into the uterine canal. *(C)* The left-handled ovoid is placed in the left lateral fornix. *(D)* The right-handled ovoid is placed in the right fornix and the handles are attached together. *(E)* The ovoids and tandem are maintained in the selected position by the packing, starting under the tandem posteriorly and in between the ovoids. Packing also fills the space, if any exists, between the ovoids and posterior fornix. *(F)* The spaces around the keeled flange are packed to minimize rotation of the tandem. Finally, the whole vagina is filled with packing.

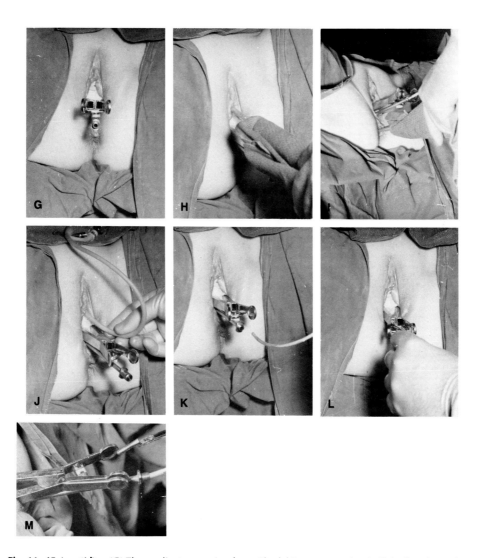

Fig. 11–45 (cont'd).   *(G)* The applicators are in place. The labia are sutured only if the fourchette does not support the packing. They are always sutured when vaginal or dome cylinders are used. *(H)* Bladder and *(I)* rectal readings can be taken in the operating room with microsources.[33] The position of the applicators is checked with orthogonal radiographs taken in the operating room. *(J)* A Foley catheter is inserted into the urinary bladder. *(K, L, and M)* The afterloading procedure is completed in the patient's room in 30 seconds.

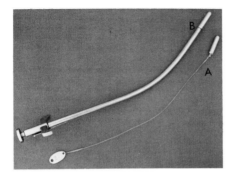

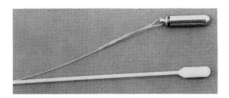

Fig. 11–46. *(A)* Regular preloadable #1 Heyman capsule attached at one end of a steel chain. A numbered tag is attached to the other end for identification. The numbers are sequentially recorded as the capsules are inserted to facilitate their removal in the reverse order. *(B)* A capsule mounted on the introducer.

Fig. 11–48. Simon–Heyman disposable afterloadable Teflon capsules compared to a preloadable #1 Heyman capsule. Simon capsules are available in several sizes and shapes.

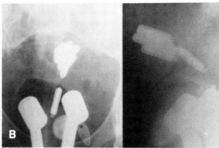

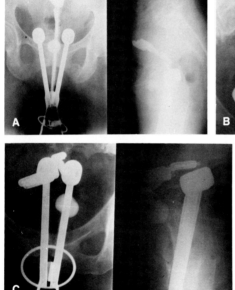

Fig. 11–47. *(A)* Modified Heyman packing as practiced at The University of Texas M.D. Anderson Hospital. The metal capsules are combined with an intrauterine afterloadable tandem that keeps the uterus in the axis of the pelvis and allows selection of the appropriate intratandem loading after the verification films have been viewed. The films are taken in the same operating room. *(B)* A Heyman packing without an intrauterine tandem. Note the gap (cold spot) between capsules. *(C)* Another example of a Heyman packing without intrauterine tandem.[5] Note the uterine anteflexion, which results in an overdose to the bladder.

11–41B) and fits the uterovaginal anatomy better in the majority of patients.

Vaginal Dilators

Plastic rods of different diameters were designed to minimize adhesions and stenosis of the vagina during and after treatment with external or intracavitary irradiation. The patient is instructed to insert a plastic dilator of the adequate diameter (there are four sizes available—Fig. 11–42)

into the vagina twice daily, for about 10 minutes at a time. This keeps the vagina open and ensures better visualization of the cervix and upper vagina on follow-up examinations.

Protective Cylinders

Plastic rods of different diameters with incorporated lead can be inserted into the vagina, allowing the shielding of selected areas of the vagina and adjacent structures,

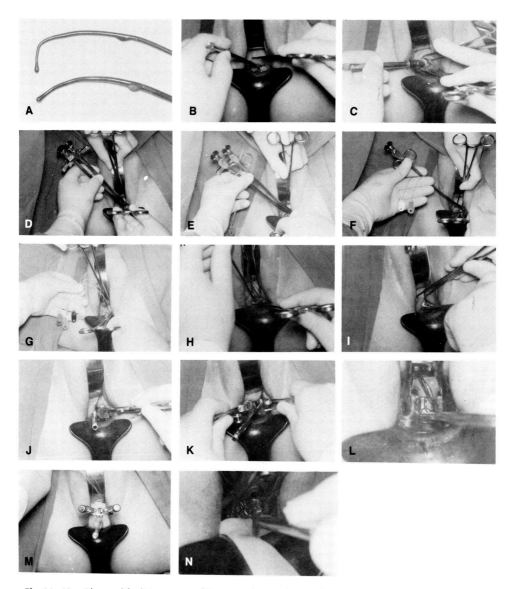

Fig. 11–49. The modified Heyman packing procedure as done at The University of Texas M.D. Anderson Hospital. *(A)* The uterine cavity is measured along the central uterine axis with a malleable hysterometer. The hysterometer tip is then bent and reintroduced into the uterine cavity. If the hysterometer rotates freely within the uterine cavity, the cavity is large enough to accommodate several capsules. *(B and C)* The uterine cervical canal is dilated without introducing the dilator all the way to the top. The dilators are calibrated as described. Start with dilator #2 and progress to #11 or #12, which is necessary for introducing two capsules beside each other. *(D)* The first capsule is introduced along the uterine canal to the fundus. Without removing the handle from the first capsule, the second capsule is introduced and positioned along the first capsule and is checked by aligning the handles. The first handle is then removed. *(E, F and G)* The same procedure is repeated with each capsule until all the capsules have been inserted. *(H)* Before inserting the tandem, and in order to minimize the possibility of dislodging the seeds during cervical dilatation, silver seeds are inserted into the anterior and posterior cervical lips to identify the cervix in the films. *(I)* After measuring the length of the uterine canal with a 5- or 6-mm dilator, the tandem with the flange set at the correct length is introduced into the canal under or along the side of the capsules. *(J, K, L, M and N)* The positioning of the afterloadable colpostats in the lateral fornices, and the packing, are done as described previously for inserting tandem and ovoids for cancer of the uterine cervix.

such as the bladder or the anorectal areas, during external irradiation. An example of such shielding is shown in Figure 11–43.

Transvaginal Treatment Equipment

Profuse cervical hemorrhage may be controlled by transvaginal irradiation with doses of 500 rad delivered 1 to 3 times daily or in alternate fractions. Exophytic lesions of the cervix and expanding endocervical tumors can be reduced in size by transvaginal irradiation without interfering with external or intracavitary irradiation. This technique may be effective in irradiating carcinoma of the cervical stump when there is no room for a satisfactory intrauterine tandem.

Figure 11–44 shows a selection of transvaginal cones (A), a cone attached to the periscope system mounted on the kilovoltage unit (B), and the gynecologic table used for transvaginal therapy with the patient in the lithotomy position (C). Makeshift plastic cones of the same diameter are available for examination and fitting purposes (Fig. 11–44D and E).

Inserting Intrauterine Tandem and Colpostats

The applicators are inserted while the patient is in the lithotomy position and under general anesthesia. A rectovaginal and bimanual examination is performed first. The patient is then prepared. When exposure by retractors is adequate, the cervix is held with the tenaculum, and the uterine cavity is probed with the hysterometer to determine its length. This is followed by cervical dilatation to 6 mm. The sequence of intrauterine tandem and colpostat placement is shown in Figure 11–45.

The Modified Heyman Packing Technique

This packing method was described by Heyman in 1934.[20] The purpose of the method is to irradiate the myometrium around wide or irregular cavities in the most effective way. Six capsules with ex-

ternal diameters varying from 5.1 mm to 10 mm are available.[19] The system is empirical, in spite of the effort made by Heyman and others to estimate the dose at the surface of the serosa of the uterus. It has proven to be a very efficient method that sterilizes tumor at any level in the uterus. When it is properly performed, significant dosage is contributed to the adjacent pelvic structures and lymph nodes.[24]

At present, the need for external irradiation in the treatment of most patients with cancer of the endometrium is questioned.[24] The Heyman packing technique has been progressively modified at M. D. Anderson Hospital. Because the procedure is so well tolerated, the dosage to the uterus has been increased from 1500–1800 rad to 2500–3000 mg hrs. The indications and doses for the Heyman technique are described in Fletcher's *Textbook of Radiotherapy*.[12] The outside diameter of the capsules is 6.3 mm (Fig. 11–46); the amount of radium in the capsule has been reduced to 5 mg. The capsules are combined with an intrauterine tandem, which has several advantages. The intrauterine tandem is afterloadable and the loading can be selected after seeing the verification films, thereby obtaining better coverage of the intrauterine canal (Fig. 11–47).[5] The tandem keeps the uterus in the midaxis of the pelvis, delivering a larger dose laterally to the pelvic structures and lymph nodes and reducing the dose to the urinary bladder.

Afterloadable Teflon capsules are now available (Fig. 11–48)[32] for small cesium-sources, completely eliminating radiation exposure to the personnel in the operating room. The Heyman packing technique sequence is demonstrated in Figure 11–49.

Protecting Personnel

The equipment used and procedures followed at M. D. Anderson Hospital when radioactive sources are handled are described in detail in Roosenbeek and Delclos' book, *The Radioactive Patient: Care, Precautions, and Procedures in Diagnosis and Therapy.*[27] Development of dexterity and skill reduces the time of each procedure, thereby minimizing the exposure.

REFERENCES

1. Chau, P.M.: Technic and evaluation of preoperative radium therapy in adenocarcinoma of the uterine corpus. *In* Carcinoma of the Uterine Cervix: Endometrium and Ovary. Chicago, Year Book Medical Publishers, 1962, p. 235.
2. del Regato, J.A., and Spjut, J.: Ackerman and del Regato's Cancer: Diagnosis, Treatment and Prognosis, 5th ed. St. Louis, C.V. Mosby, 1977.
3. Delclos, L.: Uterine cervix marker. Radiology 93:695, 1969.
4. Delclos, L.: Uterine cervix dilator designed to be used before insertion of intrauterine tandems and/or capsules. Radiology 93:1201, 1969.
5. Delclos, L., and Fletcher, G.H.: Malignant tumor of the endometrium: Evaluation of some aspects of radiotherapy. *In* Cancer of the Uterus and Ovary. Chicago, Year Book Medical Publishers, 1969, p. 62.
6. Delclos, L. et al.: Can the Fletcher gamma ray colpostat system be extrapolated to other systems? Cancer 41:970, 1978.
7. Delclos, L. et al.: Afterloading vaginal irradiators. Radiology 96:666, 1970.
8. Durrance, F.Y., and Fletcher, G.H.: Computer calculations of dose distribution to regional lymphatics from gynecological radium insertions. Radiology 91:140, 1968.
9. Fabian, C.E., and Benninghoff, D.L.: Lymphangiography as an adjunct to pelvic radium dosimetry. Am. J. Roentgenol. 96:197, 1966.
10. Fletcher, G.H.: The planning of external irradiation in pelvic cancer. Am. J. Roentgenol. 64:95, 1950.
11. Fletcher, G.H.: Cervical radium applicators with screening in the direction of bladder and rectum. Radiology 60:77, 1953.
12. Fletcher, G.H.: Textbook of Radiotherapy, 3rd ed. Philadelphia, Lea & Febiger, 1980.
13. Fletcher, G.H., and Calderon, R.: Positioning of pelvic portals for external irradiation in carcinoma of the uterine cervix. Radiology 67:359, 1956.
14. Fletcher, G.H., Shalek, R.J., Wall, J.A., and Bloedorn, F.G.: A physical approach to the design of applicators in radium therapy of carcinoma of the cervix. Am. J. Roentgenol. 68:935, 1952.
15. Green, A.E., Broadwater, J.R., and Hancock, J.A.: Afterloading vaginal ovoids. Am. J. Roentgenol. 105:609, 1969.
16. Greenhill, J.P.: Office Gynecology, 9th ed. Chicago, Year Book Medical Publishers, 1971.
17. Hammoudah, M., and Henschke, U.K.: Supervoltage beam films. Int. J. Radiat. Oncol. Biol. Phys. 2:571, 1977.
18. Henriksen, E.: The lymphatic spread of carcinoma of the cervix and body of the uterus. Am. J. Obst. Gynecol. 58:924, 1949.
19. Heyman, J.: The radiotherapeutic treatment of cancer corporis uteri. Br. J. Radiol. 20:85, 1947.
20. Heyman, J., Reuterwall, O., and Benner, S.: The Radiumhemmet experience with radiotherapy in cancer of the corpus of the uterus: Classification, method of treatment and results. Acta Radiol. 22:14, 1941.
21. Kistner, R.W.: Gynecology: Principles and Practice. Chicago, Year Book Medical Publishers, 1964.
22. Kottmeier, H.L.: Carcinoma of the Female Genitalia. Baltimore, Williams & Wilkins, 1953.
23. Lacassagne, A., Baclesse, F., and Reverde, J.: Radiotherapie des Cancers du Col de l'uterus. Paris, Masson & Cie, 1941.
24. Landgren, R.C., Fletcher, G.H., Gallager, S.H., Delclos, L., and Wharton, J.T.: Treatment failure sites according to irradiation technique and histology in patients with endometrial cancer. Cancer 40:131, 1977.
25. Meigs, J.V.: Radical hysterectomy with bilateral pelvic lymph node dissection: A report of 100 patients operated on five or more years ago. Am. J. Obstet. Gynecol. 62:854, 1951.
26. Richardson, J.E., Roosenbeek, E.V., and Morgan, J.M.: Field localization for betatron therapy. Am. J. Roentgenol. 76:934, 1956.
27. Roosenbeek, E.V., and Delclos, L.: The Radioactive Patient Care, Precautions, and Procedures in Diagnosis and Therapy. Flushing, N.Y., Medical Examination Publishing Company, 1975.
28. Rouviere, H.: Anatomie des Lymphatiques de L'Homme. Paris, Masson & Cie, 1932, pp. 406.
29. Rutledge, F., Boronow, R.C., and Wharton, J.T.: Gynecologic Oncology. New York, John Wiley & Sons, 1976.
30. Rutledge, R.H., Tan, S., and Fletcher, G.H.: Vaginal metastases from adenocarcinoma of the corpus uteri. Am. J. Obstet. Gynecol. 75:167, 1958.
31. Sharma, S.C., Gerbi, B., and Madoc–Jones, H.: Dose rates for brachytherapy applicators using Cs-137 sources. Int. J. Radiat. Oncol. Biol. Phys. 5: 1893, 1979.
32. Simon, N., and Silverstone, S.M.: Intracavitary radiotherapy of endometrial cancer by afterloading. Gynecol. Oncol. 1:13, 1972.
33. Suit, H.D. et al.: Modification of Fletcher ovoid system for afterloading using standard sized radium tubes (milligram and microgram). Radiology 81:126,1963.
34. Tod, M.C. and Meredith, W.J.: A dosage system for use in the treatment of cancer of the uterine cervix. Br. J. Radiol. 11:809, 1938.
35. Wall, J.A., and Arnold, H.: Preliminary observations on retroperitoneal lymphadenectomies. Tex. Med. 49:93, 1953.
36. Wallace, S., and Jing, B.: Clinical Lymphangiography. Baltimore, Williams & Wilkins, 1977.

Chapter 12

TREATMENT TECHNIQUES DEPENDING ON TUMOR EXTENT IN CANCER OF THE BREAST

Eleanor D. Montague

Norah duV. Tapley

William J. Spanos

Regardless of the surgical procedure that precedes irradiation, the radiotherapist may be called upon to treat part or all of the following areas in patients with breast cancer: chest wall or breast, axilla, internal mammary nodes, and supraclavicular nodes. In this chapter we present pertinent anatomic information, describe treatment areas, and suggest a variety of treatment techniques—the choice of technique depends on the prior surgical procedure and the stage of the disease.

ANATOMY OF THE BREAST

The protuberant breast extends from the second or third to the sixth or seventh costal cartilage and from the edge of the sternum to the anterior axillary line. However, mammary tissue is found as a thin layer below the clavicle to the midline and laterally to the edge of the lattissimus dorsi muscle. The thickest part of the breast is in the upper outer quadrant, which usually contains a greater bulk of mammary tissue than other parts of the breast. The axillary tail of the breast can become so large that it forms a visible axillary mass

and frequently is the site of the primary tumor.

Axilla

The axillary nodes are located in groups (Fig. 12–1). *External mammary nodes* are located beneath the lateral edge of the pectoralis major muscle, along the medial side of the axilla, following the course of the lateral thoracic artery on the chest wall from the sixth to the second rib. *Scapular nodes* are closely associated with the subscapular vessels and their thoracodorsal

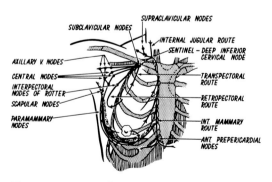

Fig. 12–1. Pattern of metastatic spread to the regional lymph nodes in carcinoma of the breast. (From Haagensen, C.D.: Diseases of the Breast. Philadelphia, W.B. Saunders Company, 1956.)

branches. *Central nodes* are in the center of the axilla and are probably the most important of the axillary nodes. *Interpectoral nodes* lie between the pectoralis major and pectoralis minor muscles along the pectoral branches of the thoracoacromial vessels. These nodes are spared when the pectoralis major muscle is not removed. *Axillary-vein nodes* are distributed along the lateral portion of the axillary vein from the tendon of the latissimus dorsi muscle to just medial to the origin of the thoracoacrominal vein. *Subclavicular nodes,* the highest and most medial group of the axillary nodes, are situated along the ventral and caudal aspect of the axillary vein where the vein disappears beneath the tendon of the subclavius muscle. These nodes lie under the skin approximately 1 cm to 1.5 cm below the midportion of the clavicle.[2]

Internal Mammary Nodes

The internal mammary lymph nodes are small, 2 mm to 5 mm in diameter, and can be either structural nodes or collections of lymphocytes in areolar tissue. They are located along the course of the internal mammary lymphatic trunks, generally within 3 cm of the lateral margin of the sternum. Rarely are nodes located under the edge of the costal cartilage; they usually lie on the endothoracic fascia in the interspaces between the costal cartilages, with the greatest concentration of nodes in the upper three interspaces. Retromanubrial connecting lymphatics between the left and right lymphatic trunks at the level of the first interspace have been described. Ultrasound has provided a means of determining the pleural reflection on which the lymph nodes are found. Lymphoscintigraphy demonstrates lymph nodes in the internal-mammary-node spaces so that their location lateral to the midline can be accurately determined; crossover is demonstrated in about 20% of patients.[5]

Supraclavicular Nodes

The lymphatics of the breast, pectoral musculature, and chest wall all empty into the confluence of the internal jugular and subclavian veins in the base of the neck. There are three primary trunks of importance: the subclavian trunk from the axilla, the jugular trunk from the neck and supraclavicular area, and the bronchomediastinal trunks.[2] All connecting trunks combine in a variety of ways to empty, on the right side, into a short common trunk called the right lymphatic duct, and on the left side, into the internal jugular vein, the subclavian vein, or the thoracic duct. The lymphatic trunks are located in the medial portion of the supraclavicular area, lying directly under the insertion of the sternocleidomastoid muscle into the clavicle. Figure 12–1 shows the pattern of metastatic spread to the regional lymph nodes in patients with carcinoma of the breast.

INDICATIONS AND TECHNIQUES OF IRRADIATION

Irradiation to the First Three Internal Mammary Nodes

The portal used to treat the first three internal mammary nodes is used for patients who have had a conventional radical or modified radical mastectomy for a T1 (<2 cm in diameter) primary tumor located in the inner or central portion of the breast and whose nodes are histologically negative. Our policy does not include bilateral internal mammary-node irradiation for the following reasons:

(1) Experience with internal-mammary-node metastases has been gained with ipsilateral surgical dissection.

(2) Adequate irradiation to nodes of both internal mammary chains would entail a portal 10 cm to 12 cm wide, which substantially increases the volume of mediastinal irradiation.

(3) Contralateral internal-mammary-

node irradiation would interfere with the future irradiation of patients who develop a contralateral breast cancer.

For either ⁶⁰Co or electrons, the patient is supine, the upper arm is abducted 90°, the forearm is supported in the upright position by a horizontal arm board, and the head is turned sharply to the contralateral side.[1]

The portal consists of a single rectangular field covering the ipsilateral internal mammary nodes of the first three interspaces and the confluence of venous drainage under the insertion of the sternocleidomastoid muscle into the head of the clavicle. The medial border is 1 cm across the midline.

With electron beams, a 5000-rad given dose is delivered over a period of 5 weeks at 5 fractions per week with an energy sufficient for approximately 90% depth dose at 3 cm. With ⁶⁰Co, a 5000-rad given dose is delivered over a period of 5 weeks at 5 fractions per week.

Irradiation to the Internal-Mammary-, Supraclavicular-, and Subclavicular-Node Areas

Irradiation to these nodal sites is delivered to patients who have central or inner-quadrant primary tumors greater than 2 cm in diameter without any grave signs, and to patients who have outer-quadrant tumors with axillary-node metastases.

Close attention must be given to the medial border of the supraclavicular field because involved nodes are usually located under the junction of the sternocleidomastoid muscle and the head of the clavicle. The upper medial border of the field should be at least 1 cm on the opposite side of the midline when the beam is sharply defined and more than 1 cm when the beam is poorly defined. The L-shaped field covers the internal mammary nodes, the nodes under the first rib, and the su-

praclavicular, subclavicular-apical, and low-jugular nodes.

⁶⁰Co Field

In the supraclavicular and axillary apex portion, the *medial border* is at the midline at the base of the xyphoid process and extends superiorly to 1 cm on the contralateral side of the level of the sternal notch. The line is continued superiorly to the thyrocricoid groove. The *superior border* extends laterally across the neck and the trapezius to the acromial process. The *lateral border* crosses the acromioclavicular joint and extends inferiorly to meet the inferior border. The *inferior border* extends laterally from the internal mammary portion of the field at the level of the first costal cartilage.

In the internal mammary chain portion, the *medial border* is the same as that of the supraclavicular portion. The *inferior border* is a horizontal line extending 6 cm laterally from the midline at the level of the xyphoid process. The *lateral border* is a vertical line 6 cm from the midline, extending from the inferior border to the level of the first costal cartilage.

Electron-Beam Fields

In electron-beam radiation, separate fields are used for the supraclavicular and internal mammary nodes because the depth of treatment determines the amount of energy to be used. The foot of the treatment table is tilted downward so that the plane of the sternum is relatively parallel to the floor (the angle of the tilt is documented for daily duplication of treatment).

In the supraclavicular and axillary apex field, the *medial border* extends superiorly from the upper medial corner of the internal mammary field 1 cm across the midline to the level of the thyrocricoid groove. The *superior border* extends laterally across the neck and the trapezius. The *lateral border* is the same as for ⁶⁰Co. The *inferior border* is a horizontal line that extends laterally at the level of the superior border of the internal mammary field. The *electron-beam energy* must be sufficient to deliver 5000 rad at a 1-cm to 2-cm depth (100%).

For the internal mammary field, the *medial border* is a vertical line 1 cm to the contralateral side of the midline of the sternum. The *superior border* is a horizontal line superior to the sternal notch, extending from the medial border above the sternal end of the clavicle. The *lateral border* is a vertical line parallel to the medial border. It is 7 cm lateral from the medial border except for the portion of the field covering the first interspace (superior to second costal cartilage) where the lateral border widens to 8 cm. The *inferior border* is a horizontal line at the level of the xyphoid process. The electron-beam energy must be sufficient for approximately 90% of the dose at a 3-cm to 4-cm depth. The doses are the same as those used for irradiation of the first three internal mammary nodes.

Peripheral Lymphatic and Chest-Wall Irradiation

Chest-wall irradiation is indicated following a modified radical mastectomy or a conventional radical mastectomy when more than 20% of the axillary nodes are histologically positive, when the primary tumor is greater than 5 cm or is associated with grave signs, and when lymphatic and perineural involvement are present. Mastectomy-scar extension on the arm, opposite breast, and the upper abdomen can be treated with electrons. Surgical drain sites are included if it is convenient; however, no recurrences have been noted at these sites. Figure 12–2 shows the electron-beam peripheral-lymphatic and chest-wall portals and pertinent energies.

[60]Co Chest-Wall Irradiation

If electrons are not available or if the mastectomy flaps are very thick, ^{60}Co is used, always with a separate internal-mammary-chain field. Figure 12–3 shows the positioning of the patient and setup with the use of a rolling ball inclinometer.

The *medial border* coincides as closely as possible with the lateral border of the internal mammary field. Because of chest-wall curvature and tangential direction, the medial border is rarely a straight line. On most patients, in order to avoid cold spots, the medial border is matched at the corners of the internal mammary field, which produces a slight overlap at the midpoint of the common border. In early breast cancer, when the breast is intact and a good cosmetic result is desired, the medial border is matched at the midportion of the common line.

The *lateral border* is at the midaxillary line. If the surgical scar extends to or beyond the midaxillary line, the lateral border is moved posteriorly to obtain adequate margins. For extremely posterior scars, adequate covering with the lateral border would require excessive lung radiation; an additional oblique cobalt or appositional electron-beam field is used for the portion of the scar beyond the midaxillary line.

The *superior border* coincides with the lower border of the supraclavicular field. For patients with Stages I and II, the contiguous line is treated with one field only; for Stages III and IV, the contiguous line is treated by both supraclavicular and chest-wall fields.

The *inferior border* is a horizontal line at the level of the tip of the xyphoid process, including the inframammary fold or scar extension with a 1-cm to 2-cm margin. For scars that extend very inferiorly, it is desirable to use electrons to treat the portion of the scar below the inframammary fold.

The ^{60}Co radiation dosage is 4500 to 5000 rad delivered over a 5-week period. Both medial and lateral fields are treated each day. The tumor percent depth dose (%DD) is determined from a contour dis-

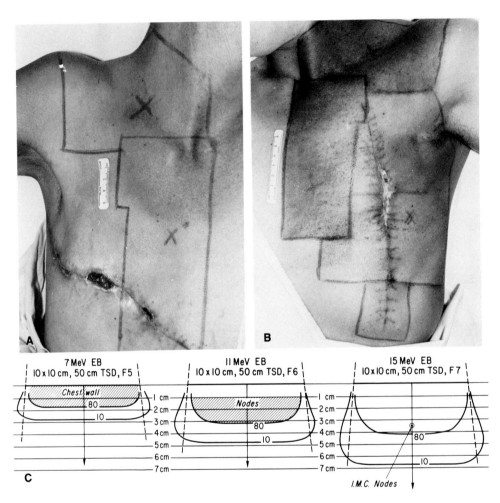

Fig. 12–2. Portals used for irradiation of peripheral lymphatics with electrons. *(A)* This 50-year-old woman had a modified radical mastectomy for a 2-cm mass in the upper inner quadrant. There was one positive axillary node of 21 nodes recovered at surgery. Electron-beam therapy was given to the supraclavicular area and the apex of the axilla, using 11 MeV electrons to deliver 5000-rad given dose in 5 weeks. The internal mammary node chain received 5000-rad given dose in 5 weeks with 15 MeV electrons. The internal mammary field is 8 cm wide at the first intercostal space and 7 cm wide for the remainder of the field. The medial margin is 1 cm across the midline. *(B)* This 38-year-old woman had a left radical mastectomy for a 1-cm upper outer quadrant mass. Seven of ten axillary nodes recovered at surgery were positive. Electron-beam therapy was given to the supraclavicular area, the apex of the axilla, the internal mammary node chain, and the chest wall. The chest wall was treated with 7 MeV electrons and received 5500-rad given dose in 5 weeks. *(C)* Isodose distributions of 7 MeV, 11 MeV, and 15 MeV electron beams. Note the field constriction at 80% dose level. For this reason the internal mammary chain field measures 7 cm in width. (From Fletcher, G.H., Montague, E.D., Tapley, N.duV., and Barker, J.L.: Radiotherapy in the management of nondisseminated breast cancer. *In* Textbook of Radiotherapy, 3rd ed. Edited by G.H. Fletcher. Philadelphia, Lea & Febiger, 1980.)

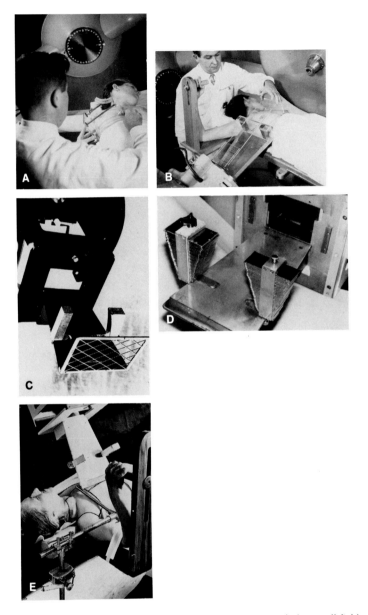

Fig. 12–3. Technique of ^{60}Co tangential chest wall irradiation. Tangential chest wall fields. Both fields must be treated every day. The patient is supine, in the same position as that used for the anterior supraclavicular and axillary field. The medial field abuts the lateral border of the internal mammary field. The breast bridge (*A* and *B*), with a rolling ball inclinometer, is fitted to the medial and lateral margins of the tangential fields to measure their separation and angles. An applicator has been designed for the tangential portals to eliminate penumbra and divergence. (*C*) A grid can be used to hold a pendulous breast in the no-bolus treatment. Because of the convexity of the sternum, the applicator may not be in contact with the skin along the total length of the medial margin. This air gap does not create a significant dosimetric problem. (*D*) Adjustable lead blocks that permit careful and uniform blocking. (*E*) Medial tangential portal. A bar prevents the breast from flopping. To avoid an unirradiated wedge of breast occurring between the internal mammary field, the medial tangential field, and the chest wall in an unusually convex rib cage or a firm full breast, it may be necessary to overlap the adjacent borders of the internal mammary field and the medial tangential fields, in which case the total dose in the area of the overlap should be taken into consideration. (*A. B.* From Fletcher, et al., AJR, *84:*761, 1960. *C. D. E.* Courtesy of L. Delclos, Professor of Radiotherapy, M.D. Anderson Hospital and Tumor Institute.)

tribution of the transverse midportion of the chest wall.

Electron-Beam Chest-Wall Irradiation

The entire chest wall is treated, if possible, with a single field; small contiguous fields are added if the scar extends beyond the usual surgical confines. The *medial border* is coincident with the lateral border of the internal mammary field. The *superior border* is coincident with the inferior border of the supraclavicular field. This remains at the level of the first costal cartilage if a conventional radical or modified (Patey) radical mastectomy has been performed and the axilla requires no irradiation. The *inferior border* is a horizontal line that includes the original level of the inframammary sulcus with a 1-cm or 2-cm margin. When scars extend lower than that level, a separate small field is added to encompass the scar extension. The *lateral border* follows the midaxillary line. If the slope of the chest wall is steep (with more than a 6-cm to 7-cm drop from the medial border) or if the chest-wall scar extends beyond the midaxillary line, it is necessary to add a second chest-wall field that abuts the first chest-wall field. This field is angled 35°–40° toward the back to avoid dose buildup at the junction.

The radiation dosage should be 5500 rad given dose over a period of 5 weeks. Treatment is 5 days per week at 220 rad per fraction. In a situation where an additional lateral chest-wall portal is used, the dosage is 5000 rad given dose over 5 weeks.

Six or 7 MeV is sufficient for most chest-wall-tissue irradiation following a conventional radical or modified (Patey) radical mastectomy. It may be necessary to use 9 MeV for unusually thick mastectomy flaps. Ultrasound is useful in determining chest-wall thickness.

Chest-Wall, Internal-Mammary, Supraclavicular, and Axillary Irradiation

The axilla requires irradiation following simple mastectomy, excision biopsy alone, or segmental mastectomy without axillary dissection, for preoperative irradiation, or in patients who have had radical mastectomy and require axillary irradiation (e.g., when axillary dissection is inadequate—most of five or six nodes recovered are positive, when extranodal axillary disease is present, when axillary disease is inoperable—nodes are greater than 3 cm in diameter, matted, or fixed.

The anterior supraclavicular-axillary field covers the low and central axilla, the subclavicular axillary apex, the supraclavicular fossa including the deep inferior-cervical and low jugular nodes, and the first internal mammary space. The *medial border* is a vertical line 1 cm across the midline extending from the second costal cartilage to the thyrocricoid groove. The *superior border* extends laterally across the neck and the trapezius as described for the peripheral lymphatic ^{60}Co field. The *lateral border* is a semivertical line at the acromioclavicular joint that is drawn across the shoulder to exclude as much of the shoulder joint as possible. The line then follows the pectoral fold, sparing a rim of pectoral fold. The *inferior border* is a horizontal line at the level of the second costal cartilage.

The beam is tilted 15° laterally to avoid irradiating part of the trachea and esophagus. The angulation additionally ensures that nodes close to the margin of the pectoral muscle are included without requiring fall-off of the beam, which would produce a moist desquamation in the axilla. Figure 12–4 shows the anterior supraclavicular-axillary field.

The dosage for the anterior supraclavicular-axillary portal is 5000 rad given over 5 weeks in 200-rad fractions 5 days per week.

For treatment of the posterior axillary field, the patient is prone. The head is turned to the contralateral side without pillows. The forearm is rotated downward, and the shoulder is in contact with

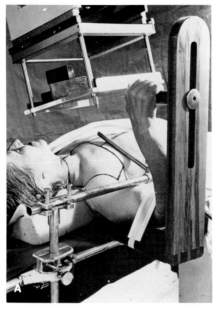
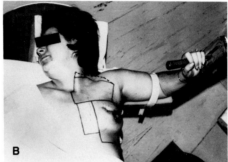

Fig. 12–4. *(A)* Irradiation technique when the axilla is treated. The inferior border of the anterior supraclavicular-axillary portal is at the level of the second costal cartilage. The medial margin of the supraclavicular fields extends 1 cm across the midline of the sternum. The lateral margin is drawn within the border of the pectoral muscle. A bar is occasionally used to keep a large breast stationary. The beam (⁶⁰Co) is tilted 15° laterally to avoid irradiating part of the trachea and esophagus while still irradiating the deep inferior cervical nodes medial to sternocleidomastoid muscle. *(B)* Patient with incisional biopsy of an upper inner quadrant tumor receiving preoperative irradiation to be followed by radical mastectomy. Supraclavicular recurrences have occurred in the posterior supraclavicular area that has been left untreated or at least marginally treated, as in this patient. The dotted line shows the correct location of the upper margin. (Courtesy of L. Delclos, Professor of Radiotherapy, M.D. Anderson Hospital and Tumor Institute.)

the table top. The back of the hand on the pelvic rim (Fig. 12–5).

The *medial superior border* follows the spine of the scapula. The *lateral superior border* bisects the humoral head. The *lower lateral border* is medial to the border of the latissimus dorsi muscle.

The *beam* is vertical.

The posterior axillary portal covers only the central and low axilla. The given dose is calculated to deliver a 5000-rad tumor dose to the central and low axillary nodes, given an approximate 2:1 ratio anterior–posterior. This is treated 2 to 3 times weekly with a 200-rad given dose at each treatment. Figure 12–6A shows the difference in the volume of irradiation between the large anterior supraclavicular-axillary portal (dotted line), used to treat the entire

axillary contents, and the smaller anterior supraclavicular portal (solid line), used for irradiation of the supraclavicular and subclavicular areas. Figures 12–6B and 12–6C are simulator films showing the difference in the volume of irradiated lung, bone, and soft tissues.

Internal Mammary Field Used with Irradiation of the Whole Axilla

With the juxtaposition of the anterior supraclavicular-axillary field and the internal mammary field over the second costal cartilage, there is a higher dose at the junction. The internal mammary field treats the internal mammary nodes from the second interspace to the base of the xyphoid process, as well as part of the chest wall.

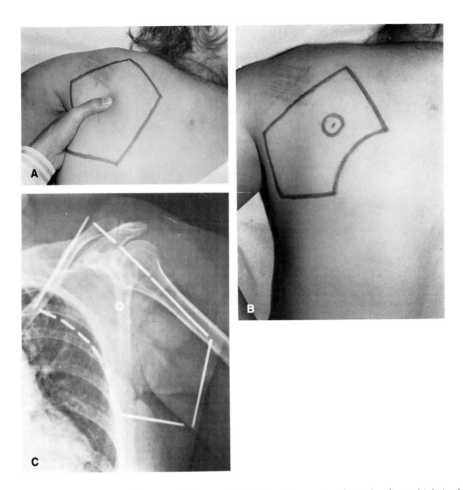

Fig. 12–5. *(A)* Posterior axillary portal drawn with the thumb opposing the index finger high in the central axilla. The field is drawn around the central axilla; final adjustments are made from the localization film. *(B)* The final adjusted posterior axillary portal. The inferior border spans the latissimus dorsi margin and is at the same level as the upper border of the tangential portals. *(C)* The adjusted localization film of the posterior axillary portal indicates the inclusion of the upper chest wall and a portion of the lung medially and soft tissues of the axilla bounded by the clavicle and humerus. (From Fletcher, G.H., Montague, E.D., Tapley, N.duV., and Barker, J.L.: Radiotherapy in the management of nondisseminated breast cancer. *In* Textbook of Radiotherapy, 3rd ed. Edited by G.H. Fletcher. Philadelphia, Lea & Febiger, 1980.)

The *medial border* is a vertical line at the midline. The *lateral border* is a vertical line 6 cm from, and parallel to, the medial border. The *superior border* is coincident with the inferior border of the supraclavicular field. The *inferior border* is a horizontal line at the base of the xyphoid process.

The dosage for irradiation of the whole axilla is 5000-rad given dose in 5 weeks, at 200-rad daily for 5 days per week. Be- cause of the greater risk of tumor infestation, patients with central and medial quadrant primary tumors with either clinically or histologically positive nodes receive additional treatment to the first three interspaces, delivering a 5000-rad tumor dose in 5 weeks at 3-cm to 4-cm depth.

Internal Mammary Field Used with Preirradiation Chemotherapy

When irradiation has been preceded by doxorubicin (Adriamycin) administra-

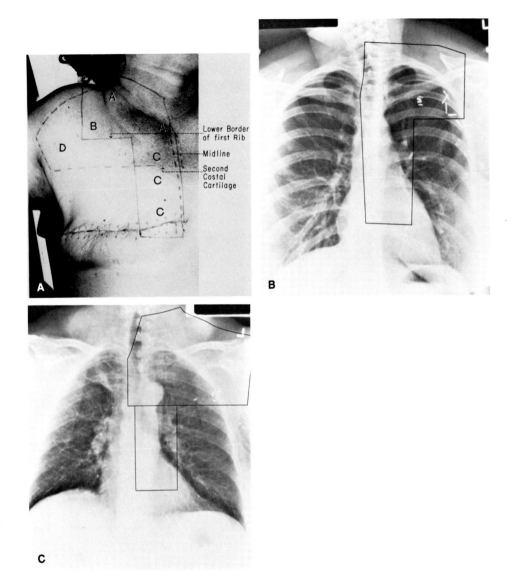

Fig. 12–6. *(A)* The medial border of the peripheral lymphatic sternal field defines the midline at the xyphoid, but slants 1 cm to the opposite side. The inferior border of the peripheral supraclavicular portal is at the level of the medial end of the first rib, incorporating the anterior supraclavicular axillary apex but excluding the axillary soft tissues. The inferior border of the anterior supraclavicular-axillary portal is at the second costal cartilage. The depth of the nodes are: A. Supraclavicular nodes—0.5–1.0 cm deep. B. Infraclavicular axillary apical nodes—1.0 cm deep. C. Internal mammary nodes—0.7–5.3 cm (average 2.0 cm) deep. D. Central axillary nodes—usually at depth of 6–7 cm, but varying with the thickness of the axilla.

Peripheral lymphatic technique portals with ^{60}Co (solid line in the supraclavicular area). The anterior supraclavicular axillary portal, used to treat the axilla, supraclavicular area, and first interspace in peripheral lymphatic technique is drawn in dotted lines to demonstrate the difference in volume irradiated. *(B)* Peripheral lymphatic portal drawn on the film of a patient who had a radical mastectomy. The small clips identify the apex of the axilla. *(C)* Portals drawn on the film of a patient who had an extended simple mastectomy. The limit of the axillary dissection is at the border of the pectoralis major muscle, which is identified with clips. (From Fletcher, G.H., Montague, E.D., Tapley, N.duV., and Barker, J.L.: Radiotherapy in the management of nondisseminated breast cancer. *In* Textbook of Radiotherapy, 3rd ed. Edited by G.H. Fletcher, Philadelphia, Lea & Febiger, 1980.)

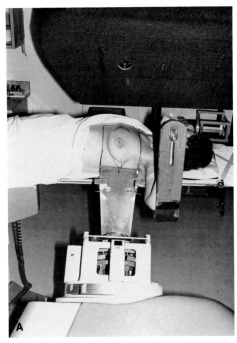

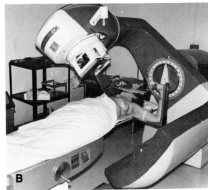

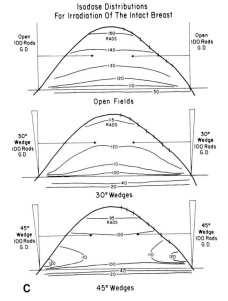

**Isodose Distributions
For Irradiation Of The Intact Breast**

Fig. 12–7. Patient, age 66, noted a mass in the upper inner quadrant of the left breast. Resection of a cystic mass revealed a 1-cm cystic structure with intracystic noninvasive carcinoma. Five-thousand-rad tumor dose was delivered in 5 weeks in 25 fractions with ⁶⁰Co. *(A)* Set-up of lateral tangential portal. *(B)* Medial tangential portal. *(C)* Isodose distributions with open fields and wedged fields, 30° and 45° for ⁶⁰Co. (From Fletcher, G.H., Montague, E.D., Tapley, N.duV., and Barker, J.L.: Radiotherapy in the management of nondisseminated breast cancer. *In* Textbook of Radiotherapy, 3rd ed. Edited by G.H. Fletcher. Philadelphia, Lea & Febiger, 1980.)

tion, the entire internal mammary chain is treated only with electrons. The field is identical to that described for electron irradiation of the peripheral lymphatic areas (see Fig. 12–2A) with the lower border at the xyphoid process because patients on Adriamycin have advanced disease and require chest-wall irradiation.

Irradiation of the Intact Breast

Irradiation is administered only to the breast of patients who have had excision or segmental mastectomy of intraductal noninvasive carcinoma and to patients who have a primary tumor in an outer quadrant of the breast with histologically negative nodes, as determined either by an axillary-node dissection or lateral node dissection (i.e., a dissection of the axilla lateral to the pectoralis minor muscle, recovering an average of 13 nodes). If no axillary histology is available, irradiation should be given to the breast, axilla, internal mammary nodes, and supraclavicular nodes as previously described.

The *medial tangential* border is at the midline. The *lateral tangential* border is at the midaxillary line or 1 cm to 2 cm beyond the confines of the breast or scar. The *inferior border* of the tangential field is at least 1 cm inferior to the inframammary sulcus or at least 1 cm beyond the scar. The *superior margin* is drawn as superiorly as can be accommodated by the lateral tangential field in the axilla. The *superior border* is generally in the first interspace. The breast tissue extending from the clavicle to the superior border of the tangential field can be treated with 7-MeV or 9-MeV electrons if the tumor is in the upper breast and close to the superior border of the tangential fields.

Infraclavicular Breast Field

The *superior border* follows the clavicle. The *medial border* is at midline. The *inferior border* is contiguous with the superior border of the tangential fields. The *lateral border* follows the curve of the pec-

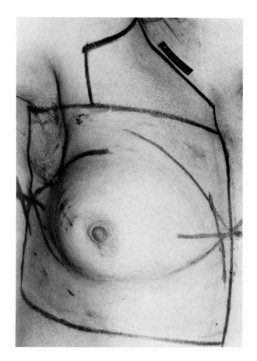

Fig. 12–8. Patient with adenocarcinoma of the outer upper quadrant measuring 1.5 cm. Fifteen axillary nodes were histologically negative. Tangential fields cover the breast proper. Superior to the tangential fields is an electron-beam field (7 MeV) treating the remainder of the breast tissue. (From Montague: Clinical experience with radiation therapy in the treatment of non-invasive or small volume invasive breast cancer. *In* Proceedings of the 19th National Conference on Breast Cancer, San Diego, California, 1981.)

toralis major muscle. Figures 12–7A and 12–7B show the portals that treat only the breast. Figure 12–7C shows the open and wedged-fields used to irradiate the breast. Figure 12–8 shows the tangential wedged-fields used to irradiate the breast and the electron-beam portal (7 MeV) treating the remaining breast tissue above the tangential fields.

The dosage for irradiation of the infraclavicular breast field is 4500 to 5000-rad given dose in 5 weeks with treatment 5 days per week.

With noninvasive or minimal breast cancer (a tumor <5 mm in greatest diameter), no boost is delivered. With larger invasive carcinoma, the field is reduced after 4500 to 5000 rad has been delivered,

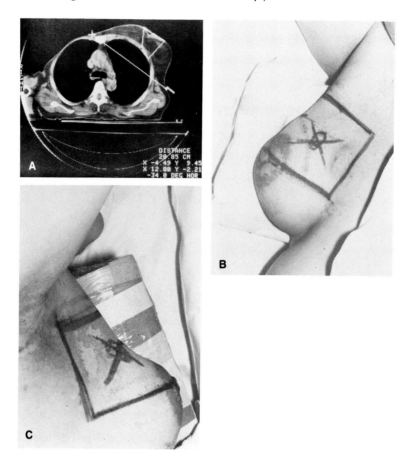

Fig. 12–9. The patient has a 3.5-cm carcinoma in the upper inner and central portions of the breast adjacent to the chest wall. It was excised with a close margin at the base. Eighteen axillary nodes were histologically negative. Because a boost of 1500-rad tumor dose at a 4.5-cm depth would necessitate a high skin dose with electrons, and because the upper half of the areola had to be included for adequate margin at the tumor site, electron irradiation was not indicated. An interstitial implant would not be effective because the tumor was adjacent to the chest wall. Therefore, after a 5000-rad tumor dose to the breast, internal mammary nodes, and supraclavicular-axillary apex nodes, a 1500-rad tumor-dose boost was delivered in 7 days by turning the patient alternately to anterior- and posterior-oblique positions, compressing the breast by its own weight on a rolled pad. *(A)* Treatment-planning CT scan showing the scar outline by a lead strip and the direct measurements from both ends of the scar to the chest wall. The medial end of the scar is 4.5 cm from the chest wall and the lateral end of the scar exceeds 5 cm. *(B)* The medial boost portal. *(C)* The lateral boost portal. (From Montague, et al.: U.T. M.D.A.H. technique for treatment of early breast cancer with conservation surgery and irradiation. *In* Proceedings of the International Conference on the Use of Conservation Surgery and Radiation Therapy in the Treatment of Early Breast Carcinoma. Cambridge, 1982.)

and an additional 1000-rad tumor dose in 5 fractions is delivered to include the site and scar of the excision biopsy (clips showing the extent of surgical excision are helpful in defining the area to be boosted). The choice of voltage depends on the thickness of the breast in treatment position; 9 MeV or 11 MeV is generally used.

An interstitial iridium implant delivering 1500 to 2000 rad is used when margins are unknown or positive.

For patients with a subareolar primary tumor or with tumors close to the chest wall, additional external irradiation is delivered by compression technique, turning the patient into the prone-oblique position

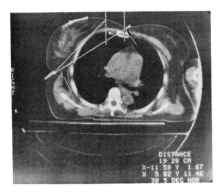

Fig. 12–10. The scar is outlined with a lead strip in a patient with an excised upper inner quadrant primary tumor. The internal mammary nodes were 3.5 cm from the midline of the sternum in the second and third interspaces on lymphoscintigraphy (solid dot). With a separate internal mammary chain field (dotted line), the base of the breast was not being irradiated. Consequently, the medial tangential field was moved 1.5 cm to the opposite side of the midline to cover the entire breast and internal mammary nodes. (Arrows) The tangential portals that were used. (From Montague, et al.: U.T. M.D.A.H. technique for treatment of early breast cancer with conservation surgery and irradiation. *In* Proceedings of the International Conference on the Use of Conservation Surgery and Radiation Therapy in the Treatment of Early Breast Carcinoma. Cambridge, 1982.)

for the lateral field and the anterior-oblique position for the medial field; an additional 1000 to 2000-rad tumor dose is delivered in 5 to 10 days (Fig. 12–9).

Breast and Internal Mammary Nodes

Following an excision or segmental mastectomy for small (≤2 cm) invasive carcinoma in the central or inner quadrant of the breast when nodes are histologically negative, only the breast and internal mammary nodes are treated. To spare mediastinal, cardiac, and pulmonary tissue, electrons (with some skin-sparing characteristics) or a combination of ^{60}Co and electrons can be used to irradiate the internal mammary nodes.

The lateral position and depth of the internal mammary nodes should be evaluated, particularly when the nodes are to be included in the tangential portals. Lymphoscintigraphy allows measurement of the distance of the nodes from the midline

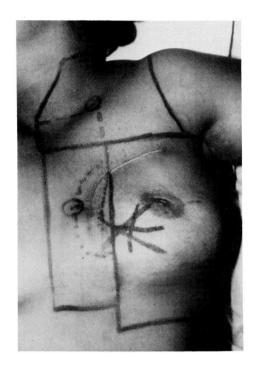

Fig. 12–11. The 44-year-old patient had a 3.5-cm upper inner quadrant carcinoma of the left breast, which was excised. A dissection of the lateral axilla revealed 18 histologically negative nodes. Because the low and central axilla had been dissected and did not require irradiation, the superior border of the tangential field was raised from its usual location at the second intercostal cartilage so that less lung would be irradiated and the tumor bed would be confined to the tangential and internal mammary portals. The posterior axillary field was not used. The breast received a 5000-rad tumor dose with ^{60}Co over a period of 5 weeks (25 fractions) with a combination of open and wedge fields. The tumor bed was then boosted with 7 MeV electrons for 1000 rad over 5 days. The internal mammary portal received a 2000-rad given dose with ^{60}Co (during which the scar extending into the straight-on portal was irradiated with bolus 3 times weekly—semicircular dotted lines within the internal mammary chain portal) and an additional 3000-rad given dose with 13 MeV electrons. The supraclavicular-axillary apex portal received a 4000-rad given dose over 4 weeks with ^{60}Co and an additional 1000-rad given dose with 9 MeV electrons. Because 9 MeV electrons deliver little or no irradiation to the internal mammary or deep medial supraclavicular nodes, the internal mammary portal was raised to include the first internal mammary space and medial supraclavicular area. The entire chain received a 4500-rad tumor dose with 13 MeV. (From Montague, et al.: U.T. M.D.A.H. technique for treatment of early breast cancer with conservation surgery and irradiation. *In* Proceedings of the International Conference on the Use of Conservation Surgery and Radiation Therapy in the Treatment of Early Breast Carcinoma. Cambridge, 1982.)

at each interspace, and ultrasound or computerized tomographic (CT) scan gives the accurate depth of the nodes.[5] When the internal mammary nodes are to be treated with a separate field, care must be taken that the entire breast receives irradiation. Figure 12–10 is a treatment-planning CT scan of a patient whose breast would be incompletely irradiated if a separate internal mammary field were used; the technique was changed to include the internal mammary nodes in the tangential fields.

The technique used for advanced local disease—the treatment of all junction lines with each field—should not be used to irradiate an intact breast with early, favorable disease; careful blocking must be used to avoid overlaps (see Fig. 12–3D).

The dosage for treatment of the breast and internal mammary nodes is 4500- to 5000-rad tumor dose, delivered in 5 weeks (25 fractions) to all areas, followed by a boost to the excision site of the breast as described above.

The internal mammary field is the same as that described previously for the electron-beam peripheral-lymphatic-irradiation technique; the breast is also treated with tangential fields using 1:1 open field 45° wedged filtered fields, as in irradiation of the retained breast.

If tumors are in the upper central or inner area, the remaining breast tissue above the tangential fields can be treated with electrons as described above.

Irradiation of the Breast, Internal Mammary, and Supraclavicular Areas

Treatment is delivered to these three sites with larger inner or central primary tumors (2–5 cm in diameter) or when the dissected axillary nodes are positive, regardless of the location of the primary tumor. The treatment technique is the same as that described under ^{60}Co Chest-Wall Irradiation. The posterior axillary field is not used in any patient who has had a low and central axillary-node dissection; it is used if there is extranodal disease or if few axillary nodes are recovered.

If patients are to be treated with cardiotoxic drugs such as doxorubicin (Adriamycin), consideration should be given to mixing photons or using only electrons for the internal-mammary-chain irradiation. Our present policy includes 2000-rad given dose with photons and 3000-rad given dose with electrons. At the same time the anterior supraclavicular-axillary field can be treated with a 4000-rad given dose with photons and 500- to 1000-rad given dose with electrons. When this is done, the internal mammary portal, irradiated with 13 MeV to 15 MeV, is raised to include the first interspace, thus bringing the total dose to a 4500-rad tumor dose (Fig. 12–11).

Throughout the various adaptations of technique for treating an intact breast, close teamwork between surgeon and radiotherapist is necessary. It is necessary to be totally informed about the surgical procedures before making any modification of the standard fields.

To gather more information about the depth of nodes, coverage of breast and pulmonary tissue, and so forth, treatment for each patient is now being planned by a computerized technique. Treatment techniques are constantly evolving, permitting the radiotherapist to achieve better cosmetic results.

REFERENCES

1. Fletcher, G.H., Montague, E.D., Tapley, N.duV., and Barker, J.L.: Radiotherapy in the management of nondisseminated breast cancer. *In* Textbook of Radiotherapy, 3rd ed. Edited by G.H. Fletcher. Philadelphia, Lea & Febiger, 1980.
2. Haagensen, C.D.: Diseases of the Breast. Philadelphia, W.B. Saunders, 1956.
3. Montague, E.D., Romsdahl, M.M., Fletcher, G.H., and Schell, S.R.: UT M.D.A.H. technique for treatment of early breast cancer with conservation surgery and irradiation. *In* Proceedings of the International Conference on the Use of Conservation Surgery and Radiation Therapy in the Treatment of Early Breast Carcinoma. Cambridge, 1982.

4. Montague, E.D.: Clinical experience with radiation therapy in the treatment of non-invasive or small volume invasive breast cancer. In *Proceeding of the 19th National Conference on Breast Cancer*, San Diego, 1981.

5. Schell, S.R., Echenique, R., Fields, R., Meoz, R., and Montague, E.D.: The clinical application of ultrasound lymphoscintigraphy and computerized tomography in radiotherapy of breast cancer. In *Proceedings of the Radiologic Society of North America*. Chicago, 1983.

Chapter 13

A TECHNIQUE FOR EXTERNAL BEAM IRRADIATION OF CARCINOMA OF THE PROSTATE

Malcolm A. Bagshaw

Successful external radiotherapy in the treatment of carcinoma of the prostate depends upon accurate definition of the histologic type, extent of the neoplasm, and the precise delivery of megavoltage radiation. The radiotherapist is usually presented with the histologic diagnosis, which is usually established by transurethral biopsy of the primary site (48% in this series). Needle biopsy is the other preferred method, with transrectal more common than transperineal. Data using the Kempson Grading System demonstrate that the incidence of lymph-node metastasis increases significantly (chi square with 2 degrees of freedom = 8.34, 0.05 > p > 0.01) as the degree of differentiation decreases.[1,2] Sixty-two percent of the poorly differentiated tumors (Grades III and IV) had lymphadenopathy. The same can be observed using the Gleason Grading System. A systematic increase in percentage of lymph-node involvement was observed as the Gleason-pattern score increased. In the data cited, no positive lymph nodes were found until the pattern score reached 5. There was a systematic progression from 15% lymph-node involvement at a pattern score of 5, to 100% lymph-node involvement at a pattern score of 10.[3] A few patients with lower Gleason scores who have positive lymph nodes have been observed; however, the risk is directly proportional to the Gleason-pattern score.

Carcinoma of the prostate is often multifocal and usually originates in the peripheral lobes;[4,5,6] samples of the neoplasm taken by transurethral resection could be misleading because transurethral resection cannot detect the full extent of disease or discover small peripheral neoplasms. It is clear that some carcinomas of the prostate are of low-grade malignacy.[5,7,8] They require years to become locally symptomatic and even longer to become disseminated and lethal. There is, however, no certain method of predicting that the disease will follow this particular course. The results of treatment are directly inversely proportional to the grade and extent of disease; it therefore seems most appropriate to me to treat aggressively at the earliest diagnostic certainty. This seems especially true in the case of younger men (40–60 years) with limited disease, in whom the

This work was supported in part by Grants CA-05838 and CA-15455 from the National Cancer Institute, National Institutes of Health, and the National Prostatic Cancer Project.

The author wishes to thank Miss Patricia Steed for the preparation of the dose calculations and the treatment plans.

burden of treatment by radiation can be kept at a minimum and treatment is well tolerated. This point of view is disputed; however, further discussion of this controversy is beyond the scope of this chapter on technique of treatment.

DIAGNOSTIC STUDIES AND THE DETERMINATION OF EXTENT OF DISEASE

Physical Examination

In addition to a thorough general history

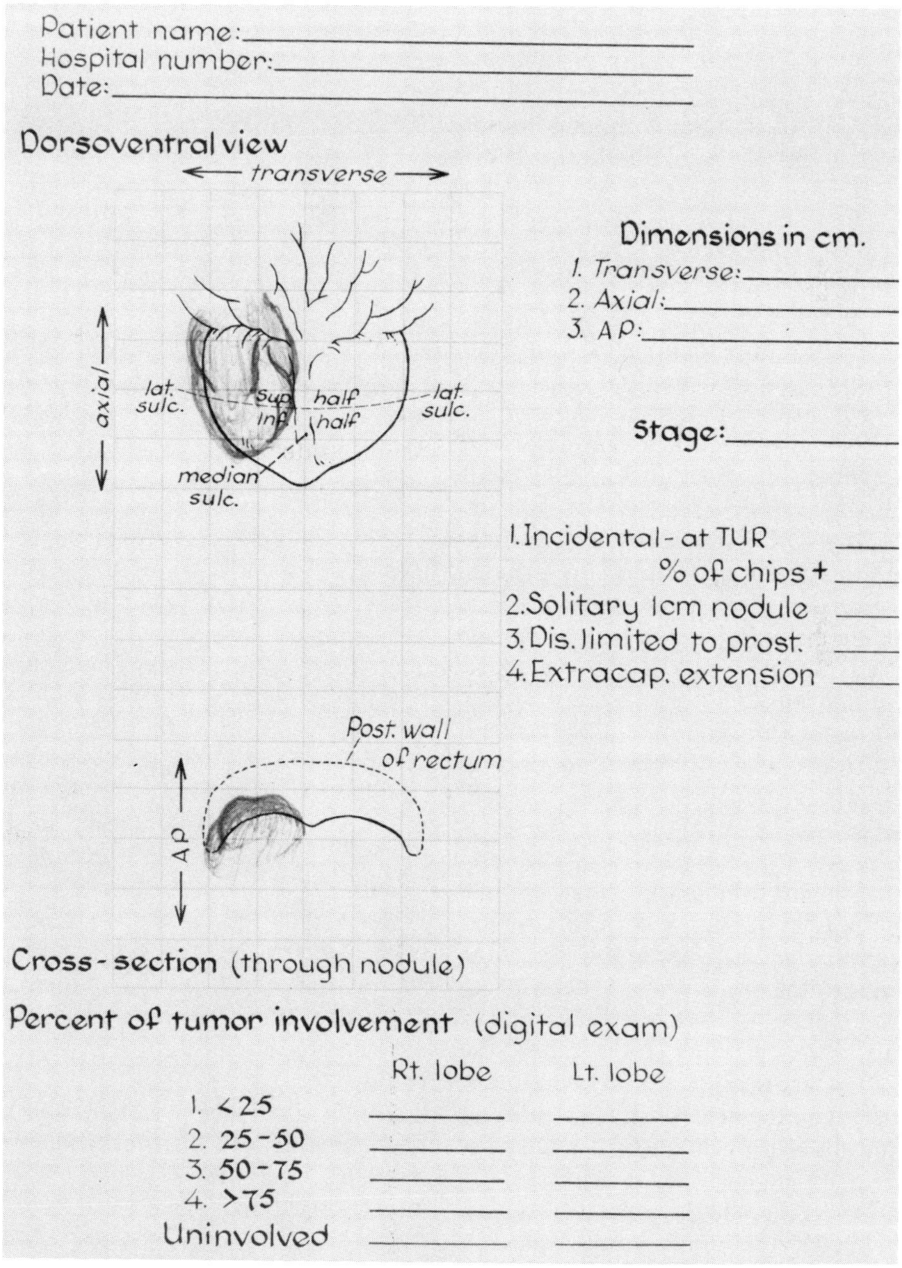

Patient name:_____
Hospital number:_____
Date:_____

Dorsoventral view
← transverse →

Dimensions in cm.
1. Transverse:_____
2. Axial:_____
3. A P:_____

axial

lat. sulc. — Sup. half — lat. sulc.
Inf. half
median sulc.

Stage:_____

1. Incidental - at TUR _____
   % of chips + _____
2. Solitary 1cm nodule _____
3. Dis. limited to prost. _____
4. Extracap. extension _____

Post. wall of rectum

AP

Cross-section (through nodule)

Percent of tumor involvement (digital exam)

	Rt. lobe	Lt. lobe
1. <25	_____	_____
2. 25-50	_____	_____
3. 50-75	_____	_____
4. >75	_____	_____
Uninvolved	_____	_____

Fig. 13–1. Suggested preprinted sheet for diagramming the position and extent of prostatic cancer.

and physical examination, specific points to evaluate include a careful review of symptoms as they pertain to the urological and skeletal systems, and an examination of the prostate with exceptional care. The physician should note by digital examination through the rectum whether the median raphe has been effaced or the lateral sulci have been distorted. The size, preferably in centimeters, and the density of the gland should be determined. A full-sized sketch of the gland should be detailed (Fig. 13–1), with nodularity indicated and a notation as to whether the tumor has penetrated the posterior capsule. Special effort should be made to palpate the region of the seminal vesicles to determine whether there has been superior extension of the neoplasm. The most convenient position for palpating the prostate is with the patient leaning forward over the end of the examining table while resting his chest on the table, and with the legs spread slightly but the toes pointed inward (pigeon-toed). The physician should be seated behind the patient; he should be able to extend one hand around the patient so that it may be placed over the patient's suprapubic region to permit bimanual palpation while the index finger of the other hand palpates the prostate transrectally. If there is any doubt concerning the superior extent of disease, the patient may assume the knee-chest position or the squating position on the examining table. Although this is rather ungainly, it is by far the best position that allows the physician to palpate the most superior extent of disease. A determination of breakout of the neoplasm through the capsule, especially in the region of the seminal vesicles, is extremely important since this and the degree of differentiation are the most significant clues to metastases to pelvic or para-aortic lymph nodes. This careful assessment of the prostate also permits staging by the popular American Urological System[9] or, preferably, by the more recently introduced International Union Against Cancer (UICC) system[10] and American Joint Committee tumor-nodes metastases (TNM) System.[11]

The physician should also examine the lymphatic system carefully with particular attention to the iliac, para-aortic, and supraclavicular lymph nodes. The skeletal system should be examined by percussion and compression in order to detect areas of tenderness.

Ancillary Procedures

[99m]Tc-labeled diphosphonate or phosphate scintiscans are probably the single, most reliable indicators of disseminated bone metastases.[12] On the other hand, this examination with modern detection equipment is exquisitely sensitive, and equivocally positive areas should be verified by radiographs or biopsy. Radiographs are probably no longer necessary as a survey tool; however, they are still indispensable for confirmation of scintiscan findings or supplementation of scintiscan information in the event the scintiscan is at variance with the physical examination. Areas of previous injury, and significant arthritic change can mimic bone metastases. Forewarned about the possibility of metastatic disease, the therapist may wish to obtain a biopsy, advocate treatment other than aggressive radiotherapy (e.g., hormonal), or treat the primary site with radiotherapy in order to forestall the serious local symptoms of obstruction, pain, and hemorrhage.

Although pulmonary metastases are unusual in early prostatic carcinoma, *chest radiographs* could provide a disincentive for radiation treatment and an indication for systemic therapy (e.g., Diethylstilbestrol).

Intravenous pyelography should be carried out in order to ascertain the presence of distal ureteral obstruction. If the obstruction is adjacent to the prostate, it probably represents obstruction due to extension of the tumor into the base of the bladder. Although not a contraindication to therapy, this finding may diminish the prognosis. If the obstruction is more cephalad, it probably represents extensive iliac-lymph-node involvement.

Sixty-seven percutaneous and 41 open-iliac-crest *bone biopsies* in patients with negative bone scintiscans failed to reveal histologic evidence of prostatic metastases. This procedure has been discontinued.

The value of *lymphography* remains controversial;[13] however, it continues to be a subject of ongoing clinical research in the program at Stanford. It is useful in identifying clearly positive studies, as an aid to the surgeon in identifying suspicious lymph nodes and to the radiotherapist in treatment planning. Spellman et al. demonstrated an overall 78% accuracy of lymphography in a group of 69 unselected patients with untreated prostatic carcinoma that, by all other physical criteria, was localized to the prostate or periprostatic region. Forty-one percent of these patients had metastases proven histopathologically for all stages. Metastases were proven for 20% of the Stage B patients, and in 64% of the Stage C patients.

Two newer methods for the determination of the extent of the local neoplasm have been studied to a limited degree. These include ultrasonography of the prostate using a transrectal probe, and computerized tomography (CT). We have had limited experience with these procedures; insufficient data is available at this time to be able to determine their ultimate efficacy. It is likely that CT will be useful both in the detection of prostatic cancer and in treatment planning.[14,15,16,17]

In addition to routine *laboratory studies*, serum-acid and alkaline-phosphatase levels should be determined. An attempt should be made to identify the prostatic fraction of the acid phosphatase, either by the use of the tartrate-inhibitable technique or the sodium thymolphthalein monophosphate (STM) substrate. If the prostatic fraction is significantly elevated,

extensive metastatic disease should be anticipated. It has not been determined at this point, however, whether modest elevations are possible as a result of lymph-node metastases alone; modest elevations in the prostatic fraction need not eliminate a patient from the treatment program. We have noted, for example, a decrease in the prostatic fraction of the acid phosphatase following lymph-node irradiation. The reliability of bone-marrow acid phosphatases also remains uncertain at this time; although several authors[18] have reported significant use of this parameter, it is not relied upon to exclude patients for radiotherapy.

During the study of the interpretation and efficacy of lymphography in prostatic carcinoma, *retroperitoneal pelvic exploration* was performed at the conclusion of the clinical evaluation.[19] Routine pelvic exploration is no longer justified because positive or equivocal lymph nodes can usually be assessed by needle biopsy. Our results to date indicate that when the para-aortic lymph nodes are involved, the chances of further dissemination approach 75%. This raises a serious question as to whether para-aortic treatment can be justified; however, longer follow-up is required to make this judgment.

At the conclusion of these studies, the radiotherapist should know whether there has been detectable distant spread of carcinoma of the prostate and whether it is confined to the prostate itself, the periprostatic region, the pelvic lymph nodes, or the para-aortic and pelvic lymph nodes.

ARRANGEMENT OF FIELDS ACCORDING TO DETERMINATION OF TUMOR EXTENT AND VOLUME

Following the pretherapeutic evaluation, the therapist is faced with the question of whether to treat the prostate only, the prostate and the pelvic lymph nodes, or the prostate, the pelvic lymph nodes, and the para-aortic lymph nodes. The irradiation is limited to the prostate in elderly patients with Gleason-pattern scores of 5 or less, and to patients in whom pelvic laparotomy fails to demonstrate involvement outside of the prostatic capsule. If involvement of the pelvic lymph nodes is identified, then treatment is justified superiorly at least to the sacropromontory. Rouvière,[20] basing his observations on the meticulous dissections of Cuneo and Marcille,[21] has described four major lymphatic pathways that drain the prostate. These include the external iliac, the hypogastric, and the posterior, or presacral nodes at the level of S2 and the sacropromontory, and the inferior lymphatic pathway that descends with the internal pudendal artery. Herman et al. have confirmed this distribution for the pelvic lymph nodes by lymphography and agree with Rouvière that the obturator node, so often involved with prostatic cancer, is anatomically in continuity with the medial chain of the external iliac group.[22] Interestingly, Rouvière has described that:

If all of the small retroprostatic intercalating nodules are withdrawn from consideration, the first lymphoid echelon for the lymphatics of the prostate is represented by the entire lymphoid girdle at the superior strait of the pelvis, viz., the external iliac, the hypogastric, and the lymph nodes of the promontory.

This is in agreement with the distribution of metastases that we have observed both by lymphography and pelvic-node dissection (Table 13–1).

Tumor Localization

We recommend the use of the isocentric technique combined with CT scanning for localization, treatment planning, and treatment. The justification and the general procedure for the isocentric system has been described elsewhere.[23] Here we present in step-by-step detail how the method may be used for the treatment of prostatic cancer. The key elements of the localization procedure include the use of contrast materials and CT scanning in order to define the boundaries of the prostate, the seminal vesicles, vital adjacent radiosensitive organs, and the regional lymph nodes. Field sizes of a predetermined dimension are not used; each plan is developed individually. The field sizes, therefore, are determined by anatomic landmarks within the treatment volume. The recent application of CT scanning, especially for assessment of seminal-vesicle involvement and tumor extent, is a substantial aid and always should be used if it is available.

Localization of the position of the prostate, both with and without the aid of CT, are described here. Although orthogonal radiographs are used for the basic localization procedure, CT permits accurate localization of the prostate and seminal vesicles without the need for the insertion of a Foley catheter. If a CT scan is not avail-

TABLE 13–1.   Incidence of Lymph-Node Involvement by Tumor.*

Lymph Node Group	Number of Patients Biopsied	Number (%) With Tumor	Percent Opacified†
Para-Aortic	74	13 (18%)	93
Common Iliac	76	13 (17%)	95
External Iliac	74	16 (22%)	94
Internal Iliac	63	15 (24%)	87
Obturator	51	16 (31%)	94

*This table represents the incidence of histopathologically-proven adenopathy in 93 patients who had both lymphography and pelvic exploration for lymph-node sampling. Over the entire series, there was not a consistent attempt to remove all involved lymph nodes; however, as the techniques evolved, more and more frequently most of the involved regional lymph nodes were removed at operation. This accounts for the fact that the denominators are not 93 in every case; the denominators indicate the number of patients in which a particular node group was biopsied; the numerators indicate the number of times a positive node was found in the biopsied group.
†*Percent opacified* refers to histologic evidence of retained contrast material within the lymph-node specimen.

able, the catheter is essential for the identification of the prostatic urethra, and it may be presumed that the seminal vesicles extend superiorly to the level of the acetabula.

Although a treatment simulator is convenient, any x-ray diagnostic unit that is capable of taking anterior-posterior (AP) and lateral films of the patient lying in a supine position can be used. The simulator assists the therapist in accurate maintenance of the source-axis (isocenter) distance (SAD) and the source-film distance (SFD) (Fig. 13–2). If ordinary radiographic equipment is used, the appropriate distances must be carefully measured for each application. The simulator employed here is a homemade, exact geometric duplicate of a 4-MeV linear accelerator (see Fig. 13–4A), the Varian Clinac 4; however, almost any isocentrically mounted simulator could be used. The simulator is

equipped with a brightly illuminated field light which exactly duplicates that of the 4 MeV linear accelerator. The central axis and central planes are identified by cross-wires interposed in both the light and x-ray beams so that they cast a shadow in the light field and a line of decreased exposure on any x-ray films exposed by the unit. (Hereafter these fiducial marks will be referred to as cross-hairs.) The simulator room is equipped with parallel-opposed incandescent or laser side lights with cross-hairs and a ceiling-mounted vertical light with cross-hairs, all of which intersect at the isocenter of the simulator. The treatment room is identically equipped.

A simple film holder at a prefixed SFD of 108 cm and an SAD of 80 cm (see Fig. 13–2) is used. Image intensification or other types of fluoroscopy is not required for the initial setup. This is not to say that image intensification equipment may not be useful; however, by following a few simple rules, a skilled technologist rapidly becomes adept at providing perfect localization films that may be reviewed by the radiotherapist and which, after approval, are used for treatment planning. The films then become an important part of the patient's record.

Technique for Prostatic Localization and Treatment Planning

Five steps are required for the complete external-radiation treatment of prostate carcinoma. These include:

I. Tumor volume localization, including information from rectal exam, markers if any, and CT scan through the prostate, seminal vesicles, pelvic, and para-aortic nodes. If a diagnostic CT is to be used for treatment planning, the table top should be converted from concave to flat by an easily constructed lucite slab. The pubic mark (step c) should be tattooed in position in advance as a reference point for the CT technologist. The CT

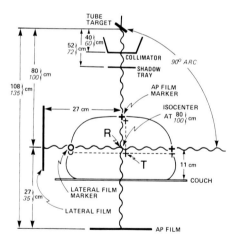

Fig. 13–2. The dimensional parameters for localization and treatment. The bold number indicates the appropriate dimension for units that have a source axis distance of 80 cm; the italicized numbers are for units having a source–axis distance (SAD) of 100 cm. By standardizing these dimensions, the magnification factor of the structures in the central plane of the localization or portal radiographs are always 1.35. For the provisional localization, the isocenter is at the setup point, R. This is always adjusted to the tumor reference point T after the treatment volume has been decided in consultation between the radiotherapist and dosimetrist. In later illustrations, R is used to designate the final tumor isocenter point.

technologist identifies this tattoo with a lead marker.

II. Verification.

III. Treatment planning.

IV. Confirmation of field arrangements.

V. Treatment.

A Place patient in comfortable supine position.

B Insert #16 Foley catheter into urinary bladder. Inflate balloon with Hypaque M, 90%, bladder with Hypaque 50%, 30 ml. This step may be omitted if localization CT scan is available.

C Place a second Foley catheter in rectum, inflate balloon with air. With traction on the catheter, snug the balloon against the internal sphincter and clamp in place with special Foley clamp gently opposed to the anus (see Fig. 13–3A & B).

D With the simulator in the vertical position, expose AP film in a 14 × 17 in. high-speed cassette, centered 4 cm superior to pubis in midline (88 kVp, 200 mA, 0.4 sec. exposure). Mark skin at central ray with temporary marking.

E Slide table craniad and center 1 cm inferior to pubis in midline. Expose film as in step D.

F Swing simulator 90° to horizontal position for orthogonal radiograph of the prostatic region.

G Adjust central axis to 10 cm above table top. Mark skin at central axis.

H Instill thin barium through rectal Foley catheter.

I Expose lateral 14 × 17 in. film (88 kVp, 200 mA, 0.8 sec. exposure).

J Slide table caudad and recenter at the same midpelvic level as indicated in D.

K Expose film using factors indicated in I.

L Using the orthogonal pairs of pelvic and prostatic set-up radiographs, the radiotherapist and simulator radiographer lay out AP and right and left lateral treatment fields, taking into account information from CT scan, digital exam, and contrast boundaries. It is recommended that posterior margins of lateral fields pass through the middle of the rectal lumen.

M Determine exact center of treatment fields as marked on set-up radiographs.

N Change set-up points 1 and 2 to reference points R_1 and R_2.

O Adjust skin marks according to the new reference points.

P Fill out physical report form.

Q Dosimetry staff obtains cross-sectional contours through isocenter planes at R_1 and R_2 and any other planes desired. If possible, these can be taken directly from the CT scans, provided a flat table top has been used and the reference point has been indicated as in "L" above.

End of first session

R Calculate treatment plan and daily dose routine.

S Prepare template for shaping the radiation fields by the addition of lead blocks to shield the corners (trim blocks).

T Obtain simulation radiograph centered at isocenter points with trim blocks in place for each of the 8 treatment fields, using a double-exposure technique.

U If para-aortic lymph nodes are not to be treated, commence treatment; otherwise proceed with localization as follows:

1. Place patient in comfortable supine position. In

order to localize the kidneys in both the AP and lateral projections, 300 ml of 25% Hypaque are given by intravenous infusion over a period of 10 minutes in order to assure sufficient density within the renal pelves for the lateral views. If CT has been obtained, it may be used to determine renal position.

2. Center field ½ the distance between 2 cm superior to the top of pelvic field and xyphoid process. Mark skin. Expose 14 × 17 in. AP film (88 kVp, 200 mA, 0.3 sec.).

3. Swing simulator 90° to lateral orthogonal position and, using the projected side light cross-hairs, establish lateral center point 10 cm above table top. Mark skin.

4. Expose film. Same exposure factors as in U2 but increase the time to 0.8 sec.

5. Radiotherapist and simulator technician lay out fields using prudence to establish the lateral margin of the AP fields sufficiently lateral to include the para-aortic lymph nodes, but sufficiently medial not to damage the kidneys. Lay out lateral field so that most of the radiation passes anterior to the renal pelvis.

6. Determine exact center of fields as marked on the films.

7. Readjust provisional skin marks to the topographic projection of the tumor point (i.e., change set-up point to reference point).

8. Fill out physical report form.

9. Obtain cross-sectional contour.

End of second session

10. Calculate treatment plan, including calculation of the gap between the superior margin of the pelvic field, which has already been established, and the inferior margin of the para-aortic field.

11. Obtain double-exposure simulation films.

V Commence treatment.

X Obtain double-exposure portal films for each field with the final treatment field configuration, using the high-energy source of the therapy machine.

Y Repeat X every time field is modified or treatment is changed.

The sequence of operations as outlined above is presented in greater detail in the following section. Boldface capital letters in parentheses indicate the step in the above outline that is being discussed in the text.

The patient is placed in a comfortable supine position **(A)** with the arms folded across chest for pelvic and prostatic treatment, or if para-aortic fields are to be treated also, with the hands clasped above the head. After appropriate sterile preparation, the urethra is anesthetized by the instillation of 2% Xylocaine Jelly and a #16 Foley catheter is inserted through the urethra into the bladder **(B)**. Omit this step if prostatic-seminal vesicle volume is to be determined by CT scan. The entire catheter is well lubricated with a half-and-half mixture of K-Y jelly and 2% Xylocaine. Occasionally the catheter does not pass, in which case a urologist is called for assistance. If the urologist is unsuccessful, the catheterization is abandoned and an intravenous pyelogram (IVP) **(U1)** is obtained to identify the position of the urinary trigone. The balloon is filled with 5 ml of high-density Hypaque, and the bladder is filled with 30 ml of conventional Hypaque. The Foley is pressed against the trigone with light pressure, and the catheter is taped to the thigh.

If CT is available, tattoo a midline point 1 cm inferior to the superior margin of the symphysis pubis. Do this before the localization procedure, at the time of initial patient examination. This point later serves as a reference for measuring craniocaudad-axis distances when transposing the prostate volume from CT scan to AP and lateral set-up radiographs. It also serves as the set-up point for the prostatic booster fields.

Schedule the pelvic CT scan, specifically requesting: the use of a flat table during the scanning procedure; a radiopaque marker placed at the level of the tattoo; a

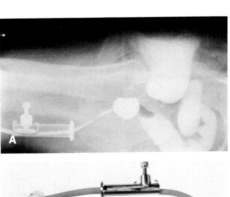

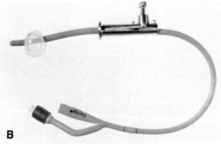

Fig. 13–3. *(A)* A lateral localization radiograph with contrast in the urinary Foley catheter (mercury), contrast in the urinary bladder (Hypaque), and contrast in the rectum (Barium). Note the metallic clamp that marks the anus and the anal canal between the rectal Foley catheter and the anal marker. *(B)* The anal marker fitted over a Foley catheter.

CT obtained and identified on the simulation radiograph at the level of the marker (tattoo); that the patient be scanned at 1-cm intervals from the ischial tuberosities to L5 or T12, depending on the clinical situation.

With the orthogonal method, a second Foley catheter **(C)** is inserted into the rectum, the balloon is inflated and gently tugged against the rectal sphincter. It is held snugly in place by the sliding clamp that is fitted over the Foley catheter and gently clamped in position against the anus (Fig. 13–3).

With the simulator vertical, the central axis of the x-ray beam is identified by the cross-hairs projected in the illuminated field. This is centered in the midline 4 cm superior to the public symphysis (Fig. 13–4); the position of the projected cross is marked on the skin **(D)** with a temporary marking, and a full 14 × 17 in. film is exposed (Fig. 13–5A). A second midline AP radiograph **(E)** is obtained at this time, centered approximately 1 cm inferior to the superior ramus of the pubis. This represents the small prostatic boost field (Fig. 13–5B).

Without moving the patient relative to the table top, the isocentrically mounted simulator is rotated 90° to the horizontal **(F)** in order to obtain a lateral localization radiograph of the small prostatic boost field (Fig. 13–5C). The table height is adjusted so that the lateral marks are 10 cm above the table top for the large pelvic fields (see Fig. 13–4). The proper positioning of these lateral marks controls the patient's position and permits the radiotherapist to minimize pelvic angulation. About 100 ml of thin Barium is instilled into the rectum through the rectal Foley catheter **(H)** and the lateral film is exposed **(I)** (see Fig. 13–5C). The Barium is not introduced prior to this because it occasionally obscures the image of the prostatic urethra on the initial AP film.

The longitudinal position of the table is then moved caudally, placing the cross-

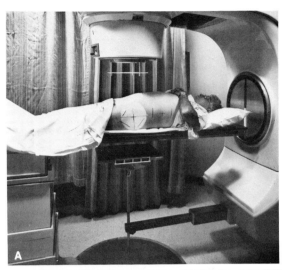

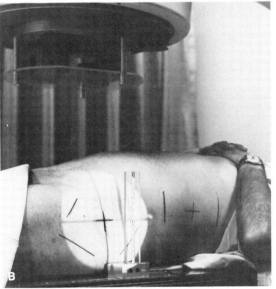

Fig. 13–4. A homemade simulator that features the precise geometry of the Varian Clinac 4. It is used to obtain isocentric orthogonal localization radiographs for the development of total pelvic irradiation of the prostate and regional lymph nodes. The key elements include a collimator system, motor-drive around the axis isocenter, a standard Clinac 4 treatment couch, a film holder adjusted at 108 cm SAD, and co-planar side lights that intersect the vertical plane at the isocenter. The round area of illumination on the patient's skin shows clearly; the shadow of the cross hairs appears not only on the skin but on the localization radiograph as well. *(A)* The simulator beam is vertical in order to define the anterior field. The central axis is centered in the midline 4 cm superior to the symphysis pubis. *(B)* A height gauge is in place in order to define the setup point for the lateral fields 10 cm above the table top. The position of the central ray is indicated on the shadow of the cross hairs projected onto the skin by the side light illuminators. The vertical arm of the cross hair projects to the same level as the central ray of the anterior field. *(C)* The simulator has been rotated 90° and centered on the central axis mark for proper exposure of the lateral localization films. The central axis mark for the anterior field is also shown. A second orthogonal pair of films is obtained at the level of the prostate centered 1 cm inferior to the pubic symphysis. When indicated, a third pair is obtained centered over the upper abdomen for treatment of the para-aortic lymph nodes. The mechanical framework and drive mechanism were manufactured in the Radiotherapy Machine Shop under the direction of C.J. Karzmark and Peter Huisman. The collimating system, fiberglass shell and treatment support assembly were supplied by Varian Associates, Inc.

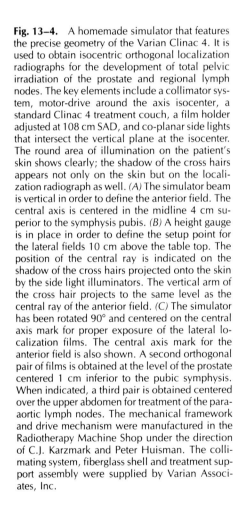

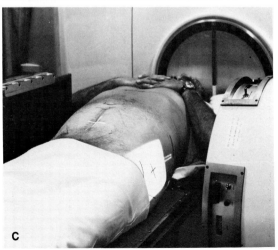

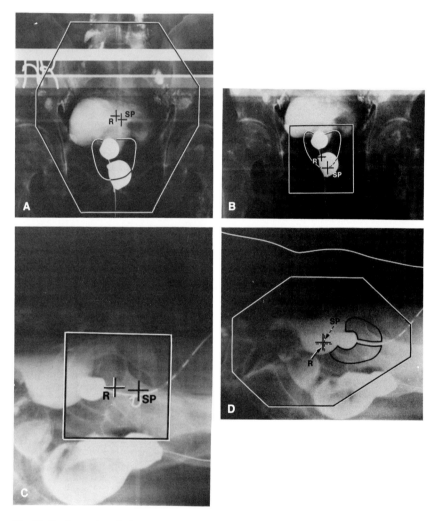

Fig. 13–5. Legend on facing page.

Fig. 13–5. *(A)* Anterior-posterior localization film. Note that the patient has had a lymphogram. Contrast material (Hypaque) has been placed in the urinary bladder, and mercury has been placed in the balloons of the Foley catheters in the bladder and rectum. The field is initially centered in the midline, 4 cm superior to the top of the symphysis, the set-up point (SP). The SP is marked on the patient's skin. The faintly visible white cross in the center of the localization films is produced by the reduction in exposure of the film by the cross hairs of the collimating system of the simulator. The point of intersection of the cross hairs is concordant with the SP. The black and white lines that depict the field perimeter are added by the radiotherapist. This is done without attention to the SP. Next, the exact center point for this treatment field is determined and designated (R). The displacement from the SP is measured and the new point, R, is marked on the patient's skin. Here it is 5 mm superior and 5 mm to the right of the SP. Now the SP is discarded and the position of R is tattooed. The bold white horizontal bars crossing the iliac crests are produced by mechanical supports in the treatment table. *(B)* Anterior-posterior localization films for prostatic boost field. Note again the Hypaque in the urinary bladder and the mercury in the Foley catheters' balloons in the bladder and the rectum. The Foley catheter is pulled downward so as to rest on the trigone of the bladder or on the fossa that is often created by a transurethral resection. The Foley catheter is taped to the inner thigh so that it does not move and continues to clearly mark the superior extent of the prostate. The presumed outline of the prostate and the field encompassing the prostate are added here. In this instance, the SP is placed too far caudad. It is adjusted to the center of the field, R, by moving it 1.5 cm superiorly and .75 cm to the right, as indicated by the black cross (R). The position of R is tattooed and becomes the isocenter point. The SP is discarded. Note that neither this field nor the lateral boost field in C are used exactly as depicted here. These fields are laid out simply to find the isocenter for the 120° lateral arc moving-beam technique that is used for the prostatic boost. *(C)* The patient is supine. The barium is visible in the rectum. The rectal marker is visible; the anal marker was not used here. The balloon of the Foley catheter and the mercury in the lumen of the catheter as it traverses the prostatic urethra are clearly visible. The Hypaque is clear in the urinary bladder. The cross hair of the illuminated radiation field is faintly visible as two intersecting lines of decreased density on the radiograph. The cross hair has been placed at the same level as the SP for the anterior field and 10 cm above the table and marked on the skin as the SP. The radiation field has been laid out by the radiotherapist. The SP has been readjusted to R. The skin marks are moved accordingly, superiorly 1.5 cm and anteriorly 0.2 cm. The reference point R becomes the isocenter point and is tattooed. The SP is discarded. *(D)* Lateral localization film for large pelvic field. The SP is placed at the level of the SP of the anterior field and 10 cm above the table top. After establishing the field outline, the reference point R remained at the same level of the SP, but was shifted 0.2 cm anteriorly.

hairs back to the level of the original localization point, which is in the midline 4 cm superior to the pubic symphysis **(J)**. This is easy to do because, with the field aperture large, the vertical arm of the cross-hairs intercepts the horizontal arm of the anterior skin mark. The lateral pelvic localization films are exposed (see Fig. 13–5D).

It should be clear that the words "treatment field" and "treatment portal" are not precisely used when applied to the isocentric technique. Historically, these words meant the portal of entry of the radiation beam through the skin. In the present context, they apply to the anatomy of the treatment region as depicted by a simulation radiograph of the target volume. Their size before trimming is indicated by the dial setting of the collimator aperture, and they are proportional but not identical to the dimensions of the "fields" or "portal" as projected upon the skin. It should be understood that if the skin portals are applied with the dimensions of the fields at the isocenter, the treatment volume will be grossly exaggerated. The true dimensions at the central planes of the isocentric fields as visualized on the localization films can be easily determined. The magnification factor has been standardized at the central plane at 1.35 for either 100-cm SAD, or 80-cm SAD (see Fig. 13–2). A series of transparent magnification rules are prepared by careful quantitative enlargement of a photograph of a transparent centimeter ruler. The sets contain 11 rulers each, which permit direct measurement of magnification factors of 1 to 1.50 at 0.05 intervals.*

---

*The 1.35 magnification factors are really true only for structures at the plane of the isocenter. By geometric calculation, one could determine the magnification at any other plane and use the corresponding ruler for direct measurement. An even simpler, perfectly accurate method for laying out structures within a cross-sectional contour is to use the inexpensive, easily constructed contour-projection device previously described.[23] In practice, however, we find that the simulator technologists and physicians prefer to work with the direct x-ray image of the treatment volume, either as described herein or, preferably, from CT cross-sections, which are now available at most radiology centers. The treatment-planning team (dosimetrists) occasionally use the orthogonal radiographs in conjunction with the contour-projection device for more precise anatomic localization. It is presumed that CT will replace these more primitive methods; however, whether more accurate treatment planning will result remains to be determined. It will undoubtedly be more costly.

With the patient positioned in this manner, the point that is at the isocenter of the simulator and in the central plane is designated the set-up point for the full pelvic treatment volume, or the set-up point for the prostatic boost volume. The topographical coordinates of these reference points have already been temporarily marked on the patient's skin from the projected cross-hair of the side lights and the central axes of the radiation fields. The radiotherapist is then presented with the orthogonal films for each pelvic and prostatic localization level **(L)**; the set-up points may be identifiable because they are coincident with the projected images of the cross hairs that designate the central planes and axes of the localization beam (see Fig. 13–5). The image quality of the projected cross hairs in the localization radiographs is variable, depending upon the size of the patient and exposure factors. Nevertheless, with appropriate adjustment of technical factors relative to the patient's physique, it can always be visualized. The position of the lymph nodes is also visualized, either because of a prior lymphogram or marking by surgical clips. If neither of these procedures has been done, the radiotherapist must make an educated guess as to the position of the lymph nodes. The position of the anus, rectum, and sigmoid are evident on the lateral views. The position of the bladder and the prostatic urethra are also visible.

The radiotherapist determines the extent and configuration of the AP and lateral fields. This requires that the therapist conceptualize the shape and extent of the treatment volume from all information at hand (i.e., CT scan, localization radiographs, physical examination, laboratory studies, and staging procedures). The therapist draws the perimeter of the treatment volume directly onto the radiographs with a wax pencil. The inferior border of the large pelvic field is generally placed at the ischial tuberosity. The superior border is placed at the top surface of L5. The lateral borders of the anterior and posterior fields are determined by the position of the common and external iliac lymph nodes, but usually lie approximately 1 cm lateral to the widest diameter of the pelvic inlet. The superior and inferior corners of the anterior and posterior fields are trimmed in order to protect as much bone marrow as possible (see Fig. 13–5A).

In Fig. 13–5D, the configuration of the lateral fields is demonstrated. Note, of course, that the superior and inferior limits are identical to those of the anterior and posterior fields. The anterior border of the lateral fields usually extends from the anteriormost aspect of the pubic symphysis. It is directly superior to a line intersecting at right angles the superior boundary of L5 or, as in the case illustrated, it is angled posteriorly to a point just anterior to the common iliac lymph nodes. The posterior margin is somewhat arbitrary and is generally established at the midlumen of the rectum. This configuration reduces the dose to the posterior wall of the rectum because there is no contribution to the dose delivered to this structure from the lateral fields. This significantly reduces rectal reactions during therapy or later on. This position of the posterior border of the lateral fields has a theoretical disadvantage in that some of the presacral lymph nodes might be missed. According to Rouvière, however, the first lymph node in the presacral chain is at S2, which is usually included in all four fields. We have encountered failure that could be directly attributed to isolated recurrence in the presacral chain on only one occasion.

In order to determine the treatment volume for the prostatic boost, the best estimate of the position of the prostate is sketched on both the frontal and the lateral prostatic localization radiograph by the radiotherapist (see Fig. 13–5B,C). In the absence of a proper CT scan, there is always some degree of arbitrariness; however, the superior aspect of the prostate is well marked by the balloon of the Foley catheter and the contrast material in the urinary bladder. The anterior surface cannot be further anterior than the posterior cortex of the pubic bone unless the neoplasm has directly invaded the pubic bone.* The posterior surface rarely bulges significantly into the rectum unless the tumor exceeds 10–12 cm in diameter. The superior margin of the field depends upon whether the seminal vesicles are involved. If so, the superior margin of the boost field is best determined by the CT scan (Fig. 13–6).

If CT is available, locate the CT level number of the cut that passes through the reference point. Find the CT level numbers that correspond to the uppermost and lowest extent of the prostate/seminal vesicle volume.

Locate the CT level reference guide (this is usually in one of the CT frames near the Vertical Reconstruction images). This guide gives the relative distances between the center of each level (in mm) and an arbitrary starting point (0 mm). Now find the levels (in mm) of the reference point, the upper prostate/seminal vesicle margin, and the lower prostate/seminal vesicle margin, using the CT level numbers.

The distance (in mm) between the reference point level and the upper level (distance A) and lower level (distance B) can now be used to locate these levels on the cone-down set-up radiographs.

If a scan is unavailable, the superior margin should extend to the superiormost concavity of the acetabulum.

The placement of the caudal margin of the prostatic boost field should provide an adequate tumor margin but remain short of the anal verge. A normal position of the prostate in the anterior view is illustrated by the gold beads of ^{125}I interstitial sources in Fig. 13–7. In most instances, these fields, measured at the isocenter, are approximately 8 cm longitudinally and 7 cm

---

*This apparently has occurred in several of our patients and has been detected by either scintiscans or roentgenograms. When this is the only metastasis, this area of assumed extension is included within the prostatic volume.

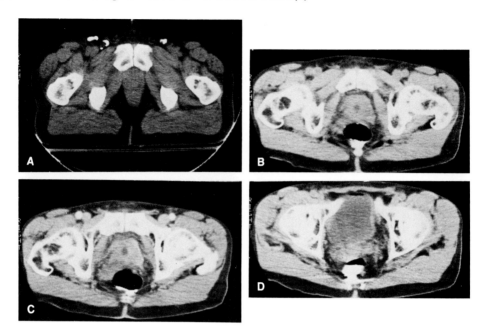

Fig. 13–6. Selected CT scans of a prostate proceeding cranially from the ischial tuberosities *(A)* to acetabulum *(D)*. *(A)* was obtained after the patient had had a lymphogram and is just caudad of the prostate at the corpus spongiosum; *(B)* is through the midprostate at midpubis; *(C)* is at the superior margin of the pubis. Note the urethral defect in the center of the prostate caused by the transurethral resection of the prostate (TURP). Note also how little of the prostate has been removed. The tumor extends posteriorly and to the right, apparently completely invading the seminal vesicles as far craniad as the acetabula. Superior CT scans showed no tumor. The patient was referred as having nodular disease and as a candidate for radical prostatectomy. Rectal examination indicated at least a Stage C (T3) but the total craniad extent had not been appreciated.

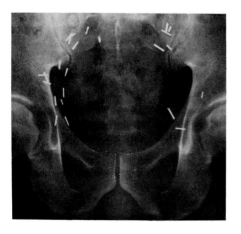

Fig. 13–7. A survey film after pelvic lymph node dissection and prostatic implant with ^{125}I seeds. The positions of the resected nodes are shown by the silver clips. The ^{125}I seeds distributed throughout the prostate are visible as tiny white dots (gold spheres).

transversely. The purpose of the localization of the caudal margin is to find the isocenter for the prostatic boost that is delivered by 120° lateral-arc technique (see Fig. 13–10). If moving-beam therapy is not available, the prostatic boost could be delivered by opposed AP and opposed lateral fields, or, more preferably, by opposing anterior and posterior oblique fields. Both the arc therapy and the oblique configuration therapy minimize the dose delivered to a suprapubic incision in patients in whom there has been either a suprapubic prostatectomy or a lymph-node dissection. When the 120° lateral-arc technique is used, the axial dimension of the boost field may be slightly increased in order to accommodate the slight edge reduction of dose produced by the penumbra at the superior and inferior edges of rotated or arced beams.

The cross-hairs that are projected on the initial localization radiographs (the set-up points) are usually not exactly in the center of the isocenter fields as they were subsequently established by the radiotherapist. In fact, it would be a coincidence if they were. The therapist should disregard the set-up points when laying out the treatment volumes. A new point R is determined **(M)** that does lie exactly in the center of the prepared radiation fields.* By direct measurement on the films using the magnification ruler, the degree of displacement of the reference point R from

---

*In more complex applications of the isocentric technique, the reference point R need not be in the center of the target volume (e.g., off-center rotations).

PHYSICAL REPORT FORM

PATIENT	PHYSICIAN	ACCELERATOR
Mr. X	Resident/Staff	LA-4

LOCATION OF ISOCENTER

DATE	SPECIFICATION	LONGITUDINAL	TRANSVERSE	SAGGITAL — (AP)
7/3/78	Set Up Point (Pelvis)	4 cm superior symphysis	Midline	10 cm above table top
	Reference Point " & Isocenter	" "	.5 cm Rt of M.L.	9.75 cm " " "
	Set Up Point (Prostate)	1 cm inferior to symphysis	Midline	10 cm above table top
	Ref. Point & Isocenter	.5 cm superior to symphysis	.75 cm Rt of M.L.	1.2 cm " " "

SPECIFICATION OF TREATMENT FIELDS

DATE 19 78	FIELD NO.	FIELD SIZE	DESCRIPTION	ANGULATIONS		WEDGE	THICK EDGE
7/3	1	19 x 16-1/2	Anterior (+Pb)			-	
	2	"	Posterior (+Pb)			-	
	3	19 x 13-1/2	Rt Lateral (+Pb)			-	
	4	"	Lt Lateral (+Pb)			-	
	5	8x7-1/2	Rt Lateral 120° arc	210°	330°	-	
	6	"	Lt Lateral 120° arc	30°	150°	-	

DOSE CALCULATION

DATE 19 78	FIELD NO.	FIELD	s	d cm	X.A.F.	RxC_i Rad/Rdl	W	D_{id} Rad	M Rdl	D_m Rad	D_{mw} Rad
7/3	1	Ant.	.307	9.0	1.02	0.868	-	61	72	93	Dmax & exit
	2	Post.	.295	9.75	1.02	0.849	-	59	71	94	= 64.4%
	3	Rt Lat.	.196	18.0	-	0.59	-	39	66	114	isocenter
	4	Lt Lat.	.202	17.6	-	0.6	-	41 / 200	68	116	
	5	Rt arc	.5	-	1.055	0.561	-	100	188		
	6	Lt arc	.5	-	1.055	0.563	-	100 / 200	187		

COMMENTS: s = fraction of the total isocenter dose delivered from a single field.
d = depth to isocenter.
X.A.F. = extra absorption factors, e.g., lucite trays which support lead trim blocks.
RxC_i = factor for converting machine monitor units to rad.
D_{id} Rad = dose in rad at isocenter.
M Rdl = monitor units
D_m Rad - dose at maximum ionization of single field.

36-11A (Rev. 4/76)

SIGN: _____

Fig. 13–8. The physical report form.

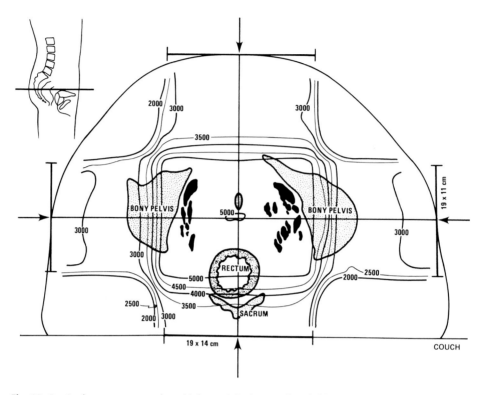

Fig. 13–9. Isodose contours at the midplane of the large pelvic field. Note that this plane is superior to any tissue that might be irradiated by the prostatic boost dose.

the projected cross-hairs is determined. Because the temporary skin marks describe the topographical position of the set-up points, the new reference points, as they are topographically projected to the skin, are determined by direct measurement; these points are tattooed in place. The physical report form is recorded **(P),** and the patient's cross-sectional contour **(Q,R)** is obtained at the central plane of both the large pelvic field and the prostate boost field (Figs. 13–8, 13–9, 13–10). An off-axis second contour is occasionally taken approximately halfway between the middle and the superior margin of the large pelvic field in order to be certain the lymph nodes fall within the 5000-rad-isodose contour and to accommodate the change in field size due to the trim blocks (Fig. 13–11). If CT is used to establish the cross-sectional anatomy, this is unnecessary (Figs. 13–12, 13–13). Figure 13–14

depicts the summated isodose patterns of the large pelvic field and the prostatic boost at the level of the prostate. The patient may be dismissed at this point and rescheduled for simulation radiographs **(T)** after the treatment plan has been completed.

Trim blocks for the anterior and posterior fields are controlled by means of templates **(S).** The shapes of these templates are traced on a piece of transparent celluloid and accurately positioned by aligning the cross-hairs of the field projection light with a cross marked on the template (Fig. 13–15). This is especially helpful in aligning the trim blocks for the posterior field which is treated with the patient supine and with the beam directed vertically upward through the Mylar window of the patient-support table. For the lateral fields, the trim marks are generally marked directly on the patient's skin because the

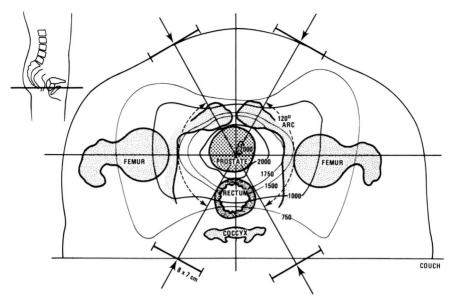

Fig. 13–10. Isodose contours through the plane of the prostate for the prostatic boost dose. The treatment in this instance was delivered by an 8 cm × 7 cm portal as measured at the isocenter. Left and right lateral arc moving-beam therapy was used. The distribution of dose would be the same if the entire treatment were given to the prostate only, except that the 2000-rad isodose line would, in the case of localized treatment, be 7600 rads delivered over a period of 7 weeks and 3 days at the rate of 200 rads per day.

skin over the hips is relatively fixed (see Fig. 13-4B). The trim blocks for the lateral fields are clamped in place by a special universal clamp that is mounted on the collimator. In our system, the blocks are suspended firmly at any required position within or at the edge of the beam cross-section. Most megavoltage machines have shadow trays upon which blocks can be locked or bolted in position. The treatment plans presented in Figures 13–9, 13–10, and 13–11 are calculated through the isocenter points for the large pelvic field, the prostatic boost, the trimmed superior portion of the large pelvic field, and the para-aortic field (Fig. 13–16).

The patient is returned to the simulator **(T)** and orthogonal verification radiographs are obtained. This time the patient is positioned with the three-point technique. The isocenter is initially placed coincident with the isocenter point R for the large pelvic fields, and then at the isocenter point R for the prostatic boost. The

three-point technique permits accurate positioning of the isocenter point by use of the horizontally directed side lights that are aligned with the lateral skin marks in conjunction with the vertical light that is aligned with the anterior skin mark.[24] The first exposure of the double-exposure verification radiographs is obtained with the fields well open. For the average-size patient, the following factors are used: 88 kVp, 200 MA, at 0.4 second for the anterior and posterior exposures, and an 0.8-second exposure for the lateral exposure. The collimator is then adjusted to the precise field size and the various trim blocks are adjusted according to the previously prepared templates. The second exposure is achieved with the same factors but one half the exposure time. It is essential that neither the patient nor the x-ray beam be moved between exposures (Fig. 13–17).

The localization procedure for the para-aortic fields is done on the second day because to accomplish the entire proce-

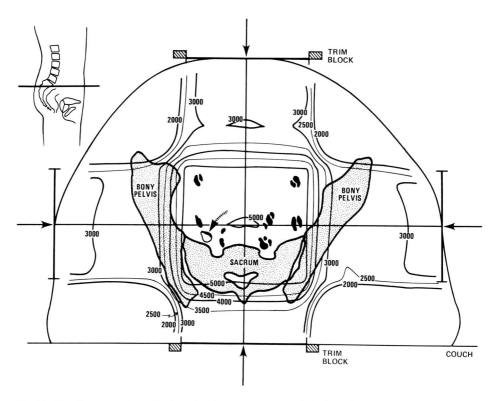

Fig. 13–11.   Demonstration of isodose distribution approximately halfway between the midplane of the large pelvic field and the superior margin of this field. It is through the upper portion of the field, illustrated in Fig. 13–5A, calculated after the addition of the trim blocks.

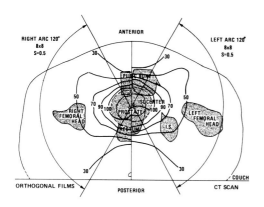

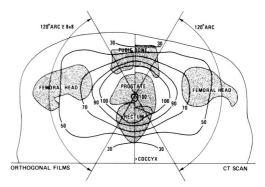

Fig. 13–12.   Right and left 120° arc moving-beam dose distributions as calculated by cross-sectional reconstruction from orthogonal films compared to distributions calculated from CT cross-sectional reconstructions. The match is not as close as in Fig. 13–13, but there is little practical difference.

Fig. 13–13.   Right and left 120° arc moving-beam dose distributions. Right side calculated from orthogonal films; left side calculated from CT scan. Excellent concordance is demonstrated by the mirror images of the dose distributions.

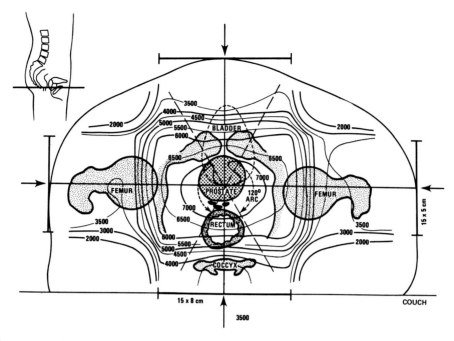

Fig. 13–14. The combined isodose pattern through the level of the prostate when the prostatic boost is added to the full 4-field box technique. A few lymph nodes are indicated lying posterior to the prostate at this level. These nodes are inconstant and poorly defined, and are referred to by Rouvière as *intercalating nodes*. They are apparently not associated with any of the specific 4 drainage pathways from the prostate.

dure during a single session is usually too fatiguing for the patient. The para-aortic treatment volume is identified by localization radiographs that are exposed after an intravenous infusion of Hypaque in order to identify the position of the kidneys **(U1)** or by the preplanning CT scan, if available. The infusion requires about 10 minutes. The anterior field is centered in the midline. Its position in the longitudinal axis is determined by the superior margin of the pelvic field. The para-aortic fields are 15 cm to 18 cm in length as measured at the anatomic site of the para-aortic lymph nodes. On many linear accelerators, the field size at the isocenter is given by the collimater dial settings. Therefore, the cross-hairs that mark the central axis **(U2)** are placed one-half the distance between 2 cm superior to the superior margin of the pelvic field and the xiphoid process. The exact dimensions of the gap are calculated by the dosimetrist and adjusted later, either by readjusting the cen-

ter point or by adding a trim block at the inferior field margin.[25] Although there is no spinal cord at the usual sites of junction of the para-aortic and pelvic treatment volumes, the proximal trunks of the nerves of the lumbar and sacral plexes, the ureters, and the bowel are at risk for radiation injury.

Because most of our patients have contrast material introduced into the para-aortic lymph nodes, the field margins are adjusted to be adequately lateral to the opacified para-aortic lymph nodes but medial to the renal pelvis (Fig. 13–18A). In some instances, the treatment volume grazes the medial aspect of the upper poles of the kidneys; however, we have never observed radiation nephritis in these patients. The upper limit of the para-aortic field is usually established at the superior margin of L1, or occasionally T12. As in the pelvis, the lateral localization radiograph is centered at 10 cm above the table top **(U3, U4)**. In Figure 13–18B there is an

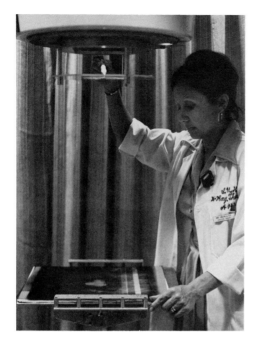

Fig. 13–15. The localization film is placed in the film holder and illuminated by the intense field light. The film holder has a white reflective surface, and the details of the film are easily seen by the radiographer. A piece of transparent celluloid is placed on the shadow tray, and the cross hair of the field illuminator is marked on the transparency after it has been aligned with the cross-hair on the localization film. By using an opaque marking pen and matching the shadow cast by the pen with the trim block lines that have been drawn on the localization radiograph by the radiotherapist, the radiographer can accurately mark the position of the trim blocks on the transparent template. This is a simple method for positioning trim blocks or for designing an aperture of complex geometry for an accessory collimator, such as might be used in the head and neck region.

ill-defined image overlying the anterior border of L1 and L2 which represents the renal pelvis. The localization radiograph clearly shows that the para-aortic lymph nodes are anterior to the vertebral bodies and, therefore, most of the renal parenchyma. The lateral verification radiograph (Fig. 13–18C) demonstrates how well the alignment is controlled by the side lights because the circle represents the skin mark on one side, and the cross-hairs demonstrate the skin mark on the other. In the final confirmation radiograph, however, it can be seen that the lateral fields have been narrowed about 1 cm and moved an-

teriorly in order to further spare the kidneys (Fig. 13–18D). The treatment plan for para-aortic irradiation is illustrated in Figure 13–16.

At the time of the initial setup, two outlines are taken around the patient, one in the center of the pelvic fields, and one in the center of the prostatic boost field. Calculations are made for the 4 pelvic fields (anterior, posterior, right and left laterals) so that their weighting assures equal (D_{max} and exit) doses at all 4 D_{max} points. If the resulting total doses at these points exceed 4000 rad, a check is made with the therapist to decide if this total is acceptable or if an alternate treatment plan should be considered.

From tumor–phantom-ratio tables, the daily accelerator monitor units, which we call "rdls", per field are calculated. Then the physical report form (see Fig. 13–8) is completed and taken to the treatment technologist. Calculations for the two 120° arcs used to treat the prostate area are made by assuring that each arc is composed of a number of evenly placed stationary fields. Six positions at 20° intervals are summated throughout the arc. The tumor–phantom ratio is found for each position and the mean used for the monitor unit calculation. Details are filled in on the physical report form, which is then transferred to the treatment technologist.

The distribution of dose for a combination of the two techniques is devised with the aid of a computer. The isodose values are produced in total treatment numbers and are in a plane containing the prostate and the four pelvic fields, as well as the two 120° arcs. A copy of this distribution is made to insert in the patient's chart. It includes not only the distribution but also the main anatomic features, such as the prostate, rectum, bladder, and femoral heads. Off-axis distributions are occasionally prepared as the need arises (see Figs. 13–9, 13–10, 13–11, 13–14). A similar calculation is prepared for the para-aortic treatment volume.

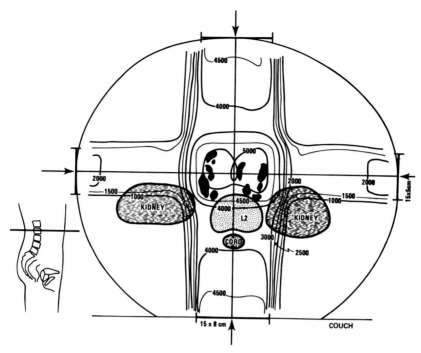

Fig. 13–16.   Treatment plan for para-aortic irradiation. Note that most of the dose is administered through AP–PA parallel opposed pair.

Although a full central plane dose distribution is plotted in every instance, an off-axis plan is occasionally needed. The dose that is recorded daily is the dose at the point of junction of the central axis of the various fields (the isocenter dose). The treatment plans, however, are adjusted so that the minimum tumor dose is never less than 95% of the maximum or isocenter dose; this 95% line is always at least 1 cm peripheral to the nearest suspected neoplasm. Space is provided on the daily treatment sheet, however, to carry additional dose points, and it is not uncommon to specify that a maximum and a minimum dose be carried on the daily treatment sheet. A point of special interest in normal tissue may also be recorded.

When the patient reports for treatment **(X)**, a double-exposure confirmation radiograph of each radiation field is obtained with the therapy beam the first time each field is treated (Fig. 13–19). Thereafter, confirmation radiographs are ob-

tained as often as necessary to assure quality control. These radiographs are of extremely low contrast, particularly in the pelvic region where bowel gas is not consistent and film contrast is often inadequate for ideal anatomic detail. Nevertheless, sufficient bone structure usually can be seen to permit comparison with the original simulation radiographs to verify the field shape and position.

Thus, for each treatment site, prostatic, pelvic, and para-aortic, three films are required. These include the initial localization radiograph, the simulator verification double-exposure, radiograph, and the therapeutic confirmation double exposure radiograph. Every time the treatment volume is modified, the confirmation radiograph is repeated.

At Stanford, the treatments for prostatic cancer are delivered with a Varian Clinac 4, with an 80-cm isocenter distance. Four MV has proved adequate for the delivery of tissue doses of up to 7600 rads in 7½

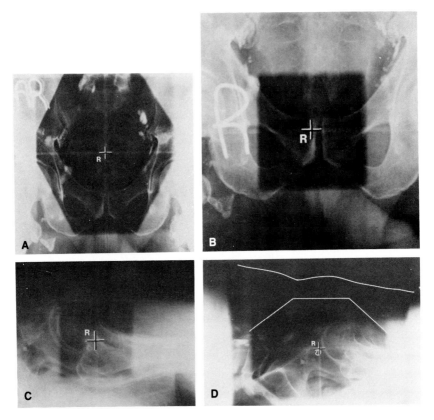

Fig. 13–17. *(A)* This is a double-exposed verification radiograph of the AP pelvic field made with the simulator, in order to verify that the new tumor position R has been properly placed and that all potentially malignant elements within the treatment volume are well covered. *(B)* Double-exposure verification radiograph of the anterior coordinate of the prostatic boost field. *(C)* A double-exposure verification radiograph of the lateral projection of the prostatic boost field is obtained with the simulator. *(D)* A double-exposure verification radiograph of the lateral large pelvic field. The position of the anterior field margins and anterior body wall are accented by the white lines.

weeks in patients with prostatic carcinoma. When working at this energy, however, at the energy of ^{60}Co, or with any accelerator up to approximately 12 MV, several precautions must be taken in order to avoid tissue injury: use the 4-field technique for the pelvic treatment, rather than a simple anterior and posterior opposed pair, and being absolutely certain that each field is treated every day. Although we have seldom encountered subcutaneous injury, suprapubic edema, or edema of the scrotum or penis that could be attributed to radiation therapy alone, such complications have been encountered by other physicians. These complications will probably increase in frequency as more men receive lymph-node dissections in addition to radiation therapy. Severe edema is a devastating complication that usually can be avoided by careful treatment planning and by treating each field each day. This is time-consuming and often is a hardship in a busy department; nonetheless, the daily tolerance is unmistakably improved and long-term injury is avoided. Another simple method to improve patient tolerance during the course of therapy is to introduce the prostatic boost dose to the prostate (Weller boost*) at approximately the midterm, rather than

---

*So named after Stephen A. Weller, M.D. who, while a resident, first suggested the technique.

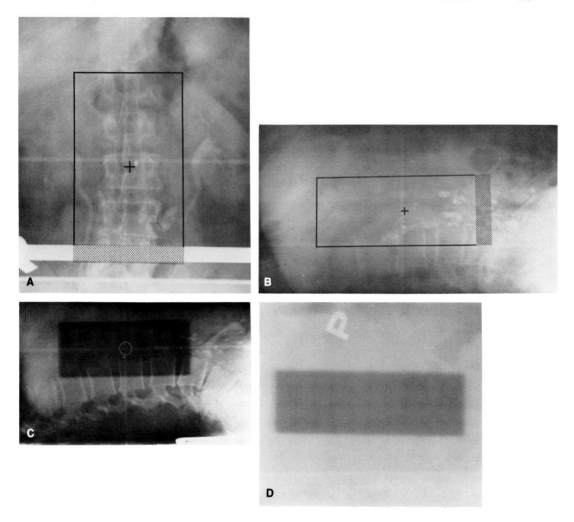

Fig. 13–18. (A) Anterior localization radiograph for para-aortic treatment fields. Note the position of the opacified lymph nodes, particularly overlying L3. Note also that the renal pelves are clearly visible, as are the proximal ureters and most of the renal parenchyma. The lateral margins of the treatment fields are between the kidneys and the para-aortic lymph nodes. The inferior margin is indicated by stippling because this is precisely determined by the dosimetrist after calculation of an appropriate gap between the superior margin of the pelvic field and the inferior margin of the para-aortic field. The SP is not labeled but is at the intersection of the cross hairs. The black cross marks the reference point R. (B) Orthogonal counterpart of (A). Although difficult to visualize, the renal pelves can be seen superimposed on the anterior margin of the inferior portion of L1 and L2 along the horizontal cross-hair line. The SP is difficult to identify and is not labeled because the vertical cross-hair line is superimposed upon the black line that indicates the posterior field margin. It was necessary to move the reference point 3 cm anteriorly and slightly inferiorly to the tumor point, which is indicated by the black cross. Note also how all of the para-aortic lymph nodes lie anterior to the vertebral bodies; thus, lateral fields in this region can be positioned so that they are anterior to most of the renal parenchyma but still encompass the para-aortic adenopathy. (C) Verification radiograph of (B). It serves to illustrate the accuracy of the side lights in achieving an even positioning of the patient; the cross-hairs show the lateral mark on one side of the patient, and the circle shows the lateral mark on the opposite side. They are perfectly opposed. On the other hand, the posterior margin of this field was not satisfactory because it overlapped too much of the kidney and gave too wide a margin on the para-aortic lymph nodes posteriorly. It was adjusted slightly by being narrowed by 1 cm and moved anteriorly another 0.5 cm, as illustrated by (D), the linear-accelerator confirmation radiograph. This confirmation radiograph represents the field dimensions upon which the dosimetry presented in Fig. 13–16 is based.

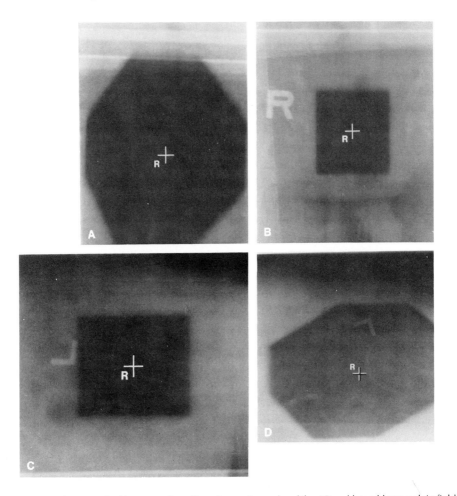

Fig. 13–19. These are double-exposed confirmation radiographs of the AP and lateral large pelvic fields and the prostate boost fields obtained with the 4-MV accelerator beam. The confirmation radiographs are difficult to interpret because of the lack of contrast range. We use cardboard cassettes with Agfa-Gevaert Curix R.P.1 x-ray film with a $\frac{1}{16}$ in. layer of steel on top of the film, placed between the film and the patient. Bony landmarks that confirm the anatomy of the soft tissues can be detected; this has been demonstrated previously on the primary localization radiographs, and the verification radiographs.

at the end, of the large-field pelvic treatment. This, in effect, is the same as using a split-course for the large pelvic volume that contains bladder, colon, and small bowel, but permits continuous treatment of the primary neoplasm within the prostate itself. We generally deliver 2600 rad at the rate of 200 rad per day to the pelvis and the para-aortic region if the para-aortic nodes are treated, then reduce the fields to the prostate continuing with lateral-arc therapy to the prostate only, for an additional dose of 2000 rad given at the rate of

200 rad per day. This permits a 2-week period of respite which is beneficial to nearly every patient. For example, if at the 2600-rad level the patient has a mild increase in diarrhea or urinary frequency, this usually subsides during the prostatic boost and usually does not recur during the last one-third of the treatment program, when the fields are again enlarged and the 4-field box therapy is resumed. The total dose, therefore, is 7000 rad delivered in 7 weeks at the prostatic isocenter, and 5000 rad delivered in 7 weeks to

the pelvic and para-aortic isocenters. The 95%-isodose line encompasses all of the pelvic adenopathy and the minimum dose to potentially involved lymph nodes is not less than 4750 rad.

Although the para-aortic nodes are treated by the 4-field technique, the initial 4000-rad dose is delivered through anterior and posterior opposed portals. This is not a sufficient dose to endanger either the terminal spinal cord or the subcutaneous tissues; it has the potential advantage of delivering approximately 4000 rad to the lumbar spine in case there should be occult metastases in this portion of the skeleton which, along with the pelvis, often appears to be the first site of bone involvement with prostate metastases.[26] The last 1000-rad dose is delivered by left and right lateral fields, which are placed anterior to most of the renal parenchyma and adequately cover the para-aortic lymph nodes.

For those patients in whom there is no evidence of extracapsular spread (i.e., patients in whom biopsy has failed to disclose either lymph-node or osseous metastases) and in whom the small-field 120° lateral-arc rotation is employed exclusively, the dose is carried to 7600 rad over a period of 7 weeks and 3 days, at the rate of 200 rad delivered at the isocenter per day. We have treated 426 patients with disease limited to the prostate (DLP). The survival rate, taking into account death due to all causes, calculated recently (1982) by the Kaplan Meier technique was 79% ±4.0%* at 5 years, and 60% ±5.4% at 5 years for the group of 349 patients with extracapsular extension (ECE). Comparable figures at 10 years were 58% ±5.8% and 36.1% ±6.0%, respectively. Although the number of patients at risk for 15 years is small (23 DLP and 14 ECE), their respective survivals are 37% ±8.2% and 22% ±7.0%.

These data are in general agreement with series reported by others and may be considered as typical of what might be achieved in external-beam radiotherapy of localized prostatic cancer.

Since 1971, patient selection has been complicated by the employment of lymphography and pelvic exploration in an effort to identify patients with pelvic or para-aortic lymph-node metastases, so that extended field radiotherapy could be administered in accordance with the extent of involvement. More than 250 additional patients have received definitive treatment; however, because they are now separated into multiple groups depending upon extent and histologic grade, and because the follow-up for some of the groups is relatively short, a rigorous analysis is not yet available. To date, the data suggest that the survival of patients who have no pathologic evidence of lymph-node involvement is about 78% at 10 years in 66 patients, whereas for those with both pelvic and para-aortic involvement, the survival in 23 patients is 15% at 10 years. In patients with positive pelvic lymph nodes only, the survival is about 20% at 10 years. It appears that knowing that the prostatic cancer is confined to the prostate is highly indicative of a good prognosis. Considerable further study is necessary in order to evaluate the efficacy of extended treatment in the face of proven adenopathy.

REFERENCES

1. Bagshaw, M.A., Pistenma, D.A., Ray, G.R., Freiha, F.S., and Kempson, R.L.: Evaluation of extended-field radiotherapy for prostatic neoplasm: 1976 progress report. Cancer Treat. Rep. 61:297, 1977.
2. Kempson, R.L. and Levine, G.: The relationship of grade to prognosis in carcinoma of the prostate. Front. Radiat. Ther. Onc. 9:267, 1974.
3. Pistenma, D.A., Bagshaw, M.A., and Freiha, F.S.: Extended-field radiation therapy for prostatic adenocarcinoma: Status report of a limited prospective trial. *In* Cancer of the Genitourinary Tract. Edited by D.E. Johnson and M.L. Samuels. New York, Raven Press, 1979.
4. Byar, D.P. and Mostofi, F.K.: Carcinoma of prostate: Prognostic evaluation of certain pathologic

---

*±2 standard errors.

features in 208 radical prostatectomies. Cancer *30*:5, 1972.

5. Rich, A.R.: On the frequency of occurrence of occult carcinoma of the prostate. J. Urol. *33*:215, 1935.

6. Franks, L.M.: Latent carcinoma of the prostate. J. Pathol. *68*:603, 1954.

7. Blackard, C.E., Mellinger, G.T., and Gleason, D.F.: Treatment of stage I carcinoma of the prostate: A preliminary report. J. Urol. *106*:729, 1971.

8. Mellinger, G.T., Gleason, D., and Bailer, J.: The histology and prognosis of prostatic cancer. J. Urol. *97*:331, 1967.

9. Rubin, P.: Cancer of the urogenital tract: prostate cancer. JAMA *210*:322, 1969.

10. TNM Classification of Malignant Tumors, 2nd ed. Geneva, Union International Contre le Cancer, 1974.

11. Amer. Joint Comm. for Cancer Staging and End Results Reporting: Classification and staging of cancer by site. Amer. Joint Comm., Chicago, 1976.

12. Pistenma, D.A., McDougall, I.R., and Kriss, J.P.: Screening for bone metastases: Are only scans necessary? JAMA *231*:46, 1975.

13. Spellman, M.C., Castellino, R.A., Ray, G.R., Pistenma, D.A., and Bagshaw, M.A.: An evaluation of lymphography in localized carcinoma of the prostate. Radiology *125*:637, 1977.

14. Asbell, S.O., Schlager, B.A., and Baker, A.S.: Revision of treatment planning for carcinoma of the prostate. Int. J. Radiat. Onc. Biol. Phys. *6*:861, 1980.

15. Lee, D., Leibel, S., Shiels, R., Sanders, R., Siegelman, S., and Order, S.: The value of ultrasonic imaging and CT scanning in planning the radiotherapy for prostatic carcinoma. Cancer *45*:724, 1980.

16. Pilepich, M.V., Prasad, S.C., and Perez, C.A.: Computed tomography in definitive radiotherapy of prostatic carcinoma. II. Definition of target volume. Int. J. Radiat. Onc. Biol. Phys. *8*:235, 1982.

17. Pilepich, M.V., Perez, C.A., and Prasad, S.: Computed tomography in definitive radiotherapy of prostatic carcinoma. Int. J. Radiat. Onc. Biol. Phys. *6*:923, 1980.

18. Chua, D.T., Veenema, R.J., Muggia, F., and Graff, A.: Acid phosphatase levels in bone marrow: Value in detecting early bone metastases from carcinoma of the prostate. J. Urol. *103*:462, 1977.

19. Bagshaw, M.A., Ray, G.R., Salzman, J.R., and Meares, E.M., Jr.: Extended-field radiation therapy for carcinoma of the prostate: a progress report. Cancer Chemother. Rep. *59*:165, 1975.

20. Rouvière, H.: Anatomy of the Human Lymphatic System. Translated by M.J. Tobias. Ann Arbor, Edwards Bros., 1938.

21. Cuneo, B. and Poirier, P.: Special study of the lymphatics in different parts of the body. *In* The Lymphatics. Edited by G. Delamere. Chicago, W.T. Keener & Co., 1904.

22. Herman, P.G., Benninghoff, D.L., Nelson, J.H., Jr., and Mellins, H.A.: Roentgen anatomy of the ilio-pelvic-aortic lymphatic system. Radiology *80*:182–193, 1963.

23. Gardner, A., Bagshaw, M.A., Page, V., and Karzmark, C.J.: Tumor localization, dosimetry, simulation and treatment procedures in radiotherapy: The isocenter technique. Am. J. Roentgen. *114*:163, 1972.

24. Martinez, A., Donaldson, S.S., and Bagshaw, M.A.: Special set-up and treatment techniques for the radiotherapy of pediatric malignancies. Int. J. Radiat. Onc. Biol. Phys. *2*:1007, 1977.

25. Page, V., Gardner, A., and Karzmark, C.J.: Physical and dosimetric aspects of the radiotherapy of malignant lymphomas. II. The inverted-Y technique. Radiology *96*:619, 1970.

26. Graves, R.C. and Militzer, R.E.: Carcinoma of the prostate with metastases. J. Urol. *33*:235, 1935.

27. Ray, G.R., and Bagshaw, M.A.: The role of radiation therapy in the definitive treatment of adenocarcinoma of the protstate. Annu. Rev. Med. *26*:567, 1975.

Chapter 14

TREATMENT TECHNIQUES OF TESTIS TUMORS

Robert L. White
John G. Maier

Testis tumors are the most common solid tumor in men between the ages of 15 and 34 years of age; however, the incidence of only 2.1 per 100,000 males makes these tumors rare. Testis tumors are rarely found in American blacks. They are also rare in Africa, Asia, and New Zealand. There is a high incidence of testis tumors found in undescended testis (1 in 20 with abdominal testes vs. 1 in 80 with inguinal testes). There is a high frequency of testis tumors in identical twins and members of the same family.

It has been shown that treatment of testicular tumors with megavoltage radiation in conjunction with surgery (and chemotherapy when indicated) improves disease-free survival and produces long-term cures. Suspected germ-cell tumors of the testis require initial treatment with inguinal orchiectomy and high ligation of the spermatic cord. The use of radiation in testicular carcinomas and seminomas is especially well documented in the early stages of the tumor, and has produced high percentages of disease-free survival and essentially no complications when treatment is properly administered. When combined with other treatment modalities (e.g., more extensive surgery and multiple-agent chemotherapy), radiation-treatment techniques take on a new air of importance. Disease-free survival is not the only parameter of importance; morbidity of treatment, mortality of treatment, quality of disease-free survival, and cost to the patient are also important. The best method of treatment is the treatment that produces the highest chance of cure, at the lowest cost, with the lowest chance of short-term or long-term side-effects and complications.

DETERMINATION OF DISEASE EXTENT AND VOLUME

It is extremely important to evaluate the extent of the disease on the first examination of the patient. This evaluation should determine prognosis as well as define the appropriate method of management. Several staging systems are available but each has some limitations. One of the earliest staging systems for testis tumors[1] was developed in Great Britain as follows:

Stage I—Tumor confined to the testis

Stage II—Tumor confined to testis and lymph nodes below the diaphragm

Stage III—Mediastinal or supraclavicular nodal metastases with primary testis tumor

Stage IV—Primary tumor with extra-lymphatic spread

A staging system used at Walter Reed General Hospital[2] combines clinical, radiologic, and surgicopathologic findings. Clinical Stage I is similar to Stage I in the British classification, but it is subdivided into IA and IB when patients undergo retroperitoneal lymphadenectomy. In this system, IA indicates the absence of microscopic metastases in the lymph nodes below the diaphragm and IB indicates the presence of microscopic metastases. This system was the first to correlate clinical and surgicopathologic staging and to allow some comparison between the results of radiation and surgical treatment. More recently, at the M.D. Anderson Hospital, Hussey et al.[3] have subdivided Clinical Stage II patients into those with small or moderate retroperitoneal metastases (Stage IIA) and those with massive retroperitoneal involvement (Stage IIB).

A tumor-nodes-metastases (TNM) definition has been offered by the Union Internationale Contre Le Cancer (UICC)[4] and the American Joint Committee on Cancer Staging and End Results Reporting (AJC).[5] A comparison of these three staging systems is shown in Table 14–1.

Although all three staging systems are useful, there are limitations to each. In the TNM system, the extent of tumor involvement in the case of seminoma often does not correlate well with ultimate prognosis. In the absence of nodal metastases or distant metastases, the prognosis is excellent regardless of the tumor stage. In the evaluation of nodal involvement, a more specific definition is needed for nonsurgical assessment, which should include lymphangiograms, CT scans, and ultrasonography. In considering distant metastases or organomegaly, the presence or absence of tumor markers (α-fetoprotein—α-FP, β-human chorionic gonadotropin—β-HCG) must be taken into account both pre- and postorchiectomy. The specific organ involved and the degree of involvement by metastatic disease is an important consid-

eration (e.g., small metastatic nodules in the lung respond very well to current chemotherapy). Bulky liver metastases have a poor prognosis. All of these factors need to be accounted for in the staging method if we attempt to compare different treatment modalities.

The physician must make a complete history and physical examination of all patients with a positive testicular examination (see Box). Preliminary tests should include complete blood-count and liver-function tests. Primary testis tumors must be distinguished from inflammatory conditions of the testis and epididymis as well as nonspecific epididymitis and orchitis. All masses suspected of tumor must undergo an inguinal orchiectomy with high ligation of the spermatic cord for final diagnosis. Needle or incisional biopsy through the scrotum is not recommended because of a 25% chance of tumor growth along the needle tract.

Diagnostic Workup for Testicular Tumor Patient

1. Complete history and physical examination
2. Complete blood count
3. Liver chemistries
4. Serum α-FP and β-HCG prior to removal of primary tumor mass
5. Serum α-FP and β-HCG 5 to 7 days after removal of primary tumor mass
6. Establishment of tumor pathology
7. Chest radiograph
8. Chest tomography where indicated
9. Intravenous pyelography
10. Bilateral pedal lymphangiography
11. Abdominal CT scan
12. Thoracic CT scan when appropriate

A chest radiograph is necessary to determine whether pulmonary or mediastinal metastasis is present. Full-lung and mediastinal tomography is of questionable value; however, one report[6] indicates that an additional 3% to 4% of patients with pulmonary metastases were found using full-lung and mediastinal tomography when none were seen in routine chest radiographs.

Diagnosis is made by inguinal orchiec-

TABLE 14–1. Staging Systems Testis Tumors

Walter Reed General Hospital	UICC		American Joint Committee	
Stage IA. Tumor confined to one testis; no clinical or roentgenographic evidence of spread by excretory or retrograde urography, lymphangiography, inferior venacavography, or chest roentgenography	T—	Primary Tumor	T—	Primary Tumor
	TX	The minimum requirements to assess fully the extent of the primary tumor cannot be met	TX	Minimum requirements cannot be met (in the absence of orchiectomy, TX must be used)
	T0	No evidence of primary tumor	T0	No evidence of primary tumor
	T1	Tumor limited to the body of the testis	T1	Limited to body of testis
	T2	Tumor extending beyond the tunica albuginea	T2	Extends beyond the tunica albuginea
	T3	Tumor involving the rete testis or epididymis	T3	Involvement of the rete testis or epididymis
	T4	Tumor invading the spermatic cord and/or scrotal wall		
	T4a	Invasion of spermatic cord	T4a	Invasion of spermatic cord
	T4b	Invasion of scrotal wall	T4b	Invasion of scrotal wall
	N—	Regional and Juxtaregional Lymph Nodes	N—	Nodal Involvement
Stage IB. Histologic evidence of metastases to the iliac or para-aortic lymph nodes	NX	The minimum requirements to assess the regional lymph nodes cannot be met	NX	Minimum requirements cannot be met
	N0	No evidence of involvement of regional lymph nodes	N0	No evidence of involvement of regional lymph nodes
Stage II. Clinical or roentgenographic evidence of metastases to femoral, inguinal, iliac, or para-aortic lymph nodes with no evidence of metastases to lymphatics above the diaphragm or to visceral organs	N1	Involvement of a single homolateral regional lymph node, which, if inguinal, is mobile	N1	Involvement of a single homolateral regional lymph node which, if inguinal, is mobile
	N2	Involvement of contralateral or bilateral or multiple regional lymph nodes, which, if inguinal, are mobile	N2	Involvement of contralateral or bilateral or multiple regional lymph nodes which, if inguinal, are mobile
	N3	A palpable abdominal mass is present or there are fixed inguinal lymph nodes	N3	Palpable abdominal mass present or fixed inguinal lymph nodes
	N4	Involvement of juxtaregional lymph nodes	N4	Involvement of juxtaregional nodes
Stage III. Clinical or roentgenographic evidence of metastases above the diaphragm or to visceral organs	M—	Distant Metastases	M—	Distant Metastasis
	MX	The minimum requirements to assess the presence of distant metastases cannot be met	MX	Not assessed
			M0	No known distant metastasis
	M0	No evidence of distant metastases	M1	Distant metastasis present
	M1	Distant metastases present	Specify sites according to the following notations:	
	M1a	Evidence of occult metastases based on biochemical and/or other tests	Pulmonary—PUL Osseous—OSS Hepatic—HEP Brain—BRA	
	M1b	Single metastasis in a single organ site	Lymph Nodes—LYM Bone Marrow—MAR	
	M1c	Multiple metastases in a single organ site	Pleura—PLE Skin—SKI	
	M1d	Metastases in multiple organ sites	Eye—EYE Other—OTH	

tomy of the involved testis through an inguinal incision resecting the entire testis as well as the distal extent of the spermatic cord. The patient requires staging with base-line-marker levels, α-FP, and β-HCG radioimmunoassay. These should be obtained both prior to and after surgery before starting chemotherapy and irradiation treatment. Lymphangiography outlines para-aortic and pelvic lymph nodes below the diaphragm; the dye can be followed through the mediastinum into the thoracic duct. The thoracic duct empties to the left of the spinal cord 90% of the time and to the right 10% of the time. The primary lymph-node receptacles are found near L2 on the left and, usually, between L1 and L3 on the right. Crossover drainage usually occurs from the right to the left, but may occur either way. Retrograde filling of the para-aortic lymph nodes has also been documented. Four to eight collecting lymphatic vessels drain from the hilum by way of the spermatic cord through the inguinal ring along the course of the right and left testicular veins. These lymphatic vessels empty into nodes related to the aorta and inferior vena cava at the levels described above. The rightmost of the draining nodes are lateral, anterior, and medial to the inferior vena cava and anterior to the aorta. On the left, most of the draining nodes are lateral and anterior to the aorta. In the normal young adult male there are 50 to 75 lymph nodes between the bifurcation of the aorta and the renal pedicles. Contralateral drainage commonly occurs above the level of the renal veins.

Intravenous pyelography is necessary in patients receiving abdominal lymph-node irradiation. It is important to document the position of the kidneys and the course of the ureters. Patients who have horseshoe kidneys, pelvic kidneys, or no kidney must be identified; appropriate changes in the dose and volume for treatment must be made.

Abdominal and thoracic CT scans have become an important part of the diagnostic workup for patients with testicular tumors. CT scans are recommended for all patients, as is lymphangiography as a complementary study. We have had experiences where lymphangiography was positive and CT scans were negative and vice versa. If the abdominal studies are negative for disease below the diaphragm, and the chest radiograph is negative, there is no need for CT scans above the diaphragm. If, however, disease above the diaphragm is suspected, CT scans are useful in determining the volume, extent of disease, and treatment planning. It must be emphasized that CT scans have not replaced the need for lymphangiography, even if CT scans are to be used for computer planning of treatment portals. Our experience has been that several patients were subsequently found to have abdominal metastasis in spite of a negative abdominal CT scan.

A history of pelvic infection or of previous pelvic surgery is important to know before treatment-volume planning is undertaken. Herniorrhaphy, orchiopexy, appendectomy, and vasectomy, as well as pelvic infection, may reroute lymph drainage through the subcutaneous lymphatic vessels of the inferior-anterior abdominal wall into contralateral iliac nodes. The epididymis drains into the ipsilateral iliac nodes; the lymph drainage of the scrotal skin and subcutaneous tissue is into inguinal and iliac nodes.

There is no need to do a bone scan, brain scan, or liver scan unless the patient has specific signs of symptoms that warrant these diagnostic studies.

TREATMENT PLAN

After all of the diagnostic and staging procedures have been performed, the treatment-planning process can begin. All of the radiographs and scans that have been made of the patient should be visible to the radiation oncologist at the time of treatment simulation. It is helpful if the patient has recently had the lymphangiogram; the contrast material in the lymphatics will appear on the simulation radiographs if they are taken immediately following the lymphangiogram. All known or suspected disease sites must be included in the treatment ports. This must be verified on simulation films. The treatment plan should follow the disease as it would progress through the lymphatic system.[7]

For a patient that has not had prior pelvic surgery or infection, the first area of lymph drainage is to the perirenal and para-aortic lymph nodes. Lymph nodes at risk of harboring microscopic disease include the ipsilateral pelvic nodes (i.e., internal and external iliac and common iliac). If the patient has had prior pelvic surgery or infection, or if there is known or suspected disease below the diaphragm, the entire ipsilateral and contralateral pelvic lymph-node system is at risk and must be treated. The lower portal margin should be located at the inferior margin of the pubis. The medial margin should be to the midline, unless the entire pelvis is to be treated. The lateral margin should be at least 1 cm or 2 cm lateral to the pelvic outlet. The exact lateral extent of the pelvic portion of the portal is determined by the location of the pelvic lymph nodes seen on lymphangiography and the CT scan. It is not necessary to irradiate the inguinal and femoral lymph nodes unless disease is suspected; nor is it necessary to irradiate the inguinal surgical incision unless it is clinically involved. It is also not necessary to include the ipsilateral scrotum, unless there are specific indications for it (e.g., history of testicular needle biopsy or of scrotal surgical approach). The treatment portal should taper as the sacrum is irradiated; the midline margin should include the contralateral common iliac nodes. The aorta bifurcates at the fourth and fifth lumbar interspace. Above the L4 level the portal can be symmetrical and can include all of the para-aortic lymph nodes. If there is no known disease below the diaphragm, the width of the para-aortic portion of the treatment portal is usually 9 cm wide; there are 4 cm beyond the midline on the contralateral side and 5 cm beyond the midline on the ipsilateral side. If the patient has known or suspected disease below the diaphragm, a 9-cm-wide portal in the perirenal, para-aortic area will not necessarily be wide enough to cover all of the areas at risk. The lymphangiogram and

the abdominal CT scan are critically important at this time in helping to determine that all suspected disease sites are irradiated even if part of the kidney must be included. The upper border of the portal should be at the top of the eleventh thoracic vertebra.

The configuration of the treatment portal below the diaphragm would be:

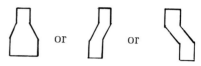

depending on the aforementioned configuration of disease or history of prior surgery or infection. Daily treatment should be given 5 days per week with both parallel-opposed portals treated each day. Daily dose fractions of 160 to 200 rad should be administered to the midline. For patients with seminoma, total doses of 2000 to 3000 rad should be given to areas of suspected or microscopic disease. If disease is known to be present below the diaphragm (from lymphangiogram or CT scan), total doses of 3500 to 4500 rad should be given to the areas of involvement using cone-down techniques. The total dose to any area of known disease should never exceed 5000 rad for patients with seminoma.

The question of prophylactic irradiation of the mediastinum and supraclavicular lymph-node areas has been discussed at length in the literature. It is our opinion that all seminoma patients should receive treatment to the areas of possible microscopic involvement.

After the patient completes the course of treatment for disease located below the diaphragm, a short rest period of no treatment can be prescribed of up to 2 weeks. The patient then should return for treatment planning for disease located above the diaphragm. When using a treatment-planning simulator, the inferior portal margin can be set to abut the inferior portal margin at the depth of the spinal cord, at the bottom of the tenth thoracic vertebra. If a simulator is not used, then a calculated gap on the skin can be used so that there is no overlap of the diaphragm portals above or below the level of the spinal cord. The usual width of the portal is 9 cm, centered over the spine. The upper border is the sternal notch. If disease is suspected, appropriately altered portals should be arranged for the patient based on findings from the chest radiographs or thoracic CT scan.

A small supraclavicular portal should also be used to treat the patient receiving mediastinal irradiation. Ninety percent of patients have drainage of the thoracic duct on the left. The drainage pattern can be documented at the time of lymphangiography if a chest radiograph is taken during the time of radiographic dye application. If the patient's thoracic duct drains bilaterally, or if the drainage pattern is unknown, then both the right and left supraclavicular areas should be irradiated. The supraclavicular portal is small, usually measuring 5 cm × 5 cm and is located lateral to the spinal cord and just above the insertion of the clavicle and the sternomastoid muscle. This field can only be treated from the anterior portal with the dose calculated to a depth of 3 cm. Because the spinal cord is not in the irradiation field, there is no need for concern about the gap between the mediastinal port and the supraclavicular port as there is about the gap between the abdominal port and mediastinal port.

When the dose is kept between 2000 and 2500 rad and techniques of daily treatment of both posterior-anterior and anterior-posterior portals are used, the adverse side-effects are minimal (i.e., limited to mild esophagitis and occasional nausea during and immediately after treatment). Patients with known disease below the diaphragm or above the diaphragm require mediastinal and supraclavicular treatment. When disease is found above the diaphragm, doses of 3500 to 4500 rad should be administered to the areas of involvement using cone-down techniques.

SPECIAL PROBLEMS

Doses for definitive treatment are higher for mixed-histology cases and for testicular carcinoma than the dose for germinoma. Doses in the para-aortic area are carried to limits of 4000 to 5000 rad. Treatment techniques should always include daily treatment of anterior and posterior fields.

When using radiation in combination with surgery or chemotherapy, several techniques appear to produce good results. Sandwich techniques, in which 2000 to 3000 rad are given prior to surgery and an additional postoperative irradiation dose is given to a combined dose of no more than 5000 rad, have produced excellent results.

Prophylactic elective mediastinal and supraclavicular irradiation is not indicated with testicular carcinomas because of the adverse side-effects seen with the higher doses of radiation necessary to sterilize these epithelial tumors.

During treatment, the patients need to have a port radiograph taken if a simulator has been used to set up the portals. During the course of treatment, it is advisable to obtain periodic verification radiographs and to check the radiographs to verify the daily reproduction of the treatment volume. Weekly complete blood counts are important because a considerable volume of bone marrow is included in the treatment volume. If the patient has a bulky tumor mass, special attention must be paid to the level of uric acid in the serum.

It is desirable to have patients treated on equipment that can encompass all areas below the diaphragm in one large contiguous portal, rather than small adjoining portals. This minimizes the risk of overlapping fields, which can result in over- or underdosing.

If one of the testicles has been excised, protection of the remaining testicle from scattered radiation is very important for testicular tumor patients, many of whom are young and desirous of fathering children. Because the definitive dose for treatment of seminoma is low, this is not usually a problem. Shielding of the remaining testicle is of marginal value because most of the scattered radiation to the testicle is along the body axis. The limitation of the thickness of the shielding material that can be physically used does little to attenuate a high-energy beam. It is still felt to be helpful, however, to shield the remaining testis.

REFERENCES

1. Smithers, D.W., Wallace, E.N., and Wallace, D.M.: Radiotherapy for patients with tumors of the testicle. Br. J. Urol. 43:83, 1971.

2. Maier, J.G. and Mittemeyer, B.T.: Carcinoma of the testis. Cancer 39:981, 1977.

3. Hussey, D.H., Luk, K.H., and Johnson, D.E.: The role of radiation therapy in the treatment of germinal cell tumors of the testis other than pure seminoma. Radiology 123:175, 1977.

4. T.N.M. Classification for Malignant Tumors. Geneva, Union Internationale Contre le Cancer, 1968.

5. Manual for staging of cancer. Chicago, American Joint Committee for Cancer Staging and End Results Reporting, 1978.

6. Sindelar, W.F., Bafley, D.H., Felix, E., Doppman, J.L., and Ketcham, A.S.: Lung tomography in cancer patients: Full tomograms in screening for pulmonary metastases. JAMA 240:2060, 1978.

7. Garnick, M.B., Prout, G.R., Jr., and Canelles, G.P.: Germinal tumors of the testis. In Cancer Medicine, 2nd ed. Edited by J.F. Holland and E. Frei III. Philadelphia, Lea and Febiger, 1982.

Chapter 15

TECHNIQUES FOR THE EXTERNAL BEAM IRRADIATION OF PATIENTS WITH CARCINOMA OF THE URINARY BLADDER

William U. Shipley
Miriam Gitterman

Modern megavoltage radiation can be curative treatment for a minority of patients with invasive carcinoma of the bladder while preserving bladder, and, in men, sexual function. The incidence of moderate to major complications in such treatment has been acceptable, although the survival rates of patients treated (with 6000–7000 rad in 6–8 weeks) is disappointingly low (19%–33% at 5 years—Table 15–1). Current reports indicate an apparent superiority of preoperative radiation therapy and cystectomy compared to radiation therapy alone in patients with muscle-invading operable bladder carcinoma.[2,3,8,16] This apparent improved survival (36%–46% at 5 years), in the one large randomized prospective trial that has been performed, was not found in patients who were over 65 years old;[16] thus, many patients who present with clinically localized invasive primary carcinoma of the bladder and who are not suitable for cystectomy (because of advanced age, of inoperability due to locally advanced tumor, or for other medical or personal reasons) should be seriously considered for definitive external-beam irradiation as the alternative curative procedure.

The technique used in radiation therapy can, as in surgery, significantly influence patient tolerance and the likelihood of an uncomplicated recovery. The radiation technique used is important both in assuring that the tumor volume is in the treatment or high-dose volume and that the treatment volume is designed to include the minimal amount of normal tissue. Tissues often unnecessarily included in the high-dose volume include the anterior abdominal-wall structures, the tissues anterior to the external iliac and common iliac lymph nodes, the anus, the posterior rectal wall, and the structures further posterior. The external-beam techniques presented in this chapter are employed in curative radiation therapy administered either preoperatively or as definitive treatment for patients with muscle-invading bladder tumors as well as in palliative irradiation for patients in whom cure is not possible but for whom the aim is to relieve symptomatic hematuria or pain.

Supported by grants from the U.S.P.H.S., National Cancer Institute (Nos. CA18032 and 15944), National Bladder Cancer Collaborative Group A, (Massachusetts General Hospital).

TABLE 15–1. Bladder Cancer: Definitive Irradiation.

Report	Treatment	Clinical Stage	No. of Patients	5-Year-Survival Rate (Determinate)	Local Failure	Complications
Houston Study[1,2]	7000 rad**	T_3 (randomized trial)	32	22%	—	—
Houston Study	7000 rad	T_3 (all patients)	75	19%	39%	15%
Stanford Study[3]	7000 rad**	T_3	218	28%*	—	—
Stanford Study	7000 rad	T_1–T_4 (including 65 Stage T_4 patients)	384	—	49%	8%
London Study[4] (randomized trial)	6000 rad**	T_3	85	23%*	not reported	not reported
Hammersmith[5] Hospital	4250 rad (20 × 212 rad)	T_3	45	28%	62%	10%
	5000 rad (20 × 250 rad)	T_3	40	33%	45%	16%

*actuarial calculation
**usually 200 rad/fraction; salvage cystectomy in selected patients

DETERMINATION OF THE TUMOR EXTENT (CLINICAL STAGING)

In addition to history and physical examination, essential diagnostic evaluations for patients with bladder carcinoma are: endoscopy, transurethral biopsy and usually fulguration, bimanual examination under anesthesia before and after transurethral resections, excretory urogram, and histologic evaluation of the tumor for the extent (depth) of the invasion. Other necessary evaluations include chest radiograph, bone scan, and histologic review of selected mucosal biopsies of clinically uninvolved areas of the bladder. Lymphangiograms and possibly computerized tomography (CT) may be helpful in evaluating possible metastatic spread in and beyond the pelvic lymph nodes. This could be important because, in patients with evidence of tumor spread to the lymph nodes at or above the bifurcation of common iliac vessels, cure by local-regional therapy (either preoperative radiation therapy and radical cystectomy or definitive radiation therapy alone) is not likely. Radiographically positive or suspicious studies should be confirmed by "skinny" needle biopsy. Even an unsubstantiated abnormal lymphogram at or above the common iliac vessels carries a very grave prognosis (10% 5-year-survival rate) for patients treated with preoperative radiation therapy and cystectomy.[15]

The American Joint Committee (AJC) Classification of the Clinical-Diagnostic Staging of the Primary Tumor is detailed in Table 15–2.[1] The AJC staging system differs slightly from the UICC system in that pathologic proof of muscle invasion is required for stages cT2–4. It is often not possible to discriminate between stages cT3a and cT3b because the tissue excised by transurethral resection often does not include perivesicle fat. Although evidence of ureteral obstruction on the excretory urogram is a poor prognostic sign, it is not

TABLE 15–2. AJC Classification of Clinical-Diagnostic Staging of the Primary Tumor.

GO	Papilloma
cTX	Minimum requirements for classification cannot be met
cTO	No evidence of primary tumor
cTIS	Sessile carcinoma *in situ*
cTa	Papillary noninvasive carcinoma
cT1	Carcinoma with microscopic evidence of invasion of the lamina propria, but not beyond. On bimanual examination prior to transurethral resection, a freely mobile mass may be felt. This mass should not be felt after complete transurethral resection of the lesion.
cT2	Microscopic evidence of invasion of superficial muscle of bladder. On bimanual examination prior to transurethral resection there may be induration of the bladder wall, which is mobile. There is no residual induration after complete transurethral resection of the lesion.
cT3	On bimanual examination prior to transurethral resection, there is induration of the bladder wall, or a nodular mobile mass is palpable in the bladder wall, which persists after transurethral resection.
cT3a	Microscopic evidence of invasion of muscle, but not beyond.
cT3b	Microscopic evidence of invasion of perivesical fat.
cT4	Tumor fixed or invading neighboring structures and there is microscopic evidence of muscle invasion.
cT4a	Tumor invading substance of prostate (histologically proven), uterus, or vagina
cT4b	Tumor fixed to the pelvic wall and/or infiltrating the abdominal wall.

The suffix 'm' should be added to the appropriate T category to indicate multiple lesions.

included in the criteria used for the TNM staging systems.

Treatment discussions and planning for patients undergoing definitive irradiation for bladder cancer are optimized if both the radiation therapist and the urologist are present at the initial endoscopic and bimanual evaluation, which is done when the patient is under anesthesia. However, the radiation therapist often is not able to be present nor to repeat the cystoscopy and therefore several additional evaluations other than the diagnostic tests listed above can be helpful in determining the tumor target volume. The first is to ask the referring urologist to complete a diagram

FEMALE

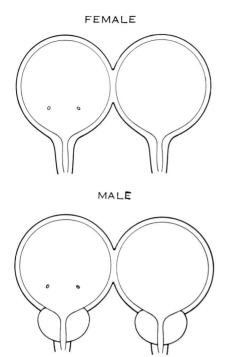

MALE

Fig. 15–1. Diagrams for tumor mapping. The bladder is bivalved in the coronal plane with hinge on the patient's left.

of his endoscopic findings and biopsy sites. Figure 15–1 is such a diagram prepared by the National Bladder Cancer Collaborative Group A (NBCCGA) for their clinical protocols.[11,12] The second evaluation is a rectal examination in men or a pelvic examination in women, which often allows identification of tumor extent either of a supraprostatic mass in the male or of a periurethral mass in the female. Thirdly, evaluation of the anterior-posterior (AP) and lateral cystogram done at the time of treatment simulation can, in conjunction with the above information, be quite helpful. With these evaluations and the use of the 4-field box technique described below, computerized tomography (CT) usually adds very little information for radiation treatment planning.[5] This, however, has not been the case for institutions that use a 3-field (one anterior and two posterior-oblique fields) technique.[6]

TREATMENT SIMULATION

Following a thorough clinical evaluation and agreement with the referring urologist on a patient's clinical stage and method of treatment, treatment simulation is the next therapeutic step. Treatment simulation is essential in determining the optimal positioning of the treatment beams with respect to the patient. The purpose of the simulation is to select the smallest possible treatment volume for the specific tumor volume. The procedure of simulation at Massachusetts General Hospital can be divided into five steps (this should take approximately 60 minutes of a physician's time, provided he has the assistance of a skilled radiographic technician).

Preparation

The patient's bladder must be catheterized to introduce a small amount of contrast medium. The patient should void just before catheterization to identify a postvoid residual, if one is present. The patient should also void just prior to daily treatment to minimize the bladder-tumor volume. Because the bladder is to be treated when it is empty, only 25 ml of iodinated dye (Cysto Contray 2, manufactured by Mallinckott, Inc.) and 20 ml of air are routinely introduced. If the patient has a significant postvoid residual, more dye is proportionally introduced. The patient is then transferred to the simulator couch and a small rectal tube inserted. The patient is placed in the supine position and adjusted so that the pelvis is straight, relative to the axes of the treatment couch. With isocentric treatment planning, the patient should not change position until the whole simulation process is finished.

Design of the Anterior and Posterior Fields

The 4-field box technique with shaping corner blocks is preferred for the treatment of all patients with bladder carcinoma. The first step in field definition is to define fluoroscopically the superior, inferior, and lateral borders of the anterior and posterior fields. These borders vary with the clinical stage of the tumor. However, once these borders are set, the isocenter has been defined in both the longitudinal and latitudinal axes. For this localization film, the isocenter is placed in the midcoronal plane of the patient. The anterior-field isocenter and margins are marked on the patient.

Design of the Paired Right and Left Lateral Fields

At this time, about 50 ml of dilute barium is introduced into the rectal catheter without motion of the patient. The simulator gantry is moved to the right lateral position and the patient is fluoroscoped to define the anterior border of the lateral field. In most patients, the air bubble can be seen in the anterior tip of the bladder. The barium in the rectum and the dye in the posterior bladder are rarely seen fluoroscopically. A field width of 12.5 cm to 13.5 cm at isocenter is selected, depending to some degree on patient and bladder shape, and a film is taken. The bladder-tumor volume is drawn on that film. The pertinent data used to draw this bladder-tumor volume include information from the pelvic and rectal examinations, the excretory urogram, the bimanual examination under anesthesia, and the diagram of the endoscopically visible lesions, as well as the histopathologic findings. The posterior border of the field should be 2.0 cm to 2.5 cm posterior to the most posterior point in the tumor volume to assure adequate coverage. After making the necessary changes in the posterior border of the field as described, the gantry is rotated 180° and a treatment simulation of the left lateral field is performed.

We have found a systematic difficulty with the position of the lateral isocenters in the anterior to posterior axis because of the difference between the treatment couch of the simulator and those of our linear accelerators. When a patient is placed on the skin-sparing window of the treatment couch (either a "tennis racket" nylon-strung grid or a mylar window), his buttocks are depressed below the plane of the table by 0.5 cm to 1.0 cm. Because this is different than the perfectly flat simulator couch, the tattooed lateral isocenters are systematically off by this amount. The solution we have used for this problem is to not place patients on the skin-sparing window when the lateral fields are treated. This is practical because very satisfactory dose distributions can be achieved by treating only 2 parallel opposed fields each treatment session; thus, a patient is, during any given treatment session, either treated by an anterior-posterior pair on the nylon grid or by a right and left lateral pair without the nylon grid.

Field Marking

Following confirmation of the positions of the desired borders of the anterior and the two lateral fields on the simulator radiograph, the isocenters of these fields are marked, with appropriate aseptic technique, by a small intradermal tattoo. The borders of the fields are drawn on the patient's surface with ink. The corner blocks are drawn on as indicated by the physician. On the anterior and posterior fields, the right and left corner blocks should be symmetrical so that, with isocentric rotation from the anterior to the posterior field, the shaping blocks do not have to be moved.

Treatment-Plan Generation

The medical physicist obtains a transverse contour through the isocenters and another one 3 cm caudad for subsequent cone-down plans. The physican draws, with appropriate demagnification from the lateral and anterior simulation films, the bladder, the bladder-tumor volume, and the rectum on the contour. Such measurements are always taken relative to the isocenter to avoid problems of parallax.

After discussion of the patient's problem with the clinical physicist, the treatment plans are generated with appropriate weighting of the (AP–PA) pairs to the lateral fields, depending on the clinical situation. Considerations of differential-field weighting are discussed in the section on the definitive treatment of patients with bladder carcinoma.

PREOPERATIVE RADIATION THERAPY

Preoperative irradiation and radical cystectomy is the present standard treatment at Massachusetts General Hospital for patients with localized, muscle-invading bladder carcinoma who are otherwise medically and psychologically suitable for this form of aggressive therapy. Recent series reporting the results of preoperative

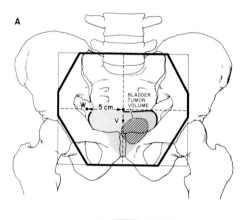

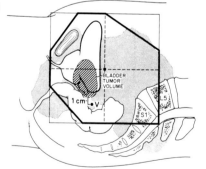

Fig. 15–2. Radiation treatment fields to the bladder-tumor volume and the pelvic lymph nodes for 4–25 MV x-rays from an isocentric linear accelerator with the 4-field box technique. *(A)* anterior and posterior fields *(B)* paired lateral fields.

irradiation and simple or radical cystectomy from either Phase-II or Phase-III trials suggest improved local tumor control and patient survival when compared to definitive radiation therapy alone.[2,3,4,8,12,16]

The rationale for preoperative radiation therapy for patients with cT2–4 operable primary bladder carcinoma is: 1) to prevent tumor seeding at the time of cystectomy, 2) to sterilize subclinical microaggregates of tumor left beyond the limits of the surgical resection, and 3) to allow pathologic down-staging as an important prognostic criterion. The radiation dose and treatment volume should not increase surgical morbidity. The target volume for the adjuvant preoperative radiation therapy should be the entire bladder-tumor volume, the pelvic lymph nodes (the hypogastric, external iliac, and distal common-iliac lymph-nodal groups), and in the male, the prostatic urethra.

The treatment fields for the 4-field box technique are shown in Figure 15–2. Point V is 1.0 cm posterior to the most posterior portion of bladder mucosa, outlined by the cystogram, or 1 cm posterior to the posterior base of the tumor volume, if it is determined to extend farther posteriorly by pelvic or rectal examination or other available diagnostic information. The pelvic sidewall (point W) is 5.0 cm lateral to the isocenter. All 4 fields extend inferiorly to the caudal pole of the obturator foramen (to include the obturator and perivesicle nodes and, in the male, the prostatic urethra) and superiorly to cover the inferior portion of L5 (about 2–3 cm above the bifurcation of the common iliac vessels). The anterior and posterior fields are shaped with inferior corner blocks, which should shield the medial border of the femoral heads. The anterior and posterior fields should extend 1.5 cm to 2.0 cm lateral to the bony margin of the pelvis at its widest point to cover the external iliac nodes. The superior corners should be shaped with blocks 2-cm to 3-cm thick on a side.

The anterior boundaries of the lateral fields should be 1.5 cm to 2.0 cm anterior to the most anterior portion of the bladder mucosa seen on air-contrast cystogram, or 1 cm anterior to the anterior tip of the symphysis, whichever is more anterior. Posteriorly, the field should extend 2.0 cm to 2.5 cm posterior to point V (see Fig. 15–2). This posterior border is usually at or just posterior to the S1-S2 junction on their anterior surface. The height of such lateral fields is usually 11.5 cm to 13.5 cm at isocenter. Inferiorly, these lateral fields should be shaped with corner blocks to block the tissues outside the symphysis and to block the entire anal canal. Superiorly, these lateral fields should be blocked anteriorly to exclude any portion of the bowel and anterior rectus fascia that are anterior to the external iliac lymph nodal groups (see Fig. 15–2). Wedges (usually 15°) should be considered as compensators for lateral fields if the transverse contour has a significant slope anteriorly.[6] The weighting of the AP–PA to lateral fields should be 1:1 for treatment energies of 4 MV to 6 MV and about 1:2 for treatment energies of 10 MV to 25 MV.

In a recent NBCCGA trial, we delivered 4000 rad as twenty 180-rad fractions and two 200-rad fractions in a 4½-week period followed by prompt (usually within 15 days) one-stage radical cystectomy and urinary diversion. Depending on the field size and the position of point V, the dose is usually prescribed to the 95% to 98% isodose line with dose normalization to 100% at the isocenter. Should the general treatment plan be other than prompt cystectomy, the dose should be at the 4500 to 5000 rad level with conventional fractionation as has been reported by several institutions.[2,8,9]

The physician must occasionally consider treating a patient with a form of "quick" preoperative irradiation prior to radical cystectomy and urinary diversion for muscle-invading bladder carcinoma. The indications for this are relatively few but include significant uncontrolled hematuria, severe irritative symptoms, or pyelonephritis in an obstructive kidney not corrected by percutaneous nephrostomy. The rationale for preoperative radiation therapy is only to prevent the possibility of tumor seeding if this is the case. A dose of 1050 rad in three 350-rad daily fractions immediately prior to surgery should therefore be given; this has been shown to achieve this important clinical goal.[14] Such minimal preoperative radiation therapy would allow additional postoperative radiation therapy to be given should the patient be found to have a high (pT3b–4 or pN1–3) pathologic stage tumor. An additional dose of 3780 rad in twenty-one 180-rad daily fractions is recommended for patients with high pathologic stage tumors who have an uncomplicated recovery from surgery.

DEFINITIVE RADIATION THERAPY

Definitive external-beam irradiation, surveillance cystoscopy, and salvage cystectomy, if necessary, is a reasonable alternative to preoperative radiation therapy and cystectomy. The individual patient may be trading a 10% to 15% decrease in probability of 5-year survival for a life whose quality would likely be improved by the absence of a major surgical operation and the presence of considerable physiologic and functional deficits. Such risk/benefit considerations in lung carcinoma have attracted patients to the nonsurgical approach.[16] Characteristics that make patients more likely to be successfully controlled by definitive radiation include: (1) an invasive cancer; (2) a tumor mass, if palpable, of less than 2 cm in diameter following transurethral resection and no hydronephrosis; (3) pre-existing adequate bladder capacity without irritative symptoms; (4) a desire to maintain bladder and, in the male patient, sexual function; (5) the absence of any significant pre-existing pelvic inflammatory diseases of the colorectum or adnexa; (6) the willingness to undergo 7½ to 8 weeks of radiation treatment; (7) the willingness to undergo surveillance cystoscopies every 3 months for 2 years, and then every 6 months thereafter to detect tumor persistence, recurrence, or evolution of a new tumor; and (8) that as complete as possible a transurethral resection of the tumor has been accomplished.

The treatment plan, which has been well tolerated by patients with tumors of stage cT2–4NXMO, includes a dose of 5040 rad (in 5½ weeks at 180 rad per frac-

XRT PLANS FOR BOOST DOSE TO BLADDER CARCINOMA

10 MV X-RAYS

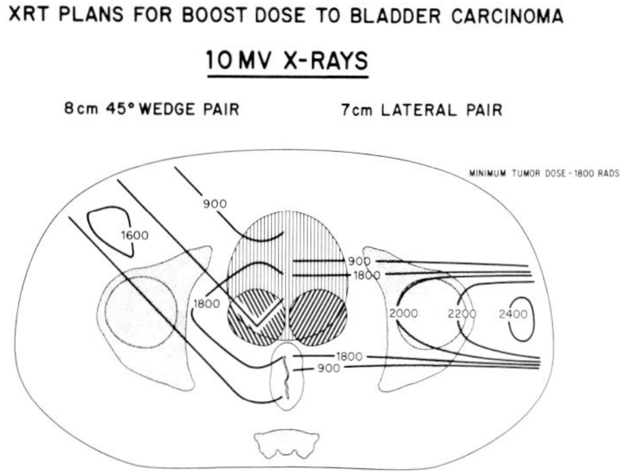

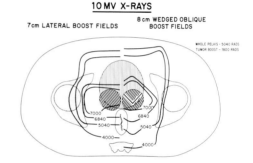

Fig. 15–5. Comparison of radiation dose distribution by 10-MV x-rays with either anterior-oblique-wedged-paired, or lateral-paired fields for boost treatment of tumor volume.

ISOCENTRIC FOUR-FIELD PELVIC XRT PLANS

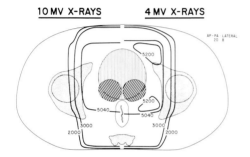

Fig. 15–3. Comparison of radiation dose distribution by 4 MV and 10 MV x-rays by an isocentric 4-field box technique for the treatment fields shown in Fig. 15–2.

LATERAL TUMOR BOOST FIELDS

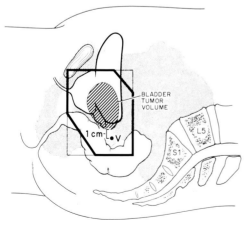

Fig. 15–4. Lateral radiation boost fields to the bladder-tumor volume with paired lateral fields by 10–45 MV x-rays.

DEFINITIVE XRT PLANS FOR T2-T3 BLADDER CARCINOMA

10 MV X-RAYS

Fig. 15–6. Comparison of the composite radiation treatment plans for the definitive irradiation by 10 MV x-rays of a T2–T3 bladder tumor with the whole pelvis treated as in Figs. 15–2 and 15–3 and the tumor boost given by either method shown in Fig. 15–5.

tion, 5 days per week), to fields as outlined in the section of this chapter on preoperative radiation therapy. Following this, a cone-down boost to the primary bladder-tumor volume is delivered at a dose of 6480 to 6840 rad in 7 to 7½ weeks. The weighting of the AP–PA and lateral field depends on the method of planned boost to the primary tumor volume in such a manner that the dose to the rectum and femoral heads is minimized. The AP–PA:lateral ratio of 20:8 seems optimal for beams of 4 MV to 10 MV if the cone-down irradiation is to be by anterior-paired oblique wedge fields, lateral arc rotation, or paired lateral fields (Fig. 15–3).

If the radiation therapist can be satisfied that the tumor is limited to one section of the bladder (usually in the trigone or posteriorly), then the boost (high-dose) volume may be designed to exclude the uninvolved areas of the bladder. This obviously requires close cooperation with the referring urologist and is greatly assisted by the diagram shown in Figure 15–1. If treatment beams of 10-MV x-rays or greater are available, cone-down irradiation by paired lateral fields is preferable because these lateral fields can have shaped corner blocks that further exclude uninvolved tissues from the high-dose region (Fig. 15–4). A comparison of the boost and composite-treatment plans for 10-MV linear-accelerator beams (Figs. 15–5 and 15–6) demonstrates that the high-dose treatment volume and the desired target volume can be closer to one another with the lateral fields. For these cone-down and composite-isodose plans, these doses have been usually normalized to the 95% to 97% line that is sufficiently outside the designated tumor volume to allow a satisfactory margin for day-to-day set-up variations in patient position. For lateral fields, this margin is 6 mm; for the oblique and lateral-arc fields, this margin is taken to be slightly greater because of the possibility of more variation in patient position and because it is more difficult to confirm field position by port films. All these plans are designed so that the composite dose to the femoral neck and femoral head is less than 5000 rad and the dose to the posterior half of the rectosigmoid is less than 6000 rad. In all these radiation dose distributions, the influence of shaping blocks is not included because such off-axis calculations would misrepresent the field width at isocenter. This specifically means that the dose expressed to the medial border of the acetabulum is less than is indicated because these are blocked on the paired anterior and posterior fields. This reduces the dose to the lateral border of the acetabulum, as ex-

pressed in these isodose distributions, by 2000 rad at a minimum (see Figs. 15–3, 15–6, 15–8 and 15–10).

Figures 15–7 and 15–8 show a comparison of the boost techniques and the composite treatment plan for treatment beams of 4 MV and 10 MV. The 120° arc rotation would seem to be the most desirable boost technique with the 4-MV accelerator. Figure 15–9 compares the lateral boost plan and the composite plan for 10-MV and 25-MV beams. Relatively little advantage is seen for the higher-energy beam when these 4-field techniques are employed (Fig. 15–10). Some advantage to the 25-

XRT PLANS FOR BOOST DOSE TO BLADDER CARCINOMA

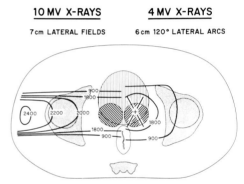

Fig. 15–7. Comparison of radiation-dose distribution for boost treatment to the tumor volume by either 10 MV x-rays (lateral fields) or 4 MV x-rays (120° lateral arc rotation).

DEFINITIVE XRT PLANS FOR T2-T3 BLADDER CARCINOMA

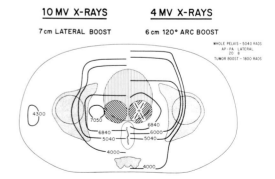

Fig. 15–8. Comparison of the composite treatment plans for the definitive irradiation of T2–T3 bladder carcinoma by 10 MV x-rays (Figs. 15–3, 15–4 and 15–7) or 4 MV x-rays (Figs. 15–3 and 15–7).

XRT PLANS FOR BOOST DOSE TO BLADDER CARCINOMA

10 MV X-RAYS   25 MV X-RAYS

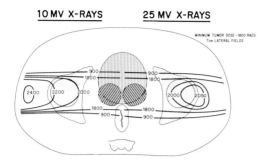

Fig. 15–9. Comparison of the radiation dose distributions for boost treatments to the bladder tumor volume with paired lateral fields (Fig. 15–4) by either 10 or 25 MV x-rays.

ISOCENTRIC FOUR-FIELD PELVIC XRT PLANS

10 MV X-RAYS   25 MV X-RAYS

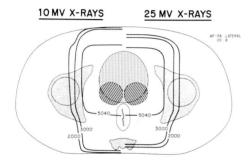

Fig. 15–10. Comparison of the radiation dose distribution for the treatment of the bladder-tumor volume and the pelvic lymph nodes with a 4-field box technique (Fig. 15–2) by either 10 or 25 MV x-rays.

MV beam would be clearly seen had the model patient been considerably larger than average.

PALLIATIVE IRRADIATION

Not infrequently, patients with advanced bladder carcinoma are referred for external-beam radiation therapy to palliate otherwise uncontrolled hematuria. For these patients, it may be necessary to treat over a Foley catheter, which is often necessary for 3-way irrigation. Under these circumstances, treatment fields that generously cover the bladder and immediate perivesical tissue are most appropriate. Doses of 300 rad per fraction for 10 daily treatments usually control the he-

maturia. Following this 2-week treatment, the patient is given a 3-week treatment break. During this interval or before, it is usually possible to remove the catheter. This is extremely desirable because the Foley catheter balloon further irritates and compromises the bladder-neck mucosa in such a way that it cannot tolerate further or higher doses of radiation therapy. After a 3-week break, during which time the patient usually recovers from some bowel hyperactivity, the treatment is resumed with the shaped 4-field box technique at 180 rad per fraction, usually for 14 or 15 treatments, to bring the total dose to about 5500 rad and the total (TDF) to about 95.

Palliation for patients who have painful metastases to bone from transitional-cell carcinoma of the bladder require a radiation dose of approximately 5000 rad with conventional fractionation, or its biologic equivalent. With these doses, control or palliation of the pain is possible in over 50% of the patients, although this often takes longer to achieve than is the case with cancer of the prostate or breast.

Acknowledgement

We thank the radiation therapists within the NBCCGA for numerous discussions of treatment techniques, they are: Mark D. Hafermann; The Mason Clinic, Seattle; Tapan A. Hazra, Medical College of Virginia, Richmond; Richard J. Johnson, Roswell Park Memorial Institute, Buffalo; Howard B. Latourette, The University of Iowa Hospital, Iowa City; M.S. Lee, Rush Presbyterian-St. Luke's Hospital, Chicago; Steven A. Leibel, Johns Hopkins Hospital, Baltimore; William T. Moss, University of Oregon Medical School, Portland; James J. Nickson, Memphis Regional Cancer Center, Memphis; and Stephen Seagren, University Hospital, San Diego.

REFERENCES

1. American Joint Committee for Cancer Staging End-Result of Reporting: A Manual for Staging of Cancer. Chicago, American Joint Committee, 1977.

2. Caldwell, W.L.: The role of irradiation in the management of clinical stage B1 (Grades II and III) and stages B_2 and C bladder cancer. Cancer Res. *37*: 2759, 1977.

3. Cummings, K.B., Shipley, W.U., Einstein, A.B., and Cutler, S.J.: Current concepts in the management of patients with deeply invasive bladder carcinoma. Sem. Oncol. *6*:220, 1979.

4. Goffinet, D.R., Schneider, N.J., Glatstein, E.J. et al: Bladder cancer: Results of radiation therapy in 384 patients. Radiology *117*:149, 1975.

5. Goitein, M., Wittenberg, J., Mendiondo, M. et al.: The value of CT scanning in radiation therapy treatment planning: A prospective study. Int. J. Radiat. Oncol. *5*:1787, 1979.

6. Hodson, N.J., Husband, J.E., MacDonald, J.S.: The role of computed tomography in the staging of bladder cancer. Clin. Radiol. *30*:389, 1979.

7. McNeil, M.C., Weichselbaum, R., Pauker, S.G.: A fallacy of the five-year survival in lung cancer. N. Engl. J. Med. *299*:1397, 1978.

8. Miller, L.S.: Bladder cancer: Superiority of preoperative irradiation therapy and cystectomy in clinical stages B_2 and C. Cancer *39*:973, 1977.

9. Miller, L.S. and Johnson, D.E.: Megavoltage radiation for bladder carcinoma: Alone, postoperative, or preoperative. *In* Seventh National Cancer Conference Proceedings. Philadelphia, J.B. Lippincott, 1973, pp. 771–783.

10. Morrison, R.: The results of treatment of cancer of the bladder clinical contribution of radiobiology. Clin. Radiol. *76*:67, 1975.

11. National Bladder Cancer Collaborative Group A: Surveillance, initial assessment, and subsequent progress of patients with superficial bladder cancer in a prospective longitudinal study. Cancer Res. *37*:2907, 1977.

12. Prout, G.R., Jr.: Classification and staging of bladder carcinoma. Sem. Oncol. *6*:189, 1979.

13. Shipley, W.U., Cummings, K.B., Coombs, L.J. et al.: 4000 rad preoperative radiation therapy followed by *prompt* radical cystectomy for bladder carcinoma with muscle invasion: A prospective study of patient tolerance in pathologic downstaging. J. Urol. *127*:48, 1982.

14. Van der werf Messing, B.: Cancer of the urinary bladder treated by interstitial radium implant. Int. J. Radiat. Oncol. *4*:373, 1978.

15. Van der werf Messing, B.: Preoperative radiation followed by cystectomy to treat carcinoma of the urinary bladder. Int. J. Radiat. Oncol. *5*:394, 1979.

Chapter 16

DETERMINATION OF TUMOR EXTENT AND TUMOR LOCALIZATION OF HODGKIN'S DISEASE AND NONHODGKIN'S LYMPHOMAS

Eli Glatstein
Henry S. Kaplan

The improvement in the results of radiotherapeutic and chemotherapeutic management of Hodgkin's disease[36] and other malignant lymphomas[35] reflects the integration of increased therapeutic efficacy, more accurate definition of disease, and the better understanding of the natural history of these disorders. When such knowledge is applied to the microscopic involvement of specific sites, the radiotherapist can design well-collimated irradiation ports that will yield maximal therapeutic benefit. Accurate determination of the extent of tumor permits individualized treatment. Invasive procedures (e.g., laparotomy with splenectomy) may be justified when the findings are expected to influence decisions concerning the details of treatment.

CLINICAL STAGING PROCEDURES

The increasing emphasis on invasive staging procedures culminated in the Ann Arbor Staging Classification for Hodgkin's disease;[3] this classification (Table 16–1), which is adaptable to nonHodgkin's lymphomas, makes a sharp distinction be-

TABLE 16–1. Hodgkin's Disease Staging Classification.*

Stage	Definition
I	Involvement of a single lymph-node region (I) or of a single extralymphatic organ (I_E).
II	Involvement of two or more lymphatic regions on the same side of the diaphragm (II), or localized extralymphatic involvement as well as involvement of one or more regional lymphatic sites on the same side of the diaphragm.
III	Involvement of lymphatic regions on both sides of the diaphragm (III); such involvement may include splenic involvement (III_S), localized extralymphatic disease (III_E), or both (III_{SE}).
IV	Diffuse or disseminated involvement of one or more extralymphatic organs or tissues, with or without nodal involvement.
	The absence or presence of unexplained fever, night sweats, or loss of 10% or more of body weight in the 6 months preceding diagnosis are designated by the suffix letters A or B, respectively. Biopsy-proved involvement of extralymphatic sites is designated by letter suffixes: bone marrow = M+; lung = L+; liver = H+; pleura = P+; bone = 0+; skin and subcutaneous tissue = D+.

*Adopted at the workshop on the staging of Hodgkin's Disease held at Ann Arbor, Michigan, in April, 1971. (From Carbone et al., Cancer Res. *31*:1860, 1971.)

This work was supported in part by USPHS Research Grants CA 05838 and CA 08122 from the National Cancer Institute, National Institutes of Health.

tween clinical staging and pathologic staging. Clinical staging refers only to the initial biopsy, physical examination, and radiologic procedures. Pathologic staging refers to any histologic attempt to identify tumor sites other than the initial biopsy. Thus, bone marrow biopsy, liver biopsy, or splenectomy specimen are designated as pathologic staging by an appropriate letter with a plus or minus sign indicating involvement. Limited extranodal extension into nonlymphoid organs or tissues is designated by the latter E, rather than by being upstaged to a Stage IV category. The letters A and B indicate the absence or presence of systemic symptoms (i.e., unexplained fever, night sweats, or significant weight loss).

Physical examination is important in determining the sites of involvement. Careful examination of lymph-node bearing areas, abdomen, and chest requires time and concentration on the part of the physician. It is important to use a mirror for the examination of the nasopharynx and Waldeyer's-ring area, especially in patients who have nonHodgkin's lymphomas.

Skin testing to determine anergy, although of interest in defining immunologic dysfunction, is not a factor in determining a patient's stage of disease, nor is it of any proved value in planning treatment.

Laboratory tests that are important to management include a complete blood count, platelet count, alkaline-phosphatase and serum-copper evaluations, corrected sedimentation rate, and urinalysis. Liver-function tests including alkaline phosphatase, Bromsulphalein (BSP), and serum glutamic-oxaloacetic transaminase (SGOT) are useful in indicating possible involvement of the liver. These tests are all nonspecific, however, and are *not* criteria for staging; the corrected sedimentation rate and serum copper levels are nonspecific, although they may corrrelate with disease activity. It is important not to use laboratory abnormalities alone as the basis for staging; histologic evidence of hepatic or marrow involvement should be obtained before classifying a patient as Stage IV in these sites.

For rational treatment planning, no examination is more important than proper evaluation of the bone marrow. It should be emphasized that any negative biopsy procedure is only as reliable as the sample itself. More marrow obtained for microscopic evaluation means more reliable information concerning the marrow of a given patient. The focal nature of involvement of the marrow in these diseases implies that a biopsy procedure, whether by Westerman-Jensen needle, Jamshidi needle, or surgical iliac-crest biopsy, would be vastly superior to bone-marrow aspiration techniques, as has been shown.[14,19,21,34] The open bone-marrow specimen, which contains more bone marrow than can be obtained by needle biopsy, is superior to the needle biopsy technique. An open biopsy of the bone marrow usually requires anesthesia, however, and is ordinarily performed at the time of a staging laparotomy. In patients with Hodgkin's disease who have a negative bone marrow needle biopsy, approximately 5% can be shown to have marrow involvement after an open specimen has been obtained.[22] In contrast, patients with non-Hodgkin's lymphoma more frequently present with advanced neoplasm; approximately 20% of such patients who have negative needle biopsies can be shown by open biopsy to have involved bone marrow.[14] The role of aspiration appears to be confined to the study of specific hematologic abnormalities in these patients; aspiration cytology may be superior to that obtained by biopsy techniques. Investigational work concerning bone marrow scanning using ^{111}In is presently underway;[13] this isotope may be useful in selecting the appropriate site for biopsy.

Patients with specific neurologic symptoms and signs may require lumbar puncture and myelography on an emergency basis to define an area of spinal cord compression, especially in patients with nonHodgkin's lymphomas. The value of cerebral spinal fluid (CFS) cytology in asymptomatic patients has not been determined.

Radiographic bone surveys in asymptomatic patients are primarily of value as a comparative baseline in patients who are expected to have long-term survival. The actual detection of asymptomatic bony lesions is not high at presentation; bone scans are probably superior for detecting early lesions. ^{99m}Tc-labelled polyphosphate appears to be an ideal isotope because of its short half-life and energy of emission;[40] bone scans using this isotope may prove to be valuable on a routine basis.

Stereo posterior-anterior (PA) and lateral chest radiographs should be obtained the first time a referred patient is seen. If any abnormality is noted, then whole-lung computerized tomography (CT) is indicated. This permits improved delineation of pulmonary parenchymal disease and better definition of the extent of mediastinal abnormalities. Within the mediastinum, a subcarinal mass is frequently difficult to identify with any technique other than CT; small superior mediastinal masses may also be quite subtle. CT is also useful in defining paravertebral abnormalities and endobronchial lesions. CT is probably the optimal method for evaluation of hilar adenopathy. If the bronchopulmonary (pulmonary hilar) nodes are enlarged on CT scans then major modifications of the treatment technique may be required.[32] In some patients, lateral lung CT scans may be necessary to define hilar adenopathy, especially when there is a large anterior mediastinal mass overlying the hilium in the posteroanterior axis.

The cardiomediastinal silhouette may be so large that the possibility of pericardial involvement by extension from a mediastinal mass must be considered. In this instance, an echocardiogram appears to be the most useful technique for determining the presence or absence of pericardial effusions. If the echocardiogram is positive for effusion, pericardiocentesis may determine whether malignant cells are present. Pericardial effusions and obstruction of the superior vena cava are more frequent in patients who have diffuse histiocytic lymphoma than in patients with Hodgkin's disease.

The presence of a pleural effusion may be detected on initial examination of the patient. Whether this represents lymphatic obstruction, tumor involvement, or some other cardiopulmonary process may be difficult to determine. At the least, thoracentesis is necessary with careful examination of the fluid including appropriate cultures, enzymes, protein, and cytology. In Hodgkin's disease, positive cytology is rarely obtained from a pleural effusion; it is far more frequent in effusions from patients with a nonHodgkin's lymphoma.

Radioisotopic scanning with ^{67}Ga has some usefulness in the evaluation of Hodgkin's disease and the lymphomas.[26,41] The absolute accuracy of ^{67}Ga has yet to be demonstrated conclusively. It does appear useful in detecting relatively large focal areas of involvement by Hodgkin's disease or diffuse histiocytic lymphoma. In the other lymphomas, the uptake of the isotope appears to be quite small. In general, ^{67}Ga appears to be more reliable in detecting disease above rather than below the diaphragm. The large normal uptake of radioactivity within the liver, spleen, and intestine contributes to the difficulty of accurate interpretation of subdiaphragmatic disorders.

In the overall evaluation and management of patients with Hodgkin's disease and the other lymphomas, the lymphangiogram is probably the most useful invasive radiographic procedure. It is important to stress that the lymphangiogram should not be done in patients who have severe underlying pulmonary disease.[10,18]

Furthermore, it should not be performed prior to whole-lung CT scan; ethiodal embolization complicates the interpretation of the tomograms. The lymphangiogram is useful even if surgery is planned. It may effectively direct the surgeon toward a single suspicious node if surgical staging is to be performed; moreover, it helps the radiation therapist in setting up treatment portals. In the post treatment period, changes within opacified nodes on follow-up films of the abdomen may be the initial sign of relapse, even in patients who are considered to have Stage IV tumors at presentation. The lymphangiogram can be safely repeated months or years later, when the status of the iliac and para-aortic nodes may still be of concern.

Liver and spleen scanning is of interest but, in our experience, has not been reliable.[29,39] Routine splenic or hepatic arteriography has not proved reliable in detecting occult subdiaphragmatic disease in these sites.[5] This unreliability presumably reflects the focal nature of involvement in these sites.

Ultrasound techniques for obtaining abdominal echograms appear safe; however, their usefulness in staging has yet to be proved. Routine barium enemas, upper gastrointestinal (GI) series, or small-bowel series have not been valuable on a routine basis in these patients. In patients who are asymptomatic, intrinsic GI lesions are surprisingly rare;[17] however, patients who have any gastrointestinal complaints or who have a positive stool guaiac should undergo these procedures. Whenever a lymphangiogram is grossly abnormal, intravenous pyelography is indicated to detect ureteral obstruction. A congenital anomaly (e.g., a horseshoe or pelvic kidney) may be detected, which markedly influences treatment planning.

As a routine staging procedure, however, the inferior vena cavagram and intravenous pyelogram have proved to be far less valuable than the lymphangiogram.[27]

LAPAROTOMY STAGING

Laparotomy with splenectomy, liver biopsy, selective lymph-node biopsy, and open bone-marrow biopsy, has become widely accepted in the staging of Hodgkin's disease; however, it remains investigational in the management of patients with nonHodgkin's lymphoma. The use of this procedure varies with the individual physician's approach to the multiplicity of clinical situations with which these patients may present. In our opinion, it should be used in patients whose treatment might be altered by the findings at surgery. The procedure is a major one and should not be undertaken by an inexperienced surgical team. In patients with Hodgkin's disease, the procedure is well-tolerated. In a series of more than 500 consecutive laparotomies in patients under 65 years of age with previously untreated Hodgkin's disease, there have been no postoperative deaths.[15] A subphrenic abscess may result, but this has been rare in our experience. On the other hand, in patients who have nonHodgkin's lymphomas, the complication rate appears to be significantly higher.[17] This probably reflects the older age of these patients and their generally more debilitated state. Patients who have massive splenic disease or hypersplenism represent a particularly high-risk group for complications. In such patients, however, the purpose of the splenectomy is usually therapeutic. The risk of postsplenectomy bacterial infections in patients with either Hodgkin's disease or the malignant lymphomas does not appear to be higher than in patients who undergo splenectomy for other reasons.[8]

In patients with Hodgkin's disease, the most important finding has been the frequency of unsuspected disease in the spleen or splenic hilar nodes. Approximately 20% of patients who have an entirely negative abdominal workup prior to surgery show focal Hodgkin's disease in these sites. In our experience, documented hepatic involvement at first examination of patients with Hodgkin's disease has always been associated with splenic involvement.

In patients with nonHodgkin's lymphomas, the most important finding at laparotomy has been the recognition of the high probability of mesenteric lymph-node involvement; such mesenteric disease cannot reliably be detected by any other clinical technique. This sharply contrasts with patients with Hodgkin's disease in whom involvement of mesenteric lymph nodes is less than 5% (Table 16–2); in Hodgkin's disease, laparotomy with splenectomy is most useful either for detecting occult disease below the diaphragm (chiefly in the spleen) or for documenting extranodal involvement in the liver. In patients with nonHodgkin's lymphomas, the primary usefulness of laparotomy with splenectomy is to define the extent of mesenteric lymph-node involvement. Knowledge of such involvement is crucial in planning appropriate radiation-therapy fields.[16]

From the viewpoint of the radiation therapist, there are additional advantages in removing the spleen. Not only does hematologic tolerance for treatment appear to be increased,[37] but left upper quadrant radiation can be confined to a smaller volume; thus, the risk of radiation injury to the left lung and kidney is minimized.

GENERAL CONSIDERATIONS OF TREATMENT

In the radiologic treatment of Hodgkin's disease and nonHodgkin's lymphomas, the usual goal is to treat, in continuity, all involved and potentially involved lymphatic chains to dose levels that offer a strong probability of tumor eradication.[12,23] This approach obviates the potential problems (i.e., overlap and overdose) inherent in matching a "patchwork" of several small fields.

The success of such a high-dose radiotherapeutic technique is dependent upon a well-collimated megavoltage-radiation beam with its significant skin-sparing and minimal penumbra. Meticulous treatment planning, with simulation and frequent verification of portal films, is a crucial factor in the success of treatment.

Whether such treatment is undertaken with a cobalt unit or with a megavoltage linear accelerator, it is essential that the radiotherapist know in detail the physical characteristics of his particular unit. Dose rate, depth-dose characteristics, and availability of large field size are all important features of such units. The flatness of the isodose distribution for large fields at long distances needs to be verified; for some

TABLE 16–2. Laparotomy Findings.

	Hodgkin's Disease	NonHodgkin's Disease
LIVER	Involvement at presentation *always* associated with splenic disease	Involvement *usually* associated with positive lymphangiogram and histologically involved spleen
SPLEEN	Often (20%) the *only* site of subdiaphragmatic involvement at presentation	When involved, usually associated with other subdiaphragmatic disease
MESENTERIC NODES	Involved in *less than* 5% of patients	Involved in *50%* or more of patients
BONE MARROW	Open biopsy is positive in 5% of patients with negative needle biopsies	Open biopsy positive in *20%* of patients with negative needle biopsies

units, such as the 4-MeV linear accelerator, a special beam-flattening filter may be required to eliminate very-high-dose regions at the lateral edges of large fields at superficial depths.[1]

Various techniques for shaping large fields have been described. The technique of compensating filters for the mantle field has been well-described elsewhere[20] and has proved useful; the treatment techniques that we describe here have proven adaptable to virtually every problem that may arise. The specific method used by a radiotherapist is probably less important than the degree of skill and care that he possesses in using any technique. If adequate skill and experience with one of these techniques are not available locally for the treatment of patients with these diseases, such patients should be referred to medical centers where sophisticated and skilled radiation therapy is available.

In terms of dose and fractionation, a total tumor dose of more than 4000 rad appears to be tumoricidal for Hodgkin's disease[23] and nonHodgkin's lymphomas.[12] For adults, a dose of 4400 rad delivered in 4 to 5 weeks, in 4 or 5 fractions per week, is normally used. Although it is ordinarily administered at a rate of 1000 to 1100 rad per week, the dose rate is reduced to 750 to 800 rads per week whenever the clinical situation requires it. Rest periods during the course of therapy are frequently employed whenever there is extensive disease that requires time to permit tumor shrinkage. We have not routinely used the nominal standard dose concept[9] in prescribing doses. When the treatment to a specific area has been protracted beyond 6 weeks, a localized small-field boost is usually administered to areas of bulky disease; the total dose to such bulky areas is usually 5000 rad.

SPECIFIC TECHNIQUES

The development of modern megavoltage equipment permits the radiotherapist to treat all major lymph-node groups above the diaphragm with a pair of large opposing fields, or mantle fields. In the usual approach to total lymphoid irradiation, the mantle and a subdiaphragmatic inverted-Y field (designed to encompass the para-aortic and iliac nodes) join or "match" at only one junction line, usually at the diaphragmatic level, approximately between the tenth and eleventh thoracic vertebrae.

The most important feature of the mantle field is the individualization that results from shaping the lung blocks to the specific contours of a given patient. By interposing such carefully shaped lung blocks between the patient and the source of the beam, the radiotherapist can effectively protect the pulmonary parenchyma from the effects of high-dose irradiation. These blocks may be shaped from solid lead or equivalent volumes of lead shot or Cerrobend in a polystyrene frame. Our own preference is the solid lead block, shaped from a prepared template and then cut out by a saw. This technique maximizes the flexibility necessary for shrinking the fields during a course of treatment. By this technique, the axillary, infraclavicular, supraclavicular, cervical, mediastinal, and hilar nodes can be exposed with ease. Slight adjustments permit treatment of the entire heart surface. By varying the thickness of the lead blocks, various calculated doses to pulmonary parenchyma can be achieved.[32]

For adult patients, rectangular fields with the midplane dimensions varying from 30 cm to 40 cm are normally used. To achieve such areas, patients are usually treated at source-to-skin distances (SSD) of approximately 130 cm; in large patients, even greater distances may be required. The need for increased SSDs makes it impossible for most patients to be treated by rotating the machine; it is usually necessary for patients to be treated in both supine and prone positions with the beam directed downward.

The mantle is a sophisticated treatment

technique and must be planned on a simulator for optimal results. The axis of the diagnostic x-ray tube in the simulator must exactly mimic that of the therapeutic beam. It is essential that the beam alignments and dosimetric calculations correspond to precise landmarks. The standard reference point for the mantle field is the suprasternal notch. When the patient is supine, localization films are taken at the necessary SSD for the supine treatment position. The beam is centered at the suprasternal notch and a small tattoo is placed on the skin of the patient exactly at this center point. Additional tattoos are placed approximately 10 cm on either side of the suprasternal notch mark; thus, there are three skin marks in a straight line, which permits maximum reproducibility on a day-to-day basis during treatment. With the patient in a supine position, a template table with a wire grid within a lucite top is centered over the patient and an AP localization radiograph is taken. To obtain truly opposing fields for the mantle, the patient turns to a prone position with the suprasternal notch visible in the center of the Mylar portion of the couch; the simulator is then rotated 180°. When the suprasternal notch is clearly identified as being coincident with the central axis of the now upward-directed simulator beam, the simulator beam is then rotated exactly 180° again so that it now points downward. Again, a tattoo is placed on the skin of the posterior chest that should exactly correspond to the anterior tattoo on the suprasternal notch. Additional lateral tattoos are placed exactly as before, permitting accurate reproducibility of the posterior field. An additional localization radiograph is taken from the posterior-anterior (PA) direction with the template table positioned over the prone patient.

Each radiograph is carefully marked to identify its direction. An outline of the precise shape of the block is made with a wax pencil for anterior and posterior blocks. The blocks need not be identical.

It is our usual policy to draw the anterior blocks as high as the level of the inferior portion of the head of the clavicle; by contrast, the posterior blocks are usually drawn to fit the inferior surface of the clavicular shaft. The reason for this difference is to permit the infraclavicular space to be adequately treated on the anterior field. If clinically significant infraclavicular adenopathy is present, the ipsilateral lung blocks can be shaved to fit even lower on the superior margin. A small, direct, anterior electron field may be used as a supplement.

Whenever it is desirable to treat the entire pericardial silhouette, special cutouts can be made of the cardiac surface. A very thin lead template is made of each block; the exact positioning, alignment, and distance are checked by another simulator radiograph. The second radiograph is taken with the thin lead template superimposed on a clear-film template carefully marked to line up with the tattoo marks on the skin. This simulator radiograph with the thin lead templates in place is then checked by the therapist. Any subsequent adjustments in the exact shape or positioning of the blocks can then be made. When the shape of the thin lead template is considered acceptable to the therapist, it can than be placed over a 5-cm-thick lead block, which is then cut to the shape of the template with a saw.

For both the anterior and posterior portals, the appropriate transparent template and its corresponding lead blocks can be placed in position on a table that supports the blocks. The table that we employ is positioned approximately 25 cm above the couch that supports the patient. This permits the lung blocks to be placed relatively close to the surface of the patient and minimizes the penumbra and error in daily positioning. Both penumbra and positioning errors would be markedly increased if the blocks were supported on the shadow tray just under the head of the beam.

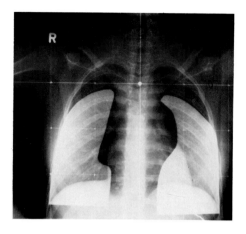

Fig. 16–1. The anterior mantle set-up field is shown wih the thin template cutouts in place. Note the dots over the left margin of the heart. The block will be cut along this line in order to permit pericardial exposure in this patient with mediastinal disease. Note that the superior margin of the anterior lung blocks is at the level of the inferior portion of the head of the clavicle.

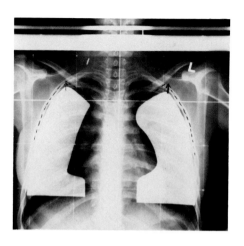

Fig. 16–3. The posterior set-up field on the patient in Fig. 16–1 shows the thin template blocks in place. The dotted lines and arrows show that the lung blocks are adequate but slightly out of position and need to be raised up to the level of the clavicle on the posterior field. The dots on the left template correspond to the cardiac margin. This is the line upon which the pericardial cutout is made.

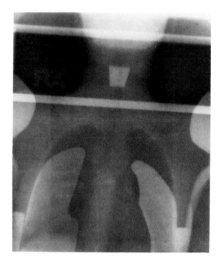

Fig. 16–2. The anterior port radiograph of the patient in Fig. 16–1 shows the blocks in place with the pericardial cutout omitted. The vocal-cord block is in place. Humeral head shields are visible at the margin of the field. Note the difference in opacity between the left lung block and the right. The right lung block represents a thin lung block and transmits a total dose to the right lung parenchyma, which is approximately 37% of the midline dose. This thin lung block is used whenever there is hilar adenopathy as there is on the right side of this patient.

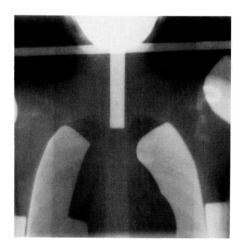

Fig. 16–4. The posterior port radiograph shows humeral blocks and the lung blocks in place with the pericardial cutout omitted. The posterior cervical spine block is present throughout the entire course of treatment. The difference in thickness of the two lung blocks is evident.

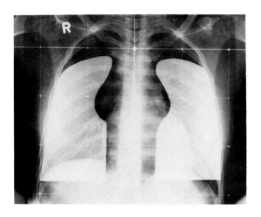

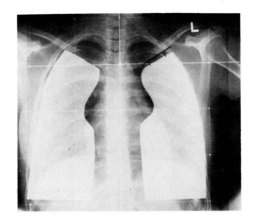

Fig. 16–5. After a treatment dose of 1500 rad, 10 days to 2 weeks have passed without treatment in order to permit tumor shrinkage. The patient is now set up for the second time with reshaping of much larger lung blocks to correspond to the shrinkage of the mediastinal mass. This second anterior setup shows no pericardial cutout because the pericardium has already been treated.

Fig. 16–7. The second setup on the posterior field for the patient in Fig. 16–1, after shrinkage of the mediastinal mass has occurred. The left lung block appears to be adequately shaped but has slipped inferiorly on the simulator radiograph with the thin template blocks in place. The right lung template has been placed approximately 0.5 cm more medially than desired.

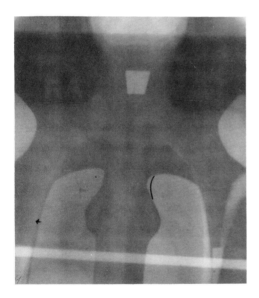

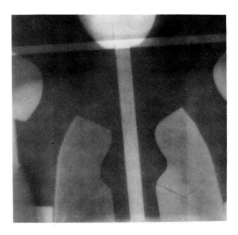

Fig. 16–6. A port radiograph taken under treatment from the anterior position. The laryngeal block and humeral blocks are seen. The right lung block has been moved slightly medially and the arrow indicates that it needs to be moved out approximately 0.5 cm to the ribcage margin. The upper medial portion of the left lung block appears to be too close to the mediastinal silhouette and a trim is necessary, as indicated by the black crayon mark.

Fig. 16–8. The port radiograph of the patient in Fig.16–1 shows the distinction between the left and right lung blocks. After 2000 rad to the midplane, a full spinal block is placed only on the posterior field for the remainder of the treatment.

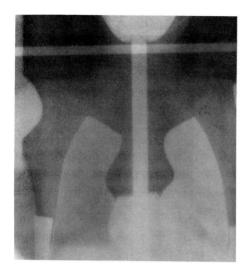

Fig. 16–9. After 3000 rad, a subcarinal block is added both anteriorly and posteriorly. The use of the subcarinal block appears to have significantly decreased the incidence and severity of radiation-induced heart disease.

Whenever hilar adenopathy is present, the lung parenchyma can be treated with modest doses of radiation by using lung blocks that are approximately 2.1-cm thick. Such thin lung blocks transmit approximately 37% of the mediastinal dose for a given exposure;[32] thus, whenever there is hilar adenopathy, the ipsilateral lung can be treated with approximately 1600 rad over the 4-week period during which the mediastinum is treated with 4400 rad (Figs. 16–1 to 16–9). The effectiveness of this technique and its relative safety have been reviewed elsewhere.[4]

Whenever there is mediastinal involvement, it is our policy to treat the entire pericardial surface with approximately 1500 rad. The rationale for this is that the margins of the tumor mass cannot be accurately distinguished from the cardiac silhouette. In patients with mediastinal involvement, the lower medial portion of the left lung block is drawn to fit the silhouette of the left lateral portion of the heart. When the block is cut by saw, this lower medial section is cut off from the main lung block and is referred to as the pericardial block (see Figs. 16–1 to 16–4).

Likewise, on the right side, the lower medial portion of the block that would ordinarily cover the right cardiac margin is also cut separately to match the border of the heart. After 1500 rad, each of these blocks is then inserted in its appropriate position and the central portion of the mediastinum is then treated with a higher dose.

When there is no known subcarinal disease, a generous 5-cm-thick lead subcarinal block may be placed from the lower border of the field to within approximately 6 cm of the carina, both anteriorly and posteriorly (see Fig. 16–9); the insertion of this block in the field after approximately 3000 rad appears to reduce significantly the incidence of radiation-induced heart disease.[4,6] More importantly, those patients who have developed radiation carditis have not manifested severe constrictive symptoms requiring pericardiectomy.[4] A 5-cm-thick lead block approximately 1 cm in width is routinely placed over the cervical spinal cord on the posterior treatment field for the entire course of treatment to protect the cord from potential radiation injury (see Fig. 16–4). After the delivery of 2000 rad, a similar posterior block is inserted to extend inferiorly to protect the entire thoracic spinal cord for the remainder of the mediastinal treatment (see Figs. 16–8 and 16–9). A small trapezoidal block is used throughout the anterior field to protect the vocal cords from the effects of the irradiation (e.g., unnecessary hoarseness—see Fig. 16–2). The humeral heads are protected by special, rounded blocks both anteriorly and posteriorly. If there is any midline disease detected on physical examination, laryngeal blocks or cervical spinal-cord blocks may be omitted. Detailed dosimetry of the mantle has been described elsewhere.[30]

One of the major advantages of this technique of treatment is the ease with which it permits shrinking the fields during split-course therapy. Whenever there is a large mediastinal mass, the initial fields are treated with approximately 1500 rad to the midplane; treatment is then discontinued for approximately 10 to 14 days. During this time, the tumor mass usually shrinks significantly and permits the delineation of an entirely new set of blocks that conform to the new size and shape of the tumor. When there is enormous mediastinal involvement, treatment may again be interrupted, followed by a third setup, at approximately 3000 rad. By this technique, progressively larger blocks are inserted to protect the pulmonary parenchyma, and maximum cell-killing in the tumor is achieved with minimum morbidity.

It is often desirable, particularly in nonHodgkin's lymphomas, to omit treatment to the mediastinum in an elderly patient if there is no overt involvement. A supramediastinal mantle is used frequently in patients with nonHodgkin's lymphomas to a full dose of 4400 rad or more. It is also useful for retreatment of axillary-supraclavicular involvement with doses of 2000 to 2500 rad with anterior and posterior spinal-cord blocks.

Two areas require special attention to prevent unnecessary recurrences after mantle-field treatment. One is the medial margin of the lung block in the region of the hilum. The hilar-cutout portion of the block may be inadequate if it fails to include the full hilar density visible on the setup radiograph. A second common area of relapse is in the axilla, which may receive decreased doses at the lateral portions of the field due to divergence of the beam. Anatomic considerations are also important; axillary nodes frequently shift medial to the rib cage when the patient is prone.[42] This could result in the axillary nodes being underdosed from shielding of the posteior lung block if some method of compensation is not used. A small sliver of lung tissue can be exposed on the posterior field at the lateral margin of the lung block or an additional boost of 600 to 800

rad can be delivered to the anterior field. We usually prefer the latter approach.

The superior margin of the mantle usually verges on the inferior border of the mandible, omitting the preauricular nodes, which are at a higher level. These nodes are frequently involved in non-Hodgkin's lymphomas and sometimes in Hodgkin's disease in patients who have high cervical adenopathy superior to the thyroid notch. In patients in whom preauricular radiation is considered desirable, a pair of small lateral-opposing fields can easily be administered (Fig. 16–10). The inferior margin of the field is matched at the midplane to the superior margin of the mantle. The superior margin of the preauricular field is above the level of the zygomatic arch and includes the floor of the sphenoid sinus. The posterior margin of the field begins at the tragus; the anterior margin of the field is usually designed to stay posterior to the molars. The morbidity of treating such fields, which are usually termed "Waldeyer's ring" fields, is signif-

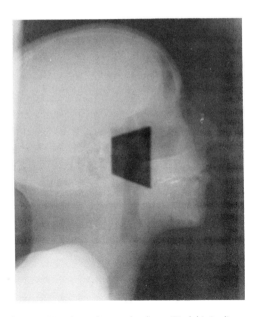

Fig. 16–10. In patients who have Hodgkin's disease with high cervical neck disease and routinely on patients with non-Hodgkin's lymphoma, the preauricular nodes are included in a small field designed to match with the superior margin of the mantle.

icant. Xerostomia is a common problem.[7] When this area is being treated on a prophylactic basis, we have usually reduced the dose of 3600 rad over approximately 4 to 5 weeks. When the Waldeyer's ring is overtly involved, a larger field is usually necessary. In such cases, we usually begin the large lateral fields well below the angle of the mandible, reducing the upper margin of the mantle field accordingly; thus, the lateral fields and mantle fields do not overlap. Marked reduction in tumor volume has usually occurred after delivery of approximately 2000 rad and a shrinking-field approach can then be used. As the Waldeyer's-ring field is reduced, the lower margin of the lateral field is moved progressively above the mandible; the superior margin of the mantle is raised accordingly.

The subdiaphragmatic portion of total lymphoid irradiation may also be highly individualized. For Hodgkin's patients, para-aortic, iliac, and femoral lymph nodes are usually treated with large opposing fields with a left upper quadrant flare to encompass the splenic hilar nodes (marked by clips at surgery) when the spleen is removed. If the spleen is intact, the left upper quadrant is treated in its entirety with a block to protect as much of the left upper kidney as possible. The patient is set up in both supine and prone positions by means of a simulator with the template table and grid centered over the abdomen. The field on the skin is marked on the basis of the relationship of opacified lymph nodes and other structures to the vertebral bodies. The kidneys are usually visualized at the time of setup by the intravenous injection of Hypaque.

In patients with Hodgkin's disease who have not had systemic symptoms and in whom surgical staging has proved entirely negative (with the most suspicious nodes having been biopsied), we usually do not treat the pelvic portion of the field. The risk of pelvic relapse after treatment of the para-aortic and common iliac nodes (a field that we refer to as a "spade" field) is approximately 4%. Whenever the patient has difficulty in tolerating the dose rate, it may be desirable to divide the subdiaphragmatic radiation into pelvic and upper-abdominal portions and treat them in sequence rather than simultaneously.

When large fields are to be treated above and below the diaphragm, an appropriate gap must be left between the fields at the surface of the skin to account for the normal divergence of the edges of the beam. The objective is to have the edges match exactly at the midplane. This can be accomplished either by shifting the position of the match on a regular predetermined basis or by calculating the gap based on simple geometric principles. Complete details of the dosimetry of inverted-Y fields[31] and of the technique for calculating the skin gap[25] have been published elsewhere.

If total lymphoid radiation is planned, it is important at the time of the initial setup to plan the approximate level of the "matchline" between the mantle and the upper abdominal fields. If splenic hilar clips are unusually high or if treatment that will require whole hepatic radiation by horizontal fields is anticipated, the exact level of the matchline is determined by the inferior margin of treatment of the initial field. Attention to this point at the time of the setup of the initial treatment field facilitates an optimal junction of the two fields.

In patients with Hodgkin's disease who have a positive spleen, it has been demonstrated that the liver is at great risk of ultimate involvement.[24] Accordingly, in patients who have positive splenic involvement, special attention should be directed toward sterilizing microscopic tumors presumably present in the liver, even if liver biopsies are negative. The radiotherapeutic technique that we use to treat the liver employs a thin block approximately 13.6 mm in thickness (for use in combination with our 6-MeV linear accelerator). This transmits 50% of the mid-

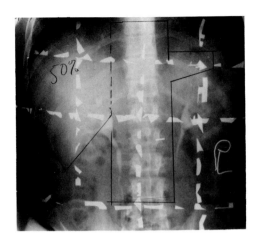

Fig. 16–11. This is an abdominal simulator field for a patient with Hodgkin's disease who has had documentation of splenic involvement. Such patients are at high risk for hepatic involvement even when the liver biopsy has proved to be negative. The right lobe of the liver is treated with a thin liver block that transmits 50% of the midline dose. Kidneys are demonstrated by intravenous pyelography at the time of setup. The para-aortic and splenic pedicle nodes receive 4400 rad over approximately 4–5 weeks, during which time the right lobe of the liver receives 2200 rad. Note clips within the splenic-pedicle portion of the field.

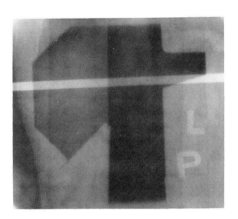

Fig. 16–12. The posterior port radiograph of the patient in Fig. 16–11. The thin liver block in place over the right lobe of the liver while the remainder of the para-aortic nodes and the splenic pedicle receive full dose.

plane dose; thus, when the para-aortic nodes are treated with 4400 rad, the midplane hepatic dose reaches 2200 rad over 4 to 5 weeks. In patients who have hepatic involvement, this treatment can be combined with intensive chemotherapy or radioactive colloidal gold for maximum tumor sterilization (Figs. 16–11 and 16–12).[38]

In treatment of the pelvis of young women, it is important to protect the ovaries from excessive doses of irradiation. At the time of surgery, an oophoropexy,[33] which sutures the ovaries in the midline anterior or posterior to the uterine body, can be performed. By using clips to mark the location of the ovaries, lead blocks approximately 10-cm-thick can be designed to shield the ovaries. Several of our young female patients have become pregnant after oophoropexy and high-dose irradiation to the pelvis,[28] and have given birth to healthy children, including one set of twins; no developmental abnormality has been detected so far.

Mesenteric lymph-node involvement is uncommon in patients with Hodgkin's disease;[22] by contrast, in patients who have nonHodgkin's lymphoma, it is a common finding, even in the absence of detectable para-aortic lymph-node abnormality. Approximately 55% of patients with nonHodgkin's lymphoma have mesenteric lymph-node involvement;[17] the therapist must consider the high risk of such involvement in formulating his treatment strategy.

The technique that we employ for the treatment of the whole abdomen is called a three-way technique.[16] The first portion of treatment consists of simple opposing AP fields from the diaphragm to the floor of the pelvis below the obturator foramina. If possible, blocks are placed over the lateral portion of each ilium in an attempt to protect the bone marrow. Using a maximum dose rate of 150 rad per day, treatment is delivered at a dose of approximately 1500 rad over 2 weeks. During this part of the treatment, the right lobe of the liver is protected by a lead block, either full thickness or half thickness, depending upon the total desired dose to the liver. It is important during the period of initial radiation that the superior border of the field correspond to the dome of the right hemidiaphragm.

The second part of the whole-abdomen therapy treats the upper abdomen separately from the pelvis. The pelvic (i.e., iliofemoral) portion of irradiation continues by an opposing AP technique; however, the upper portion of the abdomen is

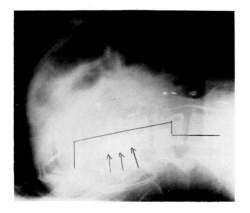

Fig. 16–13. To treat the mesenteric nodes, a portion of the radiation field is delivered by a cross-table lateral technique. With the patient recumbent on a table, the kidneys are opacified by intravenous pyelography *(arrows)*. The lead block designed to protect the kidneys from the lateral field of radiation takes advantage of their posterior position. At the same time, opacified nodes are seen in the area of the clips and the demonstrable ureter; these nodes are generally anterior to the vertebral bodies and can be irradiated at the same time the kidneys are protected.

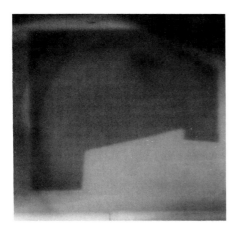

Fig. 16–14. The port film from the cross-table lateral technique shows the kidneys protected by the block and the anterior abdominal contents to be included in the high-dose radiation field.

treated by opposing cross-table-lateral fields set up by an isocentric technique. The kidneys are visualized radiographically with infusion of Hypaque (see Figs. 16–13 and 16–14). The posterior margin of the lateral radiation portal is placed anterior to the kidneys but posterior to the para-aortic nodes, which are easily visualized by lymphangiography. The anterior margin of the lateral portal extends to the anterior abdominal wall. Full-thickness lead blocks protect the kidneys posteriorly. The upper abdomen is treated with 1500 rad in approximately 2 weeks through these opposing lateral fields, bringing the dose to para-aortic lymph nodes to approximately 3000 rad. Para-aortic lymph nodes or retroperitoneal masses are occasionally noted at the time of surgery to extend to the posterior abdominal wall, thus making it impossible to shield the kidneys by this technique. In some patients, the kidneys may be located too far anterior on the lateral set-up radiographs to permit adequate protection by lateral blocks. In such cases, AP irradiation techniques are mandatory; the use of bilateral 5-cm-thick lead kidney blocks is required after 1500 rad.

The third part of the whole-abdomen technique uses a very wide inverted-Y created by opposing AP fields. Bilateral 5-cm-thick lead blocks are required to protect the kidneys from the anterior and the posterior fields. The width of the upper portion of this wide inverted-Y extends from the lateral margin of one kidney to the lateral margin of the other kidney. This is required in order to treat the full region of the mesentery.[16] The right lobe of the liver is also blocked throughout this part of the whole-abdomen technique; a total dose of 4400 rad to the central abdomen is delivered over approximately 6 to 8 weeks.

This three-way approach to whole-abdomen treatment appears to be safe. The complication rate is less than 10% and no significant radiation injury to the liver or kidneys has been detected. Radiation enteritis is possible but this protracted radiation treatment appears to be well tolerated.

Whole-body irradiation is another technique in the treatment of nonHodgkin's lymphomas, primarily of the lymphocytic or mixed-cell types. The bases of such treatment are the extreme radiosensitivity of nodular lymphocytic lymphoma and the high frequency of bone-marrow involvement. Megavoltage irradiation is used with the patient in a seated position holding his knees. Each treatment is delivered from both sides; compensating filters may be used to account for differences in tissue thickness to achieve maximum homogeneity of dose.

The ideal fractionation scheme for whole-body irradiation has not yet been established. The standard dose is usually 150 rad delivered over approximately 5 weeks, usually at the rate of 30 rad per week in 2 to 3 fractions per week; however, this program has not been carefully compared to other protracted schemas. The treatment is extraordinarily well tolerated with minimal development of complicating symptoms during the course of treatment. The major concern is thrombocytopenia, which must be carefully watched for. In patients who undergo such treatment, the absolute-platelet-count level is often not nearly as important as the rate of decline of the platelet count. The nadir of thrombocytopenia may occur 2 or 3 weeks after having interrupted the treatment, when patients begin to fail. It is essential to watch the platelet count carefully and be prepared to interrupt treatment early. Preliminary results suggest that whole-body irradiation for advanced nodular lymphocytic lymphomas is as effective as intensive combination chemotherapy.[2]

REFERENCES

1. Boge, R.J., Tolbert, D.D., and Edland, R.W.: Accessory beam flattening filter for the Varian Clinac-IV linear accelerator. Radiology *115*:475, 1975.

2. Canellos, G.P., De Vita, V.T., Young, R.C., Chabner, B.A., Schein, P.S., and Johnson, R.E.: Therapy of advanced lymphocytic lymphoma: A preliminary report of a randomized trial between combination chemotherapy (CVP) and intensive radiotherapy. Br. J. Cancer *31* (Suppl. 1):474, 1975.

3. Carbone, P.P., Kaplan, H.S., Musshoff, K., Smithers, D.W., and Tubiana, M.: Report of the committee on Hodgkin's disease staging classifications. Cancer Res. 31:1860, 1971.

4. Carmel, R.C. and Kaplan, H.S.: Mantle irradiation in Hodgkin's disease: An analysis of technique, tumor eradication and complications. Cancer 37:2813, 1976.

5. Castellino, R.A., Silverman, J.F., Glatstein, E., Blank, N., and Wexler, L.: Splenic arteriography in Hodgkin's disease. Am. J. Roentgenol. 114:574, 1972.

6. Cohn, K.E., Stewart, J.R., Fajardo, L.F., and Kaplan, H.S.: Heart disease following radiation. Medicine 46:281, 1967.

7. Daley, Thomas: Dental care in the irradiated patient. *In* Textbook of Radiotherapy. Edited by G.H. Fletcher. Philadelphia, Lea & Febiger, 1973.

8. Donaldson, S.S., Moore, M.R., Rosenberg, S.A., and Vosti, K.L.: Characterization of postsplenectomy bacteremia among patients with and without lymphoma. N. Engl. J. Med. 287:69, 1972.

9. Ellis, F.: Dose, time, and fractionation: A clinical hypothesis. Clin. Radiol. 20:8, 1969.

10. Fallat, R.J., Powell, M.R., Youker, J.E., and Nadel, J.A.: Pulmonary deposition and clearance of ^{131}I labelled oil after lymphography in man. Radiology 97:511, 1970.

11. Fuks, Z., Glatstein, E., and Kaplan, H.S.: Patterns of presentation and relapse in the non-Hodgkin's lymphomas. Br. J. Cancer *31* (Suppl. 2):286, 1975.

12. Fuks, Z. and Kaplan, H.S.: Recurrence rates following radiation therapy for nodular and diffuse malignant lymphomas. Radiology *108*:675, 1973.

13. Glatstein, E. and Goffinet, D.R.: Staging of Hodgkin's disease and other lymphomas. Clin. Haematol. 3:77, 1974.

14. Goffinet, D.R., Fuks, Z., Glatstein, E., and Kaplan, H.S.: Abdominal irradiation of non-Hodgkin's lymphomas. Cancer 37:2797, 1976.

15. Goffinet, D.R., Kim, H., Dorfman, R.F., Fuks, Z., Rosenberg, S.A., Nelsen, T.S., and Kaplan, H.S.: Staging laparotomies in unselected previously untreated patients with non-Hodgkin's lymphomas. Cancer 32:672, 1973.

16. Gold, W.M., Youker, S., Anderson, S., and Nadel, J.A.: Pulmonary function adnormalities after lymphangiography. N. Engl. J. Med. 273:519, 1965.

17. Grann, V., Pool, J.L. and Mayer, K.: Comparative study of bone marrow aspiration and biopsy in patients with neoplastic disease. Cancer 19:1898, 1966.

18. Johnson, R.E.: Clinical and technical aspects of total nodal irradiation for Hodgkin's disease. *In* Textbook of Radiotherapy. Edited by G.H. Fletcher. Philadelphia, Lea & Febiger, 1973.

19. Jones, S.E., Rosenberg, S.A., and Kaplan, H.S.: Non-Hodgkin's lymphomas. I. Bone marrow involvement. Cancer 29:954, 1972.

20. Kadin, M.E., Glatstein, E., and Dorfman, R.F.: Clinicopathologic studies of 117 untreated patients subjected to laparotomy for the staging of Hodgkin's disease. Cancer 27:1277, 1971.

21. Kaplan, H.S.: Evidence for a tumoricidal dose level in the radiotherapy of Hodgkin's disease. Cancer Res. 26:1250, 1966.

22. Kaplan, H.S.: On the natural history, treatment and prognosis of Hodgkin's disease. Harvey Lect. 64:215, 1970.

23. Kaplan, H.S.: Hodgkin's Disease. Cambridge, Harvard University Press, 1972.

24. Kay, D.N. and McCready, V.R.: Clinical isotope scanning using 67-Ga citrate in the management of Hodgkin's disease. Br. J. Radiol. 45:437, 1972.

25. Lee, B.J., Nelson, J.H., and Schwartz, G.: Evaluation of lymphography, inferior vena cavography and intravenous pyelography in the clinical staging and management of Hodgkin's disease and lymphosarcoma. N. Engl. J. Med. 271:327, 1964.

26. Lipton, M.J., De Nardo, G.L., Silverman, S., and Glatstein, E.: Evaluation of the liver and spleen in Hodgkin's disease. I. The value of hepatic scintigraphy. Am. J. Med. 52:556, 1972.

27. Page, V., Gardner, A., and Karzmark, C.: Physical and dosimetric aspects of the radiotherapy of malignant lymphomas. I. The mantle technique. Radiology 96:609, 1970.

28. Page, V., Gardner, A., and Karzmark, C.: Physical and dosimetric aspects of the radiotherapy of malignant lymphomas. II. The inverted-Y technique. Radiology 96:619, 1970.

29. Palos, B., Kaplan, H.S., and Karzmark, C.: The use of thin lung shields to deliver limited whole-lung irradiation during mantle-field treatment of Hodgkin's disease. Radiology 101:441, 1971.

30. Ray, G.R., Trueblood, H.W., Enright, L.P., Kaplan, H.S., and Nelsen, T.S.: Oophorectomy: A means of preserving ovarian function following pelvic megavoltage radiotherapy for Hodgkin's disease. Radiology 96:175, 1970.

31. Rosenberg, S.A.: Hodgkin's disease of the bone marrow. Cancer Res. 31:1733, 1971.

32. Rosenberg, S.A. and Kaplan, H.S.: Clinical trials in the non-Hodgkin's lymphomata at Stanford University. Experimental design and preliminary results. Br. J. Cancer 31 (Suppl 2): 456, 1975.

33. Rosenberg, S.A. and Kaplan, H.S.: The management of Stages I, II, and III Hodgkin's disease with combined radiotherapy and chemotherapy. Cancer 35:55, 1975.

34. Salzman, J.R. and Kaplan, H.S.: Effect of splenectomy on hematologic tolerance during total lymphoid radiotherapy with patients with Hodgkin's disease. Cancer 27:471, 1971.

35. Schultz, H.P., Glatstein, E., and Kaplan, H.S.: Management of presumptive or proven Hodgkin's disease of the liver: A new radiotherapy technique. J. Radiat. Oncol. Biol. Phys. 1:1, 1975.

36. Silverman, S., De Nardo, G.L., Glatstein, E., and Lipton, M.J.: Evaluation of the liver and spleen in Hodgkin's disease. II. The value of splenic scintigraphy. Am. J. Med. 52:362, 1972.

37. Subramanian, G., McAfee, J.G., Bell, E.G., Blair, R.J., O'Mara, R.E., and Holston, P.H.: 99Tc-labelled polyphosphate as a skeletal imaging agent. Radiology 102:701, 1972.

38. Turner, D.A., Pinsky, S.M., Gottschalk, A., Hoffer, P.B., Ultmann, J.E., and Harper, P.V.: The use of 67-Ga scanning in the staging of Hodgkin's disease. Radiology 104:97, 1972.

39. Weisenberger, T.H. and Julliard, G.: Axillary lymphangiograms in radiation therapy of lymphomas. Radiology 113:463, 1974.

Chapter 17

LOCALIZATION AND DETERMINATION OF TUMOR EXTENT IN CANCERS OF THE COLON AND RECTUM

Charles Votava, Jr.

During the past several decades there has developed an increased interest in the application of radiation therapy in the management of gastrointestinal malignancies. The presence within the treatment volume of many normal tissues vulnerable to high-dose irradiation has precluded therapy with curative intent except for lesions of the rectum. While radiation therapy remains a useful modality for palliation of symptomatic inoperable or recurrent disease, the current trend is to combine irradiation with surgery in the hope of decreasing the incidence of local and regional treatment failures, and of improving the patient's chance of long-term survival.

Determination of the extent of disease is important for making the decision as to whether to treat and what to treat. A variety of diagnostic procedures are available for this purpose (including surgical staging). An appreciation of the regional anatomy and the areas at risk for spread of disease is necessary for the proper application of the treatment ports.

ANATOMIC PATHOLOGIC CONSIDERATIONS

The potential modes of spread of tumor are direct extension, lymphatic, hematog-enous, transperitoneal, and intraoperative (surgical implantation). Because the major benefit derived from adjuvant radiation therapy is the prevention of local or regional treatment failure, this chapter emphasizes direct extension of tumor (local spread) and lymphatic metastases (regional spread).

Although some reports indicate a low incidence of local treatment failure, there is an increase in the literature claiming that a majority of patients die with or from local recurrence.[2,5,7,10] In the University of Minnesota re-operative series, Gunderson and Sosin[7] report that 48% of the failure group had local failure alone, while an additional 44% had local failure as a component of reappearance of their disease. The location of the local and regional failure in this series suggested the possibility that these sites might be covered by reasonable radiation ports (Fig. 17–1). Gilbert[5] reported 56 patients who failed following abdominal perineal resection and, of these, 57% developed symptoms from their pelvic recurrence without symptoms of distant metastases. An additional 11% developed symptoms of local pelvic recurrence; symptoms of distant metastases occurred during the terminal

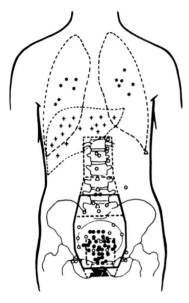

Fig. 17–1. Patterns of failure in 52 patients with evidence of carcinoma after the initial operative procedure with various superimposed radiation fields. (From: Gunderson, L.L.: Clin. Gastroenterol. 5:769, 1976.)

portion of their disease. Symptoms related to distant metastases alone occurred in only 20%. Lesions that penetrate through the bowel wall with or without positive nodes (Stages B_2 and C_2)[1] appear to have the highest incidence of local and regional failure.

DIAGNOSTIC STUDIES

Once the diagnosis of cancer of the colon or rectum is established by biopsy, or suggested by examination, the investigation is directed toward the exclusion of distant metastases and the evaluation of the extent of regional spread before definitive treatment of the primary tumor is undertaken. Although the adjacent anatomy is at risk for local spread, as are the regional lymph nodes for regional spread, the major sites for distant metastases are the liver and the lung.

The history and physical examination of the patient give important information regarding the diagnosis and the extent of disease. Digital examination may indicate the distance of the lower edge of the lesion

from the anal verge; this information must be documented. Lesions less than 8 cm from the anal verge make abdominal perineal resection the more likely operative choice. Such lesions increase the probability of pelvic and inguinal lymph-node metastases. Sigmoidoscopy and colonoscopy are used for lesions not accessible to the examining finger. Palpation of the inguinal and supraclavicular nodes, the iliac fossae, and the abdomen (especially of the liver) gives valuable clinical information regarding regional and distant spread.

A complete blood count, urinalysis, liver-function tests, and chest radiography are the minimum screening procedures for metastases. Radioisotopic liver scanning has been the main imaging test for metastases but this may not reveal small metastatic deposits. Although correlation is better if the alkaline phosphatase level is elevated, liver metastases may be present with a normal serum level of alkaline phosphatase. If alkaline phosphatase fractionation indicates a predominately liver component, then the liver may be suspect, even though the scan is normal. Radioisotopic flow studies may pick up early metastases before the static images are positive. Serum for testing the level of carcinoembryonic antigen (CEA) should be obtained before treatment. This test is not particularly useful for diagnosis, but changes in the CEA level in the serum can be used to determine the effectiveness of treatment and to detect early or asymptomatic recurrence of disease.

The barium enema is of value for diagnosis and localization of the lesion. It is also useful as an indicator of what contiguous tissues may be involved or are at risk for direct extension. Upper gastrointestinal and small-bowel series are indicated, particularly if symptoms of pain are associated with eating (Fig. 17–2). An intravenous pyelogram (IVP) determines whether obstructive uropathy is present in patients with lesions involving the rectum and sigmoid, it also demonstrates the po-

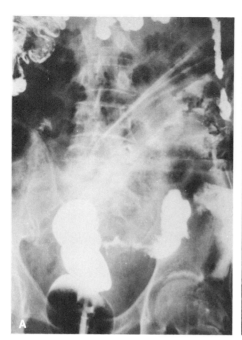
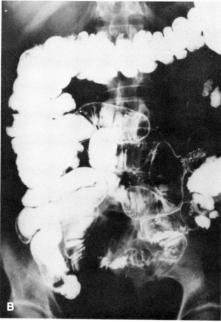

Fig. 17–2. (A) Barium enema demonstrating a carcinoma of the sigmoid colon. (B) Upper gastrointestinal series demonstrating invasion of contiguous ileum by the sigmoid lesion.

sition and function of the kidneys in patients with lesions of the ascending and descending colon who are to receive adjuvant radiation therapy. Cystoscopy with possible biopsy may be necessary if the urinalysis demonstrates microscopic hematuria, if the IVP suggests involvement of the bladder, or if the patient has suggestive symptoms. Lymphangiography is of limited practical use because the primary lymphatic drainage of the rectum and colon is to areas that are not demonstrated by lower-extremity lymphangiograms. With invasion of the anus or palpable abnormality in the inguinal or iliac nodes, the lymphangiogram may be useful prior to performing a biopsy or a definitive surgical procedure.

Ultrasound has artifact problems due to bowel gas, which restricts its value. The role of computerized tomography (CT) in this region is yet to be determined. Both modalities are limited in detecting local or regional extension, but can be used to de-

termine or supplement isotopic scanning for the presence of liver metastases.

If no definite evidence of distant metastases is revealed by the presurgical diagnostic workup, the physician can then proceed with preoperative irradiation in those patients selected for this approach. It should be realized that the actual extent of disease may be greater than appreciated preoperatively. About 11% of the patients have occult liver metastases found only at the time of operation.[6] For the patient selected for postoperative adjuvant radiotherapy, the most valuable procedure to determine the extent of disease in the pelvis and abdomen is surgical exploration. It is important that a thorough exploration be conducted, including biopsy of obvious or questionable metastases. In those patients having primary resection of their disease, but who are known to have residual or unresected disease in soft tissue or lymph nodes, description of the operative findings (including diagrams) is necessary. The placement of silver clips or other metallic markers around the area is invaluable as a guide to the radiation therapist in the placement of reduced field ports for delivery of additional dosage. Pathologic examination of the resected specimen is directed toward determining the extent of penetration of the bowel wall and the number and location of lymph-node metastases.

TREATMENT OPTIONS

Adjuvant Therapy

Although the purpose of combining radiation treatment with surgery is to eradicate occult deposits of neoplasm that have not been removed surgically, the sequence of its administration continues to be debated. Theoretically, pre- and postoperative irradiation accomplish the same purpose. Advocates of preoperative irradiation argue that the biologic and technical considerations are more optimal with this approach, while advocates of postoperative irradiation cite improved staging of disease and assessment of end results. With adequate portal coverage and dosage, there is no evidence to suggest a superiority of preoperative irradiation over postoperative irradiation in the prevention of local or regional recurrence.

Primary Therapy

Small lesions of the rectum can be irradiated with curative intent. The same considerations must be given to potential routes of spread as when adjuvant radiation therapy is used. Although disease in this area has been successfully treated with transrectal, low-kilovoltage x-rays and needle implantation,[9] it is desirable to deliver external-beam radiation therapy to cover subclinical extensions of disease outside the clinically obvious primary lesion. The local form of treatment, including boosting with a reduced external port, can be reserved for delivering a high dose to the primary lesion.

Recurrent Disease

In those patients with local failure following low anterior resection (AR), but with no presurgical evidence of metastases, surgical exploration for evaluation of the abdomen and pelvis is necessary; this should determine the feasibility of performing an abdominal perineal resection (APR). For the patient on whom resection is performed for recurrence of the tumor, postoperative irradiation should always be considered. For the patient with technically unresectable disease, but without metastases, the treatment options are preoperative irradiation and surgery or definitive irradiation.

Inoperable Disease

A tumor that is thought to be technically unresectable because of fixation may be suitable for preoperative irradiation. Under these circumstances, the use of a boost through a reduced field, to achieve a higher dose to the area of fixation, may reduce the risk of recurrence if surgical resection is not performed.

PORTAL ARRANGEMENTS

Many radiation therapists are accustomed to looking only at a two-dimensional coronal-view localization radiograph. It should be realized that there is a three-dimensional volume at risk (i.e., cephalocaudad, lateral, and anteroposterior) and that this volume must be assessed individually for each patient. Neglect of any one of these dimensions may contribute to failure to control disease, or to an increase in the risk of morbidity. The CT scan has improved our appreciation of this three-dimensional anatomy and is useful for dosimetric calculation; however, it does not, and cannot, replace orthogonal radiographic localization.

Rectum and Rectosigmoid

To prevent local and regional failure, the delivered dose must cover the volume at risk for direct extension of tumor, including the regional lymph nodes, which may contain metastatic deposits. For lesions more than 10 cm from the anal verge, the predominant lymphatic spread is cephalad along the inferior mesenteric nodes. Ports that cover the para-aortic area up to the origin of the inferior mesenteric artery have been suggested and used; however, the mesenteric chain of nodes is often adequately and easily removed with the surgical specimen. For lesions less than 8 cm to 10 cm from the anal verge, there is a greater risk of spread to pelvic (especially internal iliac) nodes, which are not easily or routinely removed by surgery and therefore must be adequately treated with radiation therapy.

In general, the volume of tissue irradiated is greater in the patient treated following APR than in those treated preoperatively or following AR. This is mainly due to the increased displacement of the inferior border of the treatment field to cover the cutaneous extent of the operation. A similar downward displacement of the lower border of the field is necessary when preoperative irradiation is given for extremely low-lying lesions that approach or invade the anus, which places the perineum and inguinal nodes at risk for involvement.

The patient may be treated in the prone or supine position, and beam direction is usually delivered through anterior-posterior and posterior-anterior (AP–PA) opposed ports or by a three-field technique (PA and two lateral ports). Whether treatment is delivered through AP–PA ports or the three-field technique, PA, AP, and cross-table lateral radiographs of the patient in the treatment position document the inferior, superior, lateral, and anterior anatomy to be treated. The cross-table-lateral radiograph with or without contrast material in the small bowel, rectum, or bladder, is a most useful projection. The radiograph outlines the contour of the patient and identifies the perineal region, the

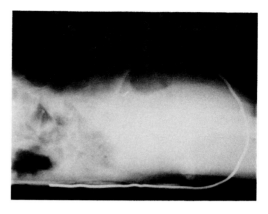

Fig. 17–3. A sagittal contour of the patient obtained by placing solder wire along the midline and taking a cross-table radiograph in treatment position. A small metallic marker is placed in the perineum and a magnification ring is placed on the dorsal surface.

clips that may be placed at surgery, and the various anatomic relationships. A simple and accurate technique for obtaining a contour is to place the patient in the treatment position with solder wire pressed against the surface in the midline of the spine posteriorly, then down along the perineum and up the anterior midline of the abdomen (Fig. 17–3). This contour can then be used for dosimetric calculation in the sagittal plane by either manual or computer technique. This is all that may be necessary if only AP–PA ports are used. A contour in the horizontal plane of the patient is required for the three-field technique. This can be obtained with the use of solder wire or by a CT image through the relevant plane.

In the patient who is receiving preoperative irradiation, or who had had a low AR and is receiving postoperative irradiation, the inferior border of the port need not be more than 5 cm below the radiographic lesion or anastomosis. This border should be at least at the level of the inferior portion of the pubic symphysis or bisecting the obturator foramina to cover the obturator lymph nodes. For the patient treated in the supine position, and in whom a localization radiograph is obtained only in the AP direction with markers on the anterior surface, there may be an inadequate inferior margin through the PA portal if treatment is directed through AP–PA opposed ports by rotating the head of the treatment unit 180° for treatment "through the table". Because of the posterior presacral location of the tumor, the divergence of the beam in the AP direction may indicate an adequate inferior margin, which may not be true if not confirmed by a PA radiograph. In the preoperative patient, it is desirable to obtain localization radiographs with barium in the rectum unless a true lateral radiograph from a diagnostic barium-enema study is available to show the level and extent of disease.

The inferior border of the portal, in the postoperative patient following APR, is at the level of the most inferior extent of the perineal incision, and may be indicated by a lead marker at the time of localization. Treatment in the prone position allows the physician to visualize and document perineal coverage; it is also helpful in placing the bolus on the perineal incision to obtain adequate surface dosage. In the obese patient, there may be sufficient anatomic bolus to assure this. If there is a great deal of opposing gluteal contact, the buttocks may be taped apart and bolus material may be substituted on the perineum. This sometimes helps to decrease the area of unwanted gluteal reaction that frequently devleops. In treating male patients in the prone position, special care must be taken to assure the maximum inferior displacement of the external genitalia to avoid acute symptomatic reactions of the scrotum and penis.

The lateral borders must cover the full width of the pelvis at the level of the lesion and, following APR, the full width of the pelvic inlet to the cutaneous surface. This is indicated by markers 1 cm to 2 cm lateral to the widest portion of the pelvic inlet to cover direct extension, and 1 cm to 2 cm lateral to the widest portion of the internal bony pelvis to cover the iliac

nodes. Shielding of the femoral heads is advised, especially in the elderly patient.

The irradiation-field margin's superior border for the rectum and rectosigmoid probably does not need to go beyond the bifurcation of the great vessels, which is around the junction of the fourth and fifth lumbar vertebra, unless disease is known to exist in the common iliac or para-aortic nodes, in which case the superior border must be extended in a more cephalad direction. The tissues of greatest concern for direct extension lie below the peritoneal reflection. Because the peritoneum covers the rectum and rectosigmoid at a more inferior level anteriorly than posteriorly, this volume can be considered to lie below a line drawn from the top of the first sacral vertebra to the top of the pubic symphysis.

In patients having APR, a small-bowel series performed prior to therapy is of value in determining the quantity and fixation of the normal small bowel, which may come to be within the treatment volume. AP views alone may be deceptive in that the small bowel may appear to lie at

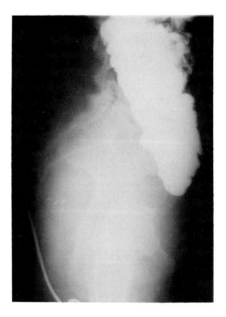

Fig. 17–4. A lateral radiograph of a small-bowel series in a patient having had an abdominal perineal resection. All of the small bowel lies above a line from the top of S1 to the top pf the pubic symphysis.

a lower level in the pelvis than is actually the case. Cross-table-lateral radiographs taken while the patient is in treatment position show the more important area, which is below the sacro-symphysis line (Fig. 17–4). With the patient in the prone position, it is possible to shield the small bowel when using lateral ports in the three-field technique. It is important that any shielding remain above the sacro-symphysis line. If the small bowel cannot be shielded or displaced out of the pelvic field by positioning of the patient, then a decision must be made by the radiation therapist and surgeon as to the benefit of treatment and relative risk of an injury occurring to this segment of the bowel (Fig. 17–5).

The posterior margin of the treatment volume in the pelvis corresponds to the anterior surface of the sacrum and coccyx.

With the use of high-energy x-ray beams, particularly in a thin person, care must be taken to avoid underdosage in this presacral region. Adding bolus material to the posterior surface of the patient may be necessary to achieve this, even at the risk of increasing the skin reaction on the posterior surface. The lateral radiograph demonstrates the continuously changing distance between the posterior surface of the patient and the anterior surface of the sacrum, knowledge of which is of vital importance for proper dosimetric calculation.

In using the three-field approach, the physician should be careful not to crowd the anterior border of the port (which is no problem in AP–PA ports) because this may lead to inadequate dosage being delivered to the anterior anatomy at risk for direct extension (Fig. 17–6).

Ascending and Descending Colon

In the left and right colon, the ports must cover the tumor bed, adjacent mesentery, and para-aortic nodes. At these sites the retroperitoneal area is at highest risk for direct extension. Portal arrangements should be directed to cover adequately the posterior portion of the involved hemiabdomen. It is not possible to shield the ipsilateral kidney from full dosage, so it is

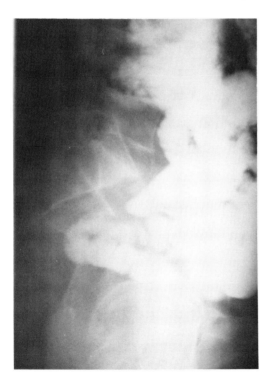

Fig. 17–5. A lateral radiograph of a small-bowel series in a patient having had an abdominal perineal resection. A loop of small bowel extends into the pelvis below the line from S1 to the public symphysis. This does not change when the patient changes position.

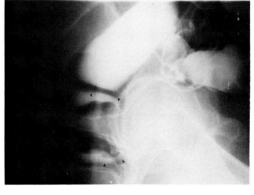

Fig. 17–6. A carcinoma involving the anterior aspect of the rectum. The lateral view from a barium enema gives valuable information regarding areas at risk for direct extension.

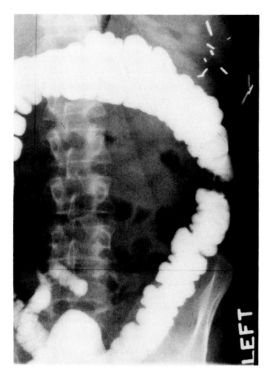

Fig. 17–7. A postoperative barium enema in a patient whose primary lesion was in the region of the splenic flexure. The postoperative configuration of the anastomosis can mimic a suture-line recurrence The line indicates the port actually treated in this patient.

important that the functional integrity of the contralateral kidney be established before treatment. On the left side, AP–PA ports can be used. On the right side, due to the presence of the liver, this may not be possible. Some beam arrangement that spares the anterior portion of the liver is necessary. Although AP and lateral radiographs can define the cephalocaudad and the medial-lateral margins, a horizontal section must be constructed, either by using solder or from a CT scan. Within this horizontal cross section, pertinent anatomy must be identified or drawn in, so that appropriate dosimetry can be performed to avoid treating sensitive structures (e.g., a contralateral kidney or the anterior portion of the liver). A postoperative barium enema determines the position of the colon and the anastomosis. This

location may not agree with its pretreatment location (Fig. 17–7).

Time–Dose Consideration

A proper time–dose relationship is crucial to avoid complications due to injury of the small and large intestine within the treatment volume. In general, a dose between 4500 and 5100 rad delivered in 5½ to 6 weeks to the volume at risk for subclinical disease produces an acceptable incidence of immediate and long-term morbidity. Shielding of the small bowel through lateral pelvic ports and surgical displacement of the bowel (out of the pelvis) have been found useful.[3,4]

For patients with residual disease (identified at surgery) who are receiving postoperative radiation therapy, an additional 500 to 1500 rad should be given to a reduced volume to increase the probability of local control.

REFERENCES

1. Astler, V.V., and Coller, F.A.: The prognostic significance of direct extension of carcinoma of the colon and rectum. Ann. Surg. 139:846, 1954.
2. Cass, A.W., Million, R.R., and Pfaff, F.A.: Patterns of recurrences following surgery alone for adenocarcinoma of the colon-rectum. Cancer 37:2861, 1976.
3. Freund, H., Gunderson L., Krause R., et al.: Prevention of radiation enteritis after abdominoperineal resection and radiotherapy. Surg. Gynecol. Obstet. 149:206, 1979.
4. Hughes, R., Brewington, K., Hanjani, P., Photopulos, G., Dick, D., Votava, C., Moran, M., and Coleman, S.: Extended field irradiation for cervical cancer based on surgical staging. Gynecol. Oncol. 9:153, 1980.
5. Gilbert, S.: Symptomatic local tumor failure following abdominoperineal resection. Int. J. Radiat. Oncol. Biol. Phys. 4:801, 1978.
6. Gunderson, L.L.: Personal Communication.
7. Gunderson, L.L. and Sosin, H.: Areas of failure found at reoperation (second of symptomatic look) following "curative surgery" for adenocarcinoma of the rectum. Cancer 34:1278, 1974.
8. Gunderson, L.L.: Radiation Therapy: Results and Future Possibilities. Clin. Gastroenterol. 5:769, 1976.
9. Papillon, J.: Intracavitary irradiation of early rectal cancer for cure: A series of 186 cases. Cancer 36:696, 1975.
10. Taylor, F.W.: Cancer of the colon and rectum: A study of routes of metastases and death. Surgery 52:305, 1962.

Chapter 18

WILMS' AND EWING'S TUMORS

Tae H. Kim

Mark E. Nesbit

Seymour H. Levitt

WILMS' TUMOR

Major improvement has been made in the management of Wilms' tumor during the last decade as a result of treatment methods developed by a national cooperative study.[1,2] The study showed that double-agent chemotherapy using vincristine (VCR) and actinomycin D (AMD) was superior to either agent alone and that postoperative radiation therapy was not necessary in patients with early-stage disease.[1] The overall survival rate has improved significantly and it appears that treatment could be refined in early-stage disease without jeopardizing tumor control so that the acute and late effects of therapy are minimized.

Clinical Signs and Symptoms

Wilms' tumor is a relatively rare tumor with the annual incidence of 7.8 per million population (ages 1 through 14 years) in the United States.[3] It has the peak incidence between 1 and 3 years of age.[4] Among the many congenital anomalies associated with Wilms' tumor, aniridia, hemihypertrophy, and urogenital anomalies are most common.

The most common presenting manifestation is a palpable abdominal mass or increasing abdominal size.[5] Abdominal pain occurs in one third of the patients. The tumor causes various nonspecific symptoms such as malaise, fever, and anorexia. Gross hematuria is seen in one quarter of the patients. Although hypertension is present in some patients with Wilms' tumor, the true incidence of hypertension is not known.

Diagnostic Workup

History

The diagnostic workup for a patient suspected of having Wilms' tumor should include a complete history, including the family history of cancer and congenital anomalies. In addition to recording the patient's height, weight, and vital signs (including blood pressure), the physician must determine the status of the lymph nodes and the size and location of the neoplasm. The tumor is fragile and should be handled gently and as little as possible.

Laboratory Study

Tests that should be included in the diagnostic workup for Wilms' tumor are routine hematologic and coagulation studies, BUN, creatine, SGOT or SGPT, and alkaline phosphatase. Urinalysis should note the presence of red and white blood cells.

Radiologic Study

Simulation radiographs should be taken from the posterior–anterior (PA) and lateral view of the chest to rule out lung metastasis. Excretory urography should be performed with special attention to the evidence of bilateral involvement. Computerized tomography (CT) is useful in making a differential diagnosis of kidney mass and detecting liver metastasis. Inferior venacavography is strongly recommended as a supplement to pyelography to determine the size of the mass and the patency of the inferior vena cava. If indicated, the catheter method from the superior vena cava should be used to rule out intracardiac extension of the tumor.

In patients with clear-cell sarcomatous-type Wilms' tumor, roentgenographic skeletal-bone survey is recommended because of the high propensity of this type of tumor to metastasize to bone.[1] CT scan of the brain is recommended in patients with rhabdoid-type Wilms' tumor because the lesion can develop brain metastasis or may be associated with central-nervous-system (CNS) malignancy.[1] Selective renal arteriography can help the physician in defining the extent of tumor as well as the status of the liver and contralateral kidney in bilateral disease.

Pathology

The analysis of the histologic specimens of the patients entered on the first National Wilms' Tumor Study (NWTS-1) showed that 11% of the patients have lesions with anaplastic foci characterized by marked cytologic atypism. These lesions were predominantly sarcomatous stroma.[6] Those patients with these lesions have a poor prognosis. Two-year-relapse-free-survival rates of favorable histology and unfavorable histology are 89% and 29%, respectively.[1]

Staging

Based on the experience of the previous two NWTSs, the third study came up with a new staging system.[7] The grouping system used for NWTS-1 and NWTS-2 is com-

pared with the new staging system for NWTS-3 in Table 18–1.

Treatment

Review of National Wilms' Tumor Study

The NWTS was begun in 1963 to answer clinical, pathologic, and epidemiologic questions in the management of Wilms' tumor.[8] Most of the major clinical cooperative study groups as well as many institutions that did not participate in one of the cooperative groups have entered patients on the study. Table 18–2 describes the schematics, design, and regimens of NWTS-1.

The study showed that routine postoperative radiation is not needed in the children with Group I disease and who are less than 24 months old. Children who were 2 years of age or older and who did not receive irradiation had a higher incidence of abdominal relapse than children who received irradiation. The overall survival rate in this group was significantly inferior to the survival rate of those children who received postoperative irradiation.

In Group II and III children, combined actinomycin-D (AMD) and vincristine chemotherapy (VCR) statistically showed significantly better relapse-free survival and overall survival (Table 18–3).

In the subsequent NWTS study,[2] postoperative irradiation was eliminated in the patients with Group-I disease and combined chemotherapy with AMD and VCR was given. Only 5 of 188 Group-I children developed a first recurrence in the abdomen. Three of these cases, all with favorable histology, had tumor in the contralateral kidney only. The fourth patient had a sarcomatous lesion; the relapse occurred in the tumor bed and there were distant metastases. Tumors in the opposite kidney are generally believed to be separate, independent neoplasms.[9] These data confirm the contention that routine postoperative irradiation is not needed in early-stage Wilms' tumor. A meticulous

TABLE 18–1. Comparison of the NWTS Staging Systems.*

	NWTS-1 and NWTS-2		NWTS-3
Group I.	Tumor limited to kidney and completely resected. The surface of the renal capsule is intact. The tumor was not ruptured before or during removal. There is no residual tumor apparent beyond the margins of resection.	Stage I.	Tumor limited to kidney and completely excised. The surface of the renal capsule is intact. The tumor was not ruptured before or during removal. There is no residual tumor apparent beyond the margins of resection.
Group II.	Tumor extends beyond the kidney but is completely resected. There is local extension of the tumor (i.e., penetration beyond the pseudocapsule into the perirenal soft tissues, or periaortic lymph-node involvement). The renal vessel outside the kidney substance is infiltrated or contains tumor thrombus. There is no residual tumor apparent beyond the margins of resection.	Stage II.	Tumor extends beyond the kidney but is completely excised. There is regional extension of the tumor (i.e., penetration through the outer surface of the renal capsule into perirenal soft tissues). Vessels outside the kidney substances are infiltrated or contain tumor thrombus. The tumor may have been biopsied or there has been local spillage of tumor confined to the flank. There is no residual tumor apparent at or beyond the margins of the treatment volume.
Group III.	Residual nonhematogenous tumor confined to abdomen. Any one or more of the following occur: a) The tumor has ruptured before or during surgery, or a biopsy has been performed. b) Implants are found on peritoneal surfaces.	Stage III.	Residual nonhematogenous tumor confined to abdomen. Any one or more of the following occur: a) Lymph nodes on biopsy are found to be involved in the hilus, the periaortic chains, or beyond. b) There has been diffuse peritoneal contamination by tumor, such as by spillage of tumor beyond the flank before or during surgery, or by tumor growth that has penetrated through the peritoneal surface.
	c) Lymph nodes are involved beyond the abdominal periaortic chains. d) The tumor is not completely resectable because of local infiltration into vital structures.		c) Implants are found on the peritoneal surfaces. d) The tumor extends beyond the surgical margins either microscopically or grossly. e) The tumor is not completely excisable because of local infiltration into vital structures.
Group IV.	Hematogenous metastases. Deposits beyond Group III (e.g., lung, liver, bone, and brain).	Stage IV.	Hematogenous metastases. Deposits beyond Stage III (e.g., lung, liver, bone, and brain).
Group V.	Bilateral renal involvement, either initially or subsequently. Not on study.	Stage V.	Bilateral renal involvement at diagnosis. An attempt should be made to stage each side according to the above criteria on the basis of extent of disease prior to biopsy.

*Staging, which is on the basis of gross and microscopic tumor distribution, is the same for tumors with favorable and with unfavorable histologic features. The patient should be characterized, however, by a statement of both criteria (e.g., Stage II, favorable histology, or Stage III, unfavorable histology). Tumors of unfavorable type are those with focal or diffuse anaplasia, or those of sarcomatous histology.

evaluation of the radiation-therapy factors of the study revealed that total dose greater than 2400 rad (200 rad/day, 5 days/week) did not yield better results, and 1800 to 2000 rad appears to be a satisfactory dose in infants under 13 months of age.[10]

Similar total-dose effect was observed by one institutional clinical trial.[16] Delay of initiation of irradiation greater than 10 days postoperatively appeared to be related to higher relapse in the flank.[10]

In case of tumor spillage, local irradiation to the renal fossa appears to be sufficient treatment. Whole-abdomen irradiation is recommended only for gross diffuse peritoneal contamination.[12]

TABLE 18–2.   Schematics of the National Wilms' Tumor Study-1 (NWTS-1).

Group I	R A N D O M I Z E		
		Regimen A	S + XRT + AMD
		Regimen B	S + AMD

Group II & III	R A N D O M I Z E		
		Regimen A	S + XRT + AMD
		Regimen B	S + XRT + VCR
		Regimen C	S + XRT + AMD + VCR

Group IV	R A N D O M I Z E		
		Regimen A	S + XRT + AMD + VCR
		Regimen B	Preoperative VCR + S + XRT + AMD + VCR

S, surgery; XRT, irradiation*; AMD, actinomycin D; VCR, vincristine.
*Irradiation:

Age	Total Tumor Dose
Birth to 18 months	1800 to 2400 rad
19 to 30 months	2400 to 3000 rad
31 to 40 months	3000 to 3500 rad
41 months or more	3500 to 4000 rad

(Adapted from D'Angio, et al., Cancer 45:1791, 1980.)

TABLE 18–3.   National Wilms' Tumor Study-2 Outcomes by Group and Regimen.

	No. of Patients	% 4-year RFS*		% 4-year Survival	
Group Regimen					
I <2 years old					
A (XRT)	38	89	} P=0.85	94	} P=0.46
B (no XRT)	41	88		90	
I ≥2 years old					
A (XRT)	42	76	} P=0.06	98	} P=0.015
B (no XRT)	42	57		81	
II/III					
A (AMD)	63	56		71	
B (VCR)	44	57	} P=0.01	71	} P=0.01
C (AMD + VCR)	63	79		84	

XRT, irradiation; AMD, actinomycin D; VCR, vincristine; P, probability of success.
*RFS = Relapse-Free Survival.

(Modified from D'Angio, et al., Cancer 45:1791, 1980.)

In the current study (NWTS-3), the maximum radiation dose for tumors with a favorable prognosis is 2000 rad. Stage-II patients are randomized between postoperative irradiation with 2000 rad and no irradiation.

Wilms' tumor of the unfavorable histologic type has a relatively higher flank-tumor recurrence rate and a very high mortality rate.[13] Total dose does not appear to be related to relapse of the disease in the abdomen. A delay of greater than 10 days in the initiation of radiation therapy from nephrectomy was suggested as a factor related to the occurrence of relapse in the abdomen in the histologic type with an unfavorable prognosis.[13]

Surgery

A generous transabdominal, transperitoneal incision is recommended for adequate incision. The primary tumor should be removed in its entirety. The contralateral kidney should be palpated and its posterior surface should be examined visually. Some surgeons recommend complete retroperitoneal lymph-node dissection; however, NWTS-3 leaves radical, or "anterior", unilateral or bilateral periaortic dissection of the node to the discretion of operating surgeons. Appropriate metal clips should be used to mark the extent of the tumor and to identify the residual tumor and any suspected tumor-involved area for postoperative radiation therapy.

Radiation Therapy

The University of Minnesota is participating in NWTS-3. The following radiation guidelines are the NWTS-3 recommendations for treatment of tumors of the favorable histologic type.

Stage I—No postoperative irradiation is indicated; chemotherapy only

Stage II—The patients are randomly chosen for either no radiation or 2000 rad given in daily fractions of 180–200 rads; babies less than 13 months of age receive 1000 rad; the

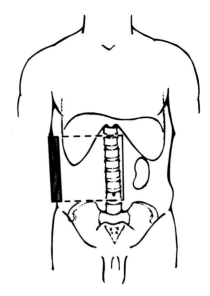

Fig. 18–1. Tumor-bed irradiation for Wilms' tumor when the tumor is on the right side. The fields extend across the midline to include the entire width of the vertebral bodies. The shaded area is to indicate the necessity of shielding the tangential abdominal wall.

tumor bed is defined as the outline of the kidney, and the associated tumor is irradiated; the radiation field is to be determined based on preoperative urography; the field extends across the midline to include the entire width of the vertebral bodies; this is an attempt to reduce possible scoliosis associated with uneven radiation to the spine (Fig. 18–1).

Stage III—The patients are randomly chosen for treatment with 2000 rad or 1000 rad; the field should include all known disease at the time of surgery; the total abdominal field is treated only when there is diffuse peritoneal seeding or gross spillage outside renal fossa prior or during surgery; the remaining kidney is shielded at 1500 rad

Stage IV—Tumor bed—2000 rad to a

Note: For Stage II and III tumors of the favorable histologic type, an additional 1000 rad may be given to bulky tumor; for all stages of Wilms' tumor of the unfavorable histologic type, an age-adjusted dose is delivered to the tumor bed as shown in Table 18–2.

treatment field, similar to Stage-II patients

Metastasis

Liver—2000 rads/2–2½ weeks for the entire liver for diffuse involvement; this may add 500 to 1000 rad additional dose to a lesser volume

Lung—1200 rad with daily fractions of 150 rads; the portal should be high enough to include apices of the lung and low enough to include posterior costophrenic angle; cross-table-lateral fluoroscopy is strongly recommended to assure that the lower margin covers the posterior costophrenic angle

Bilateral Wilms' Tumor

The reported incidence of bilateral Wilms' tumor ranges from 1.4% to as high as 14%.[14,15,22] Bishop[17] reported that 33 out of 606 children (5.4%) that were enrolled in NWTS-1 were found to have bilateral Wilms' tumor at time of diagnosis and that an additional 20 patients (3.3%) were subsequently found to have disease in the remaining kidney. Jereb[22] reported 19 cases of bilateral Wilms' tumor in 334 Wilms'-tumor patients (5.7%) in Scandinavian countries. Thirteen of these patients were found to have bilateral tumor at time of diagnosis and the remaining 6 patients were found to have disease in the remaining kidney later. This information confirms the importance of examining the opposite kidney at the time of operation, because in more than 33% of patients, bilateral disease was not suspected prior to surgery.[17]

Bilateral Wilms' tumor has a surprisingly good prognosis. An 87% (26 of 30 patients) two-year-survival rate was reported in those patients registered in NWTS. They were treated with multiagent chemotherapy, including AMD, VCR and adriamycin (ADR). All but two patients received a moderate dose of radiation. A variety of surgical procedures were used including biopsy only, nephrectomy, and partial nephrectomies. All seven patients who had all of the gross tumor removed survived; however, 19 of 22 patients with residual tumor following initial or subsequent surgery also survived. Analysis of radiation dose indicates that a dose between 1000 rad and 2000 rad usually suffices for local control.

At the University of Minnesota Hospitals, we recommend a very conservative approach as far as surgery and radiation therapy are concerned. Surgery is limited to biopsy or partial nephrectomy. Following multiagent chemotherapy with AMD, VCR, or ADR, radiation is reserved only for those patients who have persistent or progressive disease after a second exploratory operation.

EWING'S SARCOMA

A marked improvement in overall survival has been achieved in recent years in those patients with localized Ewing's sarcoma. This was the result of combined use of multiagent chemotherapy and intensive radiotherapy and surgery. The outlook for those patients with distant metastases, however, remains much less optimistic.

The marked improvement in the survival of localized Ewing's sarcoma occurred when multiagent chemotherapy, mainly AMD, cyclophosphamide, VCR, and ADR were added to radiation therapy and surgery.[18,19,20] The multi-institutional clinical study group played a major role in obtaining information on biologic behavior of the cancer and in the refinement of treatment in this relatively rare tumor.

Natural History

In 1921, James Ewing described a small, round cell of a malignant tumor of the bone, which he termed "diffuse endothelioma of bone" or "endothelial sarcoma of bone." It was thought at that time that the tumor arose from endothelial cells of medullary lymphatic and blood vessels. More than 60 years have passed since the initial description. Much has been learned in regard to the natural history, prognosis, and treatment of Ewing's sarcoma; however, the origin of the tumor cell remains controversial.[18,21] This cancer must be differentiated from the inflammatory process in bone and other small-blue-cell tumors of childhood (i.e., malignant lymphoma, neuroblastoma, medulloblastoma, embryonal rhabdomyosarcoma, and retinoblastoma).[23] The presence of glycogen in tumor cells, demonstrated by special histochemical staining in most cases, helps to differentiate Ewing's sarcoma from neuroblastoma, retinoblastoma, and malignant lymphoma.[24]

This tumor is seen mostly in children, adolescents, and young adults: 75% to 80% are diagnosed before the age of 20 years. Most series report a male to female ratio of 2:1.[25] Although the long bones, commonly in metaphysis, are most frequently affected, almost all bones in the body have been reported as the primary site at one time or another.[26] The lungs and skeletal system are the most common metastatic sites. Central-nervous-system (CNS) involvement has been reported.[27]

Review of Treatment

The traditional treatment for localized Ewing's sarcoma has been local radiation therapy or surgical removal. Although these treatments were very effective in local control of the tumor, the overall survival of these patients was dismal.[28] The poor survival rate was attributed to early hematogenous dissemination of subclinical tumor. In an attempt to prevent metastases by subclinical tumor cells, systemic chemotherapy was added to local irradiation and surgery. In their earlier report, the group at St. Jude's Hospital treated 15 patients with localized Ewing's sarcoma with 5000 rad to 6500 rad in a 5- to 8-week period using ^{60}Co.[18] With higher doses, a split-course technique was used. The ports were extended to include the entire bone and surrounding soft tissue. All patients received chemotherapy with VCR

and cyclophosphamide for 1 to 2 years. At the time it was reported in 1972, 12 patients were surviving for between 9 and 5 months.

At the National Cancer Institute (NCI),[19] 66 consecutive patients were treated with a dosage of 5000 rad over 5 weeks to the entire involved bone using megavoltage radiation for the primary lesion and with a dosage of less than 4000 rad for metastatic lesions. CNS prophylaxis was given to all patients with a 2000-rad dosage over 2 weeks to entire brain in conjunction with intrathecal methotrexate. They were all treated with ADR and VCR. Of these 66 patients, 43 patients without clinically detectable metastasis at the time of diagnosis had a 52% 5-year-survival rate.

At Memorial Sloan Kettering Cancer Center,[20] 67 consecutive patients with nonmetastatic Ewing's sarcoma were treated with adjuvant chemotherapy in addition to radiation therapy or surgery for the primary tumor. The regimen of T-2 study consisted of AMD, ADR, VCR, and cyclophosphamide chemotherapy started simultaneously with radiation therapy delivered to the primary tumor with the planned dose of 6000 to 7000 rad. A total of 19 patients were treated by the T-2 regimen. Chemotherapy was given for 18 months.

The T-6 study consisted of combination chemotherapy prior to local radiation therapy. Chemotherapy consisted of bleomycin, cyclophosphamide, AMD, VCR, ADR, Methotrexate, and BCNU. After two cycles of this treatment (each cycle takes 12 weeks, with a 3- to 4-week rest period between the first and second cycle), local treatment was given to the primary area. It consisted of either amputation, surgical resection, or radiation therapy without surgery with a planned dose of 6000 rad. A total of 30 patients were treated by the T-6 protocol.

The T-9 consists of six drugs: Cyclophosphamide, ADR, Methotrexate, bleomycin, AMD, and VCR. The local therapy is given after three cycles of chemotherapy in patients with proximal lesions (pelvis, spine, and femur) and after approximately 2½ cycles in patients with distal lesions.

When the results were reported in 1981, 53 (79%) of the 67 patients with primary Ewing's sarcoma were free of relapse for a follow-up period of 12 to 118 months (median 41 months). The disease-free survival according to local therapy is summarized in Table 18–4.

The Intergroup Ewing's Sarcoma Study was an intergroup study on Ewing's sarcoma that was initiated in June 1972, with the participation of institutions of the Cancer and Leukemia Group B, Children's Cancer Study Group, and the Southwest Oncology Group.[29] Their first study design is summarized in Table 18–5.

The results showed that an excellent tumor control rate was achieved with the radiation regimen described in Table 18–6, in combination with multiagent chemotherapy. Distant metastasis was the major cause of failure. Almost all local recurrence occurred within 3 years after therapy. In spite of the excellent local-tumor-control rate, analysis of the data failed to show any significant correlation between the dose of radiation and recurrence of the primary tumor. A similar local-tumor-control rate was achieved at the dose of radiation exceeding 4000 rad. The

volume irradiated in the bone that has primary tumor failed to show any statistically significant difference in local-tumor-control rate between those patients who were irradiated with an adequate treatment volume and those who were irradiated with a less than adequate treatment volume.

One explanation for the lack of correlation between the radiation dose and local tumor control is that approximately 50% of these patients die from metastatic disease within 3 years after the initiation of the treatment, thus precluding clinicial manifestation of local recurrence even if complete eradication of the primary tumor was not accomplished.[29] Pelvic primary Ewing's sarcoma was noted in the study as a subset of patients who have a higher local recurrence, distant metastasis, and poor disease-free survival compared to those patients who had primary lesions elsewhere.[30] The reason why this group has poor prognosis is obscure; however, one reason may be that they frequently present with a large tumor volume.[29,30]

The Intergroup Ewing's Sarcoma Study has clearly shown that high-dosage radiotherapy and multiagent chemotherapy is an effective modality in controlling local tumor and in maintaining the anatomic function of affected bones in most instances. The overall survival, however, is not satisfactory. Further investigation is

TABLE 18–4.   Disease-Free Survival According to Local Therapy (Ewing's Sarcoma).

Local Therapy	No. of Patients		No. Failing Local Therapy		No of Patients with Disease-Free Survival	
Radiation therapy*	34†	(51%)	7	(21%)	26	(76%)
Surgery‡	13	(19%)	0	—	10	(77%)
Surgery + radiation therapy§	20	(30%)	0	—	17	(85%)
TOTAL	67	(100%)	7	(10%)	53	(79%)

*4500–7000 rad
†Includes two patients who had amputation after persistent tumor was demonstrated following completion of radiation therapy
‡Amputation
§Surgical resection followed by radiation therapy (3000 rad) to the remaining bone and tumor bed

(From: Rosen, et al.: Cancer 47:2204, 1981.)

TABLE 18–5. Intergroup Ewing's Sarcoma Study: Study Design.

Group 1 Institutions	RANDOMIZE	Regimen I	Radiotherapy to primary tumor plus cytoxan + vincristine + actinomycin + adriamycin
		Regimen II	Radiotherapy to primary tumor plus cyclophosphamide + vincristine + actinomycin D
Group 2 Institutions	RANDOMIZE	Regimen II	Radiotherapy to primary tumor plus cyclophosphamide + vincristine + actinomycin D
		Regimen III	Radiotherapy to primary tumor plus cyclophosphamide + vincristine + actinomycin D + bilateral pulmonary radiotherapy

Radiation Dose (rad): Age	Whole Bone	Boost	Total Dose
Under 5 years	4500	1000	5500
5–15 years	5000	1000	6000
Older than 15 years	5500	1000	6500

Lung Irradiation: 1500 rad/10 fractions without correction for lung transmission factor

(From Perez, et al.: Int. J. Radiat. Oncol. Biol. Phys. 7:141, 1981.)

TABLE 18–6. Local Tumor Control (Ewing's Sarcoma).*

Regimen	No. of Patients	No. of Patients Who Achieved Local Tumor Control	No. of Patients Alive and Free of Disease
I	113	113 (92.9%)	85 (72.4%)
II	73	62 (84.9%)	26 (35.6%)
III	85	75 (88%)	47 (55.3%)

*Median follow-up is 2 years after the initiation of radio-therapy.

(Adapted from Perez, et al.: Int. J. Radiat. Oncol. Biol. Phys., 7:141, 1981.)

needed to improve the survival and refinement of treatment (i.e., radiation dose and volume of treatment is needed to minimize the late effects and improve the quality of life of the affected patient).

Diagnostic Workup

PA and lateral radiographs of the primary tumor should be taken with or without soft-tissue technique. CT scan or an arteriogram of the primary lesion is mandatory to delineate the extension of the tumor to the surrounding soft tissue.[20,29] Other diagnostic procedures include PA and lateral radiographs and CT scan of the chest, lactic dehydrogenase, bone scan with ^{99}Tc, a biopsy on extraosseous Ewing's sarcoma, without violating the boney lesion (if possible), bone-marrow biopsy, and other baseline studies (e.g., CBC, urinalysis, renal function).

Treatment Technique of Nonmetastatic Ewing's Sarcoma

At the University of Minnesota Hospitals, the majority of patients are treated within the guidelines of the Intergroup Ewing's Sarcoma Study, in which we are actively participating.

Surgical Resection

In order to alleviate the late effects of high-dosage radiation therapy and chemotherapy, surgical resection is recommended for expendable bones. These include bones of the foot, fibula, rib, forearm bones, the clavicle, and the scapula. Complete surgical resection implies ablation of the biopsy site and of the entire tumor with the surrounding normal tissue with a resection margin that is microscopically free of tumor. These patients do not receive postoperative radiation therapy. They are treated with multiagent chemotherapy, including VCR, ADR, AMD, and cyclophosphamide. Surgical resection of the aforementioned bones is indicated only when it is thought that there will be no major functional deficit following the surgery.

Radiation Therapy

The following is an outline of the radiation treatment of nonmetastatic Ewing's sarcoma according to the site of the neoplasm.

Long Bones. If the primary lesion is lo-

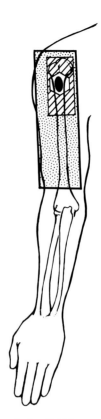

Fig. 18–3. The radiation field for treatment of Ewing's sarcoma at the middle of the long bone. Both epiphyseal plates are included in the first field, which receives 4500 rad.

calized within the half of the end of a long bone, the other metaphysis and epiphyseal plate are spared from irradiation; otherwise, the entire shaft is treated. The dosage is 4500 rad delivered over 4½ weeks, in 200-rad daily fractions, treating two fields per day. The field should have 5-cm margins of soft-tissue infiltration. The field is then reduced twice, giving a 5-cm margin around the tumor and a 1-cm margin around the tumor each time receiving 500 rad. The total dosage to the tumor area is 5500 rad in 5½ weeks (Figures 18–2 and 18–3). A strip of bolus is applied to the biopsy scar in order to bring the skin surface dose up to the level adequate for treatment. Every effort is made to block a strip of soft tissue from radiation. It is very important to prevent disturbance of lymphatic drainage secondary to excessive

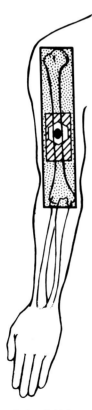

Fig. 18–2. The radiation field for treatment of Ewing's sarcoma, localized within the half of the end of the long bone. The other metaphysis and epiphyseal plate are spared from irradiation.

subcutaneous fibrosis caused by irradiation.

Pelvis. Because of the poor prognosis of patients with pelvic Ewing's sarcoma, aggressive surgery is attempted. If possible, the tumor is resected after 7 weeks of chemotherapy with VCR, Cytoxan, AMD, and ADR. If the tumor is completely resected, no postoperative irradiation is given.

If surgery is not adequate, or if the tumor is entered at the time of surgery, radiation is given to the hemipelvis and the tumor-bed area with a dosage of 5000 rad over 6 weeks. The last 500 rad is given through a small field with a 1-cm margin around the tumor. If surgery is not performed, a total of 5500 rad is given over a period of 5½ weeks. The treatment is similar to that delivered to the lesions in long bones except that the initial volume includes a 2-cm margin around the pelvis and soft-tissue extension instead of a 5-cm margin, as in the long-bone lesions.

A pelvic CT scan is extremely important in the treatment of pelvic Ewing's sarcoma because of the frequency and the large volume of soft-tissue extension of the tumor. The CT scan should be repeated before the field size is reduced in order to ensure that all the known tumor is included in the field.

Rib. The radiation dosage and volume is the same as with treatment for Ewing's sarcoma of long bones; however, we use an arc-rotation electron beam in order to minimize damage to the lesions beneath the rib.

The appropriate electron energy is chosen depending on the thickness of the chest wall, which is determined by the chest CT scan that is taken while the patient is in treatment position. A special cast for mounting the lead shield is made to reproduce the daily positioning of the patient. An example of an isodose curve taken for one of our patients is shown in Figure 18–4.

Other Bones. Although it is very rare,

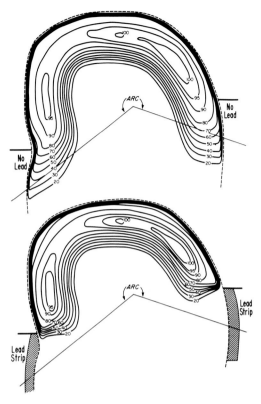

Fig. 18–4. Isodose distribution in arc rotation with and without lead strips at the ends of the arc, using a section of an Alderson Rando phantom closely simulating an actual patient cross section. Arc angle = 236°; average radius of curvature = 10 cm; beam energy = 10 MeV; lead strip thickness = 6 mm; field size at the surface = 4.2 cm × 8.5 cm.

Ewing's sarcoma of the vertebral column presents an interesting problem because of its location in relation to the spinal cord, the major radiation-dose-limiting organ. Although most of the proximal vertebral lesions are treated with a lower dosage (4000–5000 rad) compared to distal vertebral lesions, they have excellent prognosis (86%).[31] It is thought that poor prognosis in distal vertebral Ewing's sarcoma is because of the more advanced size of the lesion. For the proximal lesion, a dose of less than 5000 rad is recommended. For early lesions, doses between 4000 and 4500 rad may be adequate.[30] For distal vertebral lesions, a more aggressive surgical procedure is recommended, as discussed in regard to pelvic primary tumors.

Because patients with Ewing's sarcoma are usually children, the emphasis of treatment should be placed not only on the cure of the tumor but also on maintaining the maximum function and cosmetic effect. The therapy must be individualized, depending on the age of the patient, the primary site, and the degree of soft-tissue and boney involvement.[32]

REFERENCES

1. D'Angio, G.J., Beckwith, J.B., Breslow, N.E., et al.: Wilms' tumor: An update. Cancer 45:1791, 1980.
2. D'Angio, G.J., Evans, A., Breslow, N., et al.: The treatment of Wilms' tumor: Results of the second National Wilms' Tumor Study. Cancer 47:2302, 1981.
3. Third National Cancer Survey: Incidence data. NCI Monograph 41. Bethesda, National Cancer Institute, 1975.
4. Sutow, W.W., Vietti, T., Fernboch, D.: Clinical pediatric oncology. St. Louis, C.V. Mosby, 1977.
5. Holland, P.: Clinical and biochemical manifestations of Wilms' tumor. In Wilms' Tumor. Edited by C. Pochedly and D. Miller. New York, John Wiley & Sons, 1976.
6. Beckwith, J.B., Palmer, N.F.: Histopathology and prognosis of Wilms' tumor. Cancer 41:1937, 1978.
7. Farewell, V.T., D'Angio, G.J., Breslow, N., et al.: Retrospective evaluation of a new staging system for Wilms' tumor. Cancer Clin. Trials 4:167, 1981.
8. D'Angio, G.J., Beckwith, J.B., Bishop, H.C., et al.: The National Wilms' Tumor Study: progress report. Proc. Natl. Cancer Conf. 7:627, 1973.
9. D'Angio, G.J.: Radiation therapy in Wilms' tumor revisited. Int. J. Radiat. Oncol. Biol. Phys. 6:737, 1980.
10. D'Angio, G.J., Tefft, M., Breslow, N., et al.: Radiation therapy of Wilms' tumor: According to dose, field, postoperative timing and histology. Int. J. Radiat. Oncol. Biol. Phys. 4:769, 1978.
11. Hustu, J.O., Pinkel, D., Pratt, C.B.: Treatment of clinically localized Ewing's sarcoma with radiotherapy and combined chemotherapy. Cancer 30:1522, 1972.
12. Tefft, M., D'Angio, G.J., Grant, W.: Postoperative radiation therapy for residual Wilms' tumor: Review of Group III patients in the National Wilms' Tumor Study. Cancer 37:2768, 1976.
13. Tefft, M., D'Angio, G.J., Beckwith, B., et al.: Patterns of intra-abdominal relapse (IAR) in patients with Wilms' tumor who received radiation: anal-ysis by histopathology. A report of National Wilms' Tumor Study I and II. Int. J. Radiat. Oncol. Biol. Phys. 6:663, 1980.
14. Abeshouse, B.S.: The management of Wilms' tumor as determined by national survey and review of the literature. J. Urol. 77:792, 1957.
15. White, J.J., Galloday, S., Kaizer, H., et al.: Conservatively aggressive management with bilateral Wilms' tumor. J. Ped. Surg. 11:859, 1976.
16. Jeal, P.N., Jenkin, D.T.: Abdominal irradiation in the treatment of Wilms' tumor. Int. J. Radiat. Oncol. Biol. Phys. 6:655, 1980.
17. Bishop, H., Tefft, M., Evans, A., et al.: Survival in bilateral Wilms' tumor: Review of 30 National Wilms' Tumor Study cases. J. Pediatr. Surg. 12:631, 1977.
18. Hou-Jensen, K., Priori, E., Dmochowski, L.: Studies in the ultrastructure of Ewing's sarcoma of bone. Cancer 29:280, 1972.
19. Pomeroy, T.C., Johnson, R.E.: Integrated therapy in Ewing's sarcoma. Front. Radiat. Oncol. 10:152, 1975.
20. Rosen, G., Caparros, B., Nirenberg, A., et al.: Ten year experience with adjuvant chemotherapy. Cancer 47:2204, 1981.
21. Kadin, M.E., Bensch, K.G.: On the origin of Ewing's tumor. Cancer 27:257, 1971.
22. Jereb, B.: Bilateral nephroblastoma: Clinical review of 19 cases. Acta Radiol. 10:417, 1971.
23. Dehner, L.: Pediatric Surgery Pathology. St. Louis, C.V. Mosby, 1975.
24. Schajowica, F.: Ewing's sarcoma and reticulum sarcoma of bone, with special reference to the histochemical demonstration of glycogen as an aid to differential diagnosis. J. Bone Joint Surg. 41-A:349, 1959.
25. Larsson, S., et al.: The incidence of malignant primary bone tumors in relation to age, sex, and site. J. Bone Joint Surg. 56–B:534, 1974.
26. Dehner, L.: Tumors of the mandible and maxilla in children. II. A study of 14 primary and secondary malignant tumors. Cancer 32:112, 1973.
27. Metha, Y., Hendrickson, F.R.: CNS involvement in Ewing's sarcoma. Cancer 33:859, 1974.
28. Falk, S., Alpert, M.: Five year survival of patients with Ewing's sarcoma. Surg. Gyn. Obstet. 124:319, 1967.
29. Perez, C.A., Tefft, M., Nesbit, M., et al.: The role of radiation therapy in the management of non-metastatic Ewing's sarcoma of bone: Report of the Intergroup Ewing's Sarcoma Study. Int. J. Radiat. Oncol. Biol. Phys. 7:141, 1981.
30. Tefft, M., Razek, A., Perez, C.A., et al.: Local control and survival related to chemotherapy in non-metastatic Ewing's sarcoma of pelvic bones. Int. J. Radiat. Oncol. Biol. Phys., 5:367, 1978.
31. Pilepich, M.S., Vietti, T., Newbit, M., et al.: Ewing's sarcoma of the vertebral column. Int. J. Radiat. Oncol. Biol. Phys. 7:27, 1981.
32. Donaldson, S.: History of continuing success: Radiotherapy for Ewing's sarcoma. Int. J. Radiat. Oncol. Biol. Phys. 7:279, 1981.

Index

Page numbers in italics indicate figures; numbers followed by "t" indicate tables.